AF184045

Aortic Valve Disease - Recent Advances

Edited by P. Syamasundar Rao

Published in London, United Kingdom

Aortic Valve Disease - Recent Advances
http://dx.doi.org/10.5772/intechopen.107754
Edited by P. Syamasundar Rao

Contributors
Ali Yasar Kilinc, Mustafa Ucar, Alexander Zotov, Oleg Shelest, Emil Sakharov, Alexander Troitskiy, Robert Khabazov, Hafez Golzarian, Sidra R. Shah, Sandeep M. Patel, P. Syamasundar Rao, Gian-Manuel Jimenez-Rodriguez, Mariana Chaire-Hernandez, José-Luis Elizalde-Silva, Jesus Diaz-Marin, Guering Eid Lidt, Gustavo Rojas Velasco, Philip Hutchens, Poonam Velagapudi, Muhammad Asim Shabbir, Nidhish Tiwari, David Freiholtz, Per Eriksson, Hanna M. Björck, Abdumadjidov Khamidulla Amanullaevich, Urakov Shukhrat Tukhtaevich, Sunil Ohri, Manoraj Navaratnarajah, Amit Modi, Rita Milewski, Syed Usman Bin Mahmood, Prashanth Vallabhajosyula, Massimo Mancone, Gennaro Sardella, Gianluca Di Pietro, Improta Riccardo, Lucia Ilaria Birtolo, Colantonio Riccardo, Emanuele Bruno, Marco Tocci

© The Editor(s) and the Author(s) 2024
The rights of the editor(s) and the author(s) have been asserted in accordance with the Copyright, Designs and Patents Act 1988. All rights to the book as a whole are reserved by INTECHOPEN LIMITED. The book as a whole (compilation) cannot be reproduced, distributed or used for commercial or non-commercial purposes without INTECHOPEN LIMITED's written permission. Enquiries concerning the use of the book should be directed to INTECHOPEN LIMITED rights and permissions department (permissions@intechopen.com).
Violations are liable to prosecution under the governing Copyright Law.

Individual chapters of this publication are distributed under the terms of the Creative Commons Attribution 3.0 Unported License which permits commercial use, distribution and reproduction of the individual chapters, provided the original author(s) and source publication are appropriately acknowledged. If so indicated, certain images may not be included under the Creative Commons license. In such cases users will need to obtain permission from the license holder to reproduce the material. More details and guidelines concerning content reuse and adaptation can be found at http://www.intechopen.com/copyright-policy.html.

Notice
Statements and opinions expressed in the chapters are these of the individual contributors and not necessarily those of the editors or publisher. No responsibility is accepted for the accuracy of information contained in the published chapters. The publisher assumes no responsibility for any damage or injury to persons or property arising out of the use of any materials, instructions, methods or ideas contained in the book.

First published in London, United Kingdom, 2024 by IntechOpen
IntechOpen is the global imprint of INTECHOPEN LIMITED, registered in England and Wales, registration number: 11086078, 5 Princes Gate Court, London, SW7 2QJ, United Kingdom
Printed in Croatia

British Library Cataloguing-in-Publication Data
A catalogue record for this book is available from the British Library

Additional hard and PDF copies can be obtained from orders@intechopen.com

Aortic Valve Disease - Recent Advances
Edited by P. Syamasundar Rao
p. cm.

This title is part of the Cardiology and Cardiovascular Medicine Book Series, Volume 1
Topic: Cardiovascular Surgery
Series Editor: Kaan Kırali
Topic Editor: Takashi Murashita

Print ISBN 978-1-83769-153-1
Online ISBN 978-1-83769-154-8
eBook (PDF) ISBN 978-1-83769-155-5
ISSN 3033-361X

We are IntechOpen, the world's leading publisher of Open Access books

Built by scientists, for scientists

6,800+
Open access books available

184,000+
International authors and editors

200M+
Downloads

156
Countries delivered to

Our authors are among the
Top 1%
most cited scientists

12.2%
Contributors from top 500 universities

WEB OF SCIENCE™

Selection of our books indexed in the Book Citation Index
in Web of Science™ Core Collection (BKCI)

Interested in publishing with us?
Contact book.department@intechopen.com

Numbers displayed above are based on latest data collected.
For more information visit www.intechopen.com

For EU product safety concerns:
IN TECH d.o.o., Prolaz Marije Krucifikse Kozulić 3, 51000 Rijeka, Croatia,
info@intechopen.com or visit our website at intechopen.com.

IntechOpen Book Series

Cardiology and Cardiovascular Medicine

Volume 1

Aims and Scope of the Series

Today, since molecular science on structural causes of oncological pathologies and their molecular treatments are developing at an unbelievable rate, the primary medical cause of death in the twenty-first century will be cardiovascular disease. Neither pandemics that threaten all humanity nor deterioration in the ecosystem will be able to change this fact. Especially, this century seems poised to witness an incredible struggle against atherosclerotic disease, which develops in the arterial walls and results in narrowing and occlusion of the arterial lumen. In addition to this disease, there has been an increasing prevalence of heart rhythm problems, deterioration of heart valves due to aging, and heart failure. Serious vascular pathologies such as stenosis and occlusion, dissection and rupture, and aneurysmal enlargement are also major concerns. Medical and invasive treatment methods may work to save human lives, but they will never provide a real solution. All kinds of medical, technological, and genetic engineering developments obtained in these processes have not yet been sufficient to alleviate or eliminate cardiovascular disease. This book series, Cardiology and Cardiovascular Medicine, includes three topics. The first, Cardiovascular Diseases and Health, reviews important cardiovascular diseases and the developments in their prognosis. The second topic, Cardiovascular Electrophysiology, illuminates the abnormal functioning of the cardiac conduction system, which is caused by all heart pathologies and negatively affects prognosis. The third topic in this series, Cardiovascular Surgery, details treatment for cardiovascular pathologies and how to regulate normal physiological functions with percutaneous or extracorporeal interventions.

Meet the Series Editor

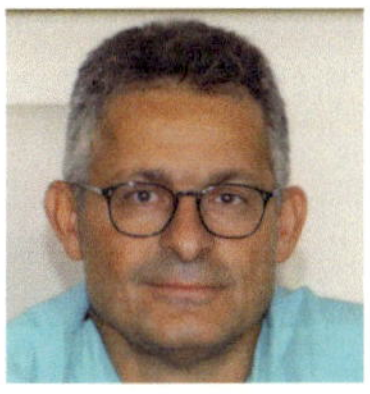

After completing his studies at the Medicine Faculty of Istanbul University in 1990, Prof. Kaan Kırali fulfilled his mandatory medical service and commenced his residency training at Koşuyolu Heart and Research Hospital in 1992. Following five years of assistant education, he pursued further training in England and the USA in 1998. Specializing in laparoscopic and minimally invasive cardiac surgery, he earned the titles of consultant cardiovascular surgeon in 1998, Assistant Professor in 1999, Associate Professor in 2002, and Chief in 2005 at the same hospital. Prof. Kırali also developed an interest in preventive medicine, obtaining an MSc in Public Health from Istanbul University in 2000. Over the past two decades, he has concentrated his scientific pursuits on cardiovascular repairs requiring specialized experience. With his expertise in coronary artery surgery, minimally invasive cardiac surgery, valve repair, and aortic root surgery, he has established new methods for awake coronary bypass revascularization, a new surgical approach for AVR during first and re-operations, aortic valve-sparing procedure, and radiofrequency ablation. Notably, he pioneered awake complete coronary artery bypass grafting (CABG) with bilateral internal mammary arteries (BIMA) and played a crucial role in advancing aortic root surgery with a new aortotomy incision, simplifying aortic valve interventions. Since the year 2000, Prof. Kırali has expanded his interests to heart transplantation, and in recent years, to left ventricular assist devices. He has served as the head of the transplantation department since 2015 and currently continues his work as the director of Koşuyolu High Specialization Education and Research Hospital in Istanbul, Turkey. In his prolific career, he has authored numerous papers in SCI journals, contributed to various book chapters, and served as an editor and reviewer for multiple academic journals. Additionally, he has edited several international books in the field of cardiovascular medicine.

Meet the Volume Editor

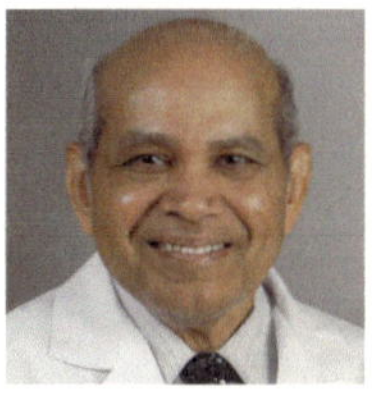

Dr. P. Syamasundar Rao, MD, DCH, FAAP, FACC, FSCAI, is a Professor of Pediatrics and Medicine and Emeritus Chief of Pediatric Cardiology, University of Texas-Houston Medical School, USA. He received his medical degree from Andhra Medical College, India, and subsequently received post-graduate training both in India and the United States before joining the faculty at the Medical College of Georgia, USA, in 1972. His subsequent positions were Chairman of Pediatrics at King Faisal Specialist Hospital and Research Center, Saudi Arabia; Professor and Director of the Division of Pediatric Cardiology, University of Wisconsin-Madison, USA; and Professor and Director of the Division of Pediatric Cardiology, Saint Louis University School of Medicine, Missouri, USA. He has authored 430 papers, 16 monographs/books, and 150 book chapters. Dr. Rao is a recipient of several honors and awards.

Contents

Preface

This book presents some of the advances that have occurred in the diagnosis and management of aortic valve disease over the last 50 years for healthcare personnel involved in the care of infants, children, and adults with aortic valve abnormalities.

The book is divided into seven sections. Section 1 introduces the book. In the introductory chapter, I review the normal anatomy of the aortic valve apparatus, the prevalence of different types of aortic valve diseases and ascending aortic aneurysm, and topics not adequately dealt within the other chapters in the book, including clinical features, echocardiographic diagnosis, and aortic valve surgery other than valve replacement.

In Section 2 on the pathology of the aortic valve, Dr. Abdumadjidov Khamidulla Amanullaevich and Urakov Shukhrat Tukhtaevich address issues associated with acquired heart disease in Chapter 2. The author identifies these issues as an assortment of pathological abnormalities that develop during the life of a patient. Because there is already a high prevalence of rheumatic heart disease in the developing regions of the world, the added burden of aortic valve disease is substantial. The prevalence of aortic valve disease in the elderly in the author's region (Republic of Uzbekistan) is estimated to be greater than 10%. Aortic stenosis (AS) is more prevalent, with aortic insufficiency (AI) coming second. The chapter includes excellent illustrations of the surgical anatomy of the aortic valve, including surgical photographs and pathologic specimens. The chapter concludes that acquired aortic valve disease is of high scientific and practical importance in the region.

In Chapter 3, Dr. Freiholtz et al. review the relationship of aortic valve phenotypes to ascending aortic aneurysms (AAAs). They state that the bicuspid aortic valve (BAV) is a major risk factor for the development of AAA. There appear to be different mechanisms for aneurysm development in bicuspid vs. tricuspid aortic valves (TAVs). The authors assert that AAA associated with BAV is pathologically distinct from that associated with TAV. They go on to describe molecular mechanisms of AAA in both these groups; BAV aortopathy is associated with endothelial instability and endocardial-to-mesenchymal transition, presumably embryonic in origin, whereas TAV aortopathy manifests medial degeneration, inflammation, and fibrosis.

In Section 3 on the technique of transcatheter aortic valve replacement, Dr. Ali Yasar Kilinc and Mustafa Ucar, in Chapter 4, discusses the technique of transcatheter aortic valve replacement (TAVR) with a focus on current approaches. Since the description of TAVR by Cribier in 2002, it has been increasingly used to treat calcific AS in the elderly. The author classifies the types of available transcatheter aortic valves into self-expandable valves and balloon-expandable valves. He then names and characterizes each of them as well as reviews details of the technique of the procedure.

In Section 4 on the management of AS, I discuss, in Chapter 5, transcatheter interventions in the management of congenital aortic valve stenosis. I review the procedure of balloon aortic valvuloplasty (BalAV) and its results. BalAV offers good relief of aortic valve obstruction and serves as a substitute for surgery. It is considered a favored option in the management of AS in all age groups, namely, fetuses, neonates, infants, children, adolescents, and young adults. However, BalAV in elderly patients with calcific AS offers only temporary relief of aortic valve obstruction. While there is conclusive data for the provision of pressure gradient relief both acutely and at follow-up as well as deferral of any surgery after BalAV, the development of AI at long-term follow-up is an important drawback of this procedure. Notwithstanding the issue of AI, BalAV is presently believed to be a therapeutic procedure option in the treatment of valvar AS in pediatric and young adult patients. Methodical follow-up to identify the reappearance of aortic obstruction and the development of substantial AI is suggested.

In Chapter 6, Dr. Shah et al. address catheter-based therapies in the management of patients with severe AS. They detail the indications and contraindications for aortic valve replacement and discuss pre-procedural work-up. They also present a detailed description of the available devices (both balloon-expandable and self-expanding valves) for TAVR. This is followed by a discussion of the techniques of the TAVR procedure, followed by a review of post-procedure management.

In Chapter 7, Dr. Navaratnarajah et al. describe valve-in-valve TAVR (ViV-TAVR) to address recurrence following a prior surgical aortic valve replacement (SAVR) or TAVR. Repeat SAVR or ViV-TAVR are the available options. The authors compare these options and conclude that ViV-TAVR shows better short-term mortality, but that both procedures have similar mortality rates at mid-term. ViV-TAVR is also associated with higher rates of patient–prosthesis mismatch, post-procedural AI, and elevated transvalvular gradients. Given the limitations of these meta-analysis studies, the authors recommend randomized control studies. They conclude that ViV-TAVR is preferred at most institutions around the world and that ViV-TAVR is a safe and effective treatment option to address failed bioprosthetic aortic valves, however, they suggest retaining the repeat SAVR strategy.

In Chapters 8 and 9, Di Pietro et al. and Jiménez-Rodríguez et al. and their associates review the risk of stroke during TAVR and state that prevention is better than cure. Strokes are linked with high mortality with an impact on cognitive function. Cerebral embolic protection devices (CEPDs) may help capture the embolic debris and their use appears to be safe and effective for decreasing the risk of stroke. The authors classify CEPDs as deflectors (TriGUARD, Embrella, Point-Guard, and ProtEmbo) and filters (Sentinel, Emboliner, and Emblok). They describe the use of some of these devices and conclude that use of CEPDs is a novel strategy for preventing strokes during TAVR and that they help decrease the frequency of disabling strokes.

In Chapter 10, Dr. Zotov et al. review the surgical treatment of aortic valve disease in patients who also have atrial fibrillation (AF). The authors state the incidence of AF is much higher (4% to 30%) in patients with severe AS than in the general population and that AF adversely affects long-term survival. The authors review the surgical and transcatheter procedures to treat AF that have been developed over the years. They present two options in the management of these patients, namely, a complete

MAZE-IV operation and a non-MAZE procedure (pulmonary vein isolation, box-lesion, and their variations). Then they describe the operative procedure in detail. They assert that performing ablation of the arrhythmogenic substrate during aortic valve surgery does not adversely affect in-hospital mortality and does not increase the length of hospital stay. Accordingly, it is recommended that these procedures should be performed in all patients diagnosed with AS and AF. The authors propose an original approach of combined treatment of AS and arrhythmia using the Perceval-S suture-less valve and the Gemini-S clamp ablator.

In Section 5 on the management of AI, Dr. Velagapudi et al. review transcatheter therapies for AI in Chapter 11. AI is classified into stages A through D according to its severity. The author states that stage D AI with severe symptoms is a Class I indication for SAVR. TAVR may be used on an off-label basis for patients who are at a prohibitive risk for SAVR. He then enumerates challenges for TAVR in patients with AI, namely, lack of calcification of valve leaflets and perivalvular apparatus dilatation, which may compromise optimal anchorage of the valve prosthesis with the consequent risk of valve embolization and perivalvular leak. Oversizing the valve by 10%–15% (but no more than 20%) may overcome some of these difficulties. Current data indicate satisfactory results for off-label use of Medtronic Evolut and Edwards Sapien 3. Results of clinical trials with specially designed JenaValve to address TAVR for native AI are awaited. The author suggests cautious selection of AI subjects for off-label use of TAVR until the results of randomized control trials become available.

In Section 6 on surgical therapy for BAV syndrome, Milewski et al., in Chapter 12, review current therapeutic strategies to address BAV syndrome. Patients with BAV exhibit a range of aortic valvar and ascending aortic and aortic root aneurysmal pathology. This varying pathology requires designing different surgical techniques to develop a tailored approach to BAV syndrome. The authors review embryologic and genetic bases for BAV syndrome with associated aortic aneurysms. They also describe genetic syndromes associated with BAV. Then, they discuss issues related to surveillance of BAV syndrome depending upon symptomatology and magnitude of pathology. Then they review evidence-based surgical therapeutic strategies including aortic valve repair, replacement of the aortic valve, and replacement of supra-coronary ascending aorta, Bentall procedure, and valve-sparing aortic root reimplantation. The authors conclude that BAV syndrome manifests aortic valvar disease (AS and AI) and ascending aortic and aortic root aneurysms. This varying spectrum of pathologies mandates the development of individualized approaches to manage these conditions.

Finally, in Section 7 on patient perspective, Dr. Hutchens, who had TAVR, describes his perspective as a patient in Chapter 13. He was in touch with several patients who either had TAVR or are being considered for TAVR. Most of these patients were concerned about the high cost and safety of the procedure, their longevity after TAVR, and the longevity of the replaced aortic valve. Dr. Hutchens points to improved quality of life after TAVR. He also presents his life-long story of his aortic valve problems. He concludes with the hope that his story of heart valve experience will be of comfort to future patients and physicians.

The last five decades have witnessed a great many advances in the diagnosis and management of aortic valve disease, which resulted in increased survival of neonates, infants, children, and adults with diseases of the aortic valve. This book discusses some of these advances and is a useful resource on diagnostic and therapeutic methods for healthcare professionals in providing quality care to their patients with aortic valve and aortic root diseases.

P. Syamasundar Rao, MD, DCH, FAAP, FACC, FSCAI
Children's Heart Institute,
Children's Memorial Hermann Hospital and McGovern Medical School,
University of Texas Health Sciences Center at Houston,
Houston, TX, USA

Section 1

Introduction

Chapter 1

Introductory Chapter: Aortic Valve Disease – Recent Advances

P. Syamasundar Rao

1. Introduction

The title of the book "Aortic Valve Disease" was selected with the intent to discuss etiologic, diagnostic, and therapeutic aspects of aortic valve disease with a focus on recent advances. Selected clinicians and investigators were invited to submit chapter proposals, once received, suitable proposals were accepted. The purpose of this chapter is to introduce the subject, describe the normal anatomy of the aortic valve apparatus, review the prevalence of different types of aortic valve diseases, and address topics not adequately dealt with in the other chapters in the book.

Several advances in the understanding of the anatomy of the aortic valve, the development of investigative tests to diagnose and quantitate the magnitude of aortic valve disease, and multiple modalities to treat the aortic valve disease have occurred over the last five decades. The objective of this book was to bring some of these advances to the attention of the reader. While surgical therapy of aortic valve disease has been in vogue since the early 1950s, catheter-based interventional techniques introduced in the early 1980s became initial management options at many institutions. This book will address the anatomy of the normal and diseased aortic valve; explore the utility of diagnostic tests such as echocardiogram, Doppler interrogation, magnetic resonance imaging, computed tomography, cardiac catheterization, and selective cine angiography; and review the relative usefulness of catheter-based vs. surgical techniques in addressing the aortic valve disease. Finally, a discussion of both short-term and long-term results of catheter interventional and surgical therapeutic modalities was included.

2. Normal anatomy of the aortic valve apparatus

The functional unit of a normal aortic root is made up of three aortic sinuses of Valsalva. They are formed by the aortic wall and the aortic valve leaflets, which are attached to the corresponding sinus. This establishes three pocket-like spaces. They are divided by commissural spaces and interleaflet triangles, the so-called trigone [1, 2]. The sum of the zones of the valve leaflets is larger than the cross-sectional region of the aortic root and this in addition to valve leaflet tissue pliability permits for a competent valve closure during the diastolic phase and unhindered valve opening to allow forward flow during the systolic phase of the cardiac cycle. While tricuspid valve leaflets are the most common morphologic structure of the aortic valve, unicuspid, bicuspid, and quadricuspid morphologic variants are also seen, the later in aortic valve or truncal disease states.

IntechOpen

3. Prevalence

3.1 Congenital valvar AS

The incidence of congenital valvar aortic stenosis (AS) is 5–6% of all congenital heart defects (CHDs). Given the prevalence of CHDs in 0.8% of live births [3, 4], the population prevalence of AS is estimated to be 0.5–0.6% (5 to 6 per 1000) of live births. AS's occurrence is more frequent in males than in females.

3.2 Bicuspid aortic valve

The prevalence of bicuspid aortic valve is generally thought to be 1–2% of population [5, 6]. More recent studies indicated a slightly lower prevalence. A study that reviewed echocardiograms of 24,265 subjects with a gender distribution of 47% males and 53% females revealed a 0.6% prevalence of bicuspid aortic valves [7]. Screening echocardiograms of 1742 teenage athletes with male preponderance (67% male and 33% female) revealed a 0.5% incidence of bicuspid aortic valves [7]. In another study of 2273 competitive athletes, aged 8–60 years, bicuspid aortic valves were present in 2.5% [8], higher than seen in the previous study. An echocardiogram of 1075 neonates revealed a prevalence of 0.46%; there was a higher (0.71%) prevalence in male babies than in female infants (0.19%) [9]. Studies do confirm a high level of accuracy of echocardiography in diagnosing bicuspid aortic valve [10]. Variations from 0.5 to 2.5% in the prevalence of bicuspid aortic valve appear to be related to the types of study cohorts selected in each study.

3.3 Calcific AS

In a study published in 2013, the prevalence of calcific AS in the elderly has ranged between 2.8 and 4.6% [11]. In a more recent study examining the global epidemiology of valvular heart disease, calcific AS among adults is age-dependent, older the subject, and more frequent, is its prevalence; the highest is in the older adults: 1000 per 100,000 (1%) in 75–79 year-olds and 1400 per 100,000 (1.4%) in 80–85 year-olds [12]. These prevalences are lower than those described in the above study [11]. There was nearly an equal gender distribution [12]. By contrast, rheumatic heart disease is more common in low-income countries with prevalence rates of 400–500 per 100,000 with similar distribution among all adult age groups [12]. The gender distribution of rheumatic heart disease is also similar in all age groups [12].

3.4 Aortic insufficiency

In the Framingham heart study involving 1696 men and 1893 women aged 54 ± 10 years, the prevalence of aortic insufficiency (AI) was found to be 13% in men and 8.5% in women; the subjects were assessed by echocardiography [13].

3.5 Ascending aortic aneurysm

The prevalence of ascending aortic aneurysms is 5 per 100,000 patient-years; this is based on population-based studies [14].

DOI: http://dx.doi.org/10.5772/intechopen.112887

4. Clinical features

4.1 AS in the pediatric patient

Most children with valvar AS are asymptomatic and the AS is usually detected because of a cardiac murmur heard on routine auscultation [15–17]. Patients with severe AS may exhibit symptoms such as dyspnea, easy fatigability, or chest pain. Syncope may be a presenting complaint in some children with very severe AS. On physical examination, the left ventricular impulse is increased (left ventricular heave) in all but mild cases. A thrill may be felt at the right upper sternal border and/or in the supra-sternal notch. The first heart sound is usually normal. The second heart sound is also normal unless the AS is extremely severe when there may be a paradoxical splitting of the second heart sound. An ejection systolic click is heard best at the apex and left mid and right upper sternal borders and the click does not vary with respiration. An ejection systolic murmur of grade II–V/VI intensity is heard best at the right upper sternal border with radiation into both carotid arteries. The arterial pulses are usually normal.

4.2 Critical AS in neonates

The term critical AS is used to describe very severe aortic valve stenosis who have high peak systolic pressure gradients across the aortic valve, signs and symptoms of congestive heart failure (CHF) are present, and/or a ductal-dependent systemic circulation exists. The pressure gradient across the aortic valve may not be high in some babies because of poor left ventricular function. They usually present during the first 24–48 hours after birth with symptoms of tachypnea, respiratory distress, cyanosis, pallor, lethargy, metabolic acidosis, and oliguria. Physical examination reveals signs of CHF and poor pulses in all four extremities. Ejection systolic click at the apex and ejection systolic murmur at the right upper sternal border may be heard, but not as prominent as non-critical AS patients.

4.3 Mild, moderate, and severe AS in the adult

The clinical features are essentially like those seen in pediatric patients described above, although, the findings are less discernable in obese adult subjects.

4.4 Calcific AS in the elderly

Patients with milder forms of calcific AS are asymptomatic and are usually detected because of a cardiac murmur heard on routine physical examination or by an echocardiographic study performed for an unrelated reason. Moderate to severe forms may present with symptoms of dyspnea on exertion or exercise intolerance. Rarely, the presenting symptoms such as syncope, chest pain, or signs of CHF may appear. Physical examination reveals increased left ventricular impulse; slow upstroke of the pulse (pulsus tardus) and small pulse volume (pulsus parvus), both are better perceived in carotid than in radial and brachial pulses; ejection systolic click at the apex, unless the aortic valve is immobile because of marked calcification; soft aortic component of the second heart sound; and an ejection systolic murmur, heard at the right upper sternal border, radiating to the carotid arteries. Higher grades of the murmur (grade IV) and late peaking in systole suggest more severe obstruction.

4.5 Aortic insufficiency

Most patients with mild to moderate AI are asymptomatic and are detected because of a cardiac murmur. Severe AI patients present with symptoms of easy fatigability, dyspnea on exertion, or chest pain. On physical examination, while the peripheral pulses are normal in mild AI, they are increased and "bounding" in patients with moderate and severe AI. The pulse pressure is increased secondary to increased systolic blood pressure with a concurrent decrease in diastolic pressure. Peripheral signs of AI such as water-hammer pulse (rapid increase and decrease of pulse when palpating the forearm), Corrigan's pulse (strikingly augmented carotid pulses), Duroziez's murmur [bruits both in systole and diastole auscultated in the femoral artery region while it is partially occluded], pistol shot sounds (systolic and diastolic vibrations of the arterial wall—Traube's sign), and Quinke's pulse (flushing and blanching alternatively of the capillary beds of the tips of finger) are seen in subjects with moderate to severe AI; however, these signs do not inevitably categorize that the AI is severe. The left ventricular impulse is prominent to hyperdynamic. The diastolic thrill of AI is rarely felt. In general, there are no abnormal cardiac sounds. If the AI is due to a bicuspid aortic valve, an aortic systolic click is auscultated. A systolic ejection murmur is heard at the upper right or at mid-left sternal borders; this may be related to the increased volume of blood that has to be pumped back via the aortic valve. Alternatively, the systolic component may be due to associated aortic valve stenosis. An early diastolic decrescendo murmur is auscultated at the right upper and left mid sternal borders. The murmur has a high pitch and is heard better with the diaphragm than the bell of the stethoscope. The murmur begins with the aortic component of the 2nd sound and is better heard when the patient sits up, leans forward, and holds the breath at end-expiration. It may transmit inferiorly to the left lower sternal border. An Austin-Flint type of mid-diastolic murmur may be appreciated at the apex.

5. Echocardiographic diagnosis

5.1 Congenital AS in the pediatric patient

Echocardiographic studies are very useful in the diagnosis of the type of AS (valvar, sub-valvar, and supra-valvar), in characterizing the aortic valve morphology, and in quantitating the degree of obstruction.

5.1.1 Types of AS

Obstruction of the left ventricular outflow tract may be seen at valvar (**Figure 1**), sub-valvar (subaortic membranous stenosis [**Figure 2**] and hypertrophic cardiomyopathy [**Figure 3**]), and supra-valvar (**Figure 4**) locations [15–17]. Examples are shown in **Figures 1–4**.

5.1.2 Characterization of aortic valve morphology

The normal aortic valve is tricuspid as shown in **Figure 5**. In congenital AS, most commonly, the aortic valve is bicuspid (**Figures 6** and 7),

The aortic valve leaflets are thickened (**Figures 1A**, **B** and 7**A, B**) and dome during systole (**Figures 1B** and 7C) in most patients.

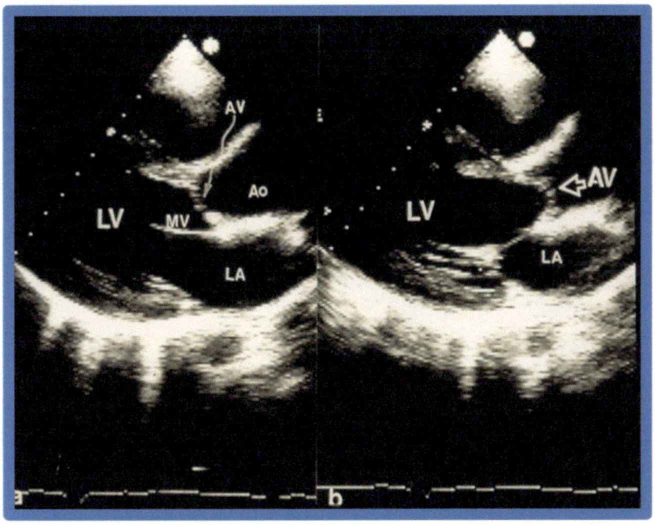

Figure 1.
Echocardiographic frames from precordial long axis view of the left ventricle (LV) demonstrating valvar AS. Note the thickened and domed aortic valve (AV). Ao, aorta; LA, left atrium; LV, left ventricle. Reproduced from reference [17].

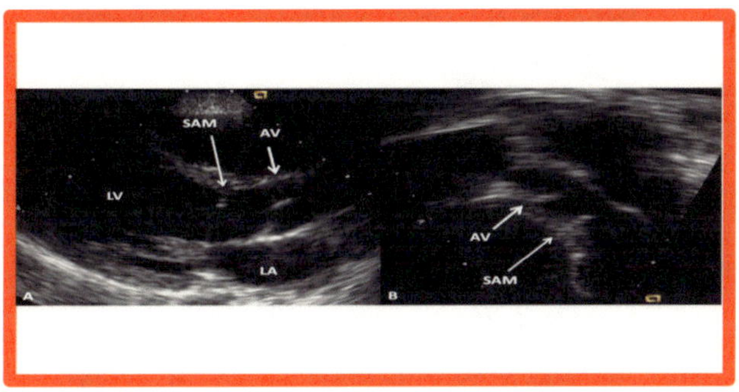

Figure 2.
Echocardiogram in parasternal long axis (A) and apical five-chamber (B) projections demonstrating the subaortic membrane (SAM). The position of the aortic valve (AV) is shown. Continuous wave and color Doppler studies demonstrated elevated Doppler flow velocity across SAM but are not shown in these echo frames. LA, left atrium; LV, left ventricle. Reproduced from reference [18].

5.1.3 Quantification of the degree of obstruction

The flow velocity magnitude across the aortic valve, measured by Doppler, is increased (**Figures 7E** and **8C**) which is used to calculate the systolic pressure gradient across the aortic valve by a modified Bernoulli equation:

$$\text{Peak instantaneous gradient} = 4V^2 \quad (1)$$

Where V is the peak Doppler velocity across the aortic valve in meters/sec.

The Doppler velocity measurements are made in parasternal, suprasternal notch, and apical views. Most important, however, is to achieve a close alignment of the Doppler signal to the aortic flow. It should be understood that the Doppler peak

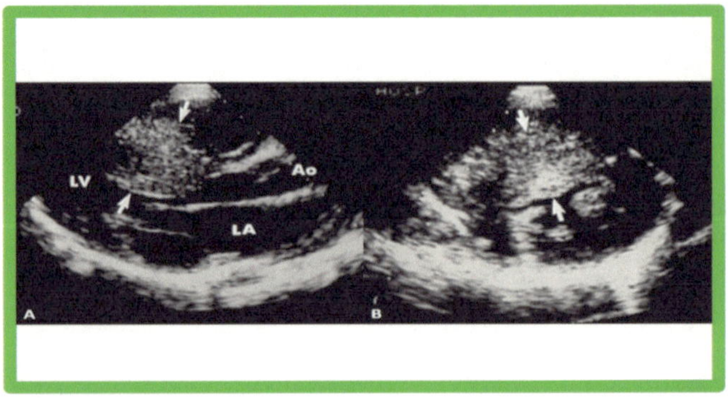

Figure 3.
Echocardiograms in parasternal long (A) and short (B) axis projections illustrating severe thickening of the inter-ventricular septum (arrows), suggestive of hypertrophic cardiomyopathy. Continuous wave and color Doppler studies demonstrated elevated Doppler flow velocity across the left ventricular outflow tract at the level of thickened inter-ventricular septum. Ao, aorta; LA, left atrium; LV, left ventricle. Modified from reference [17].

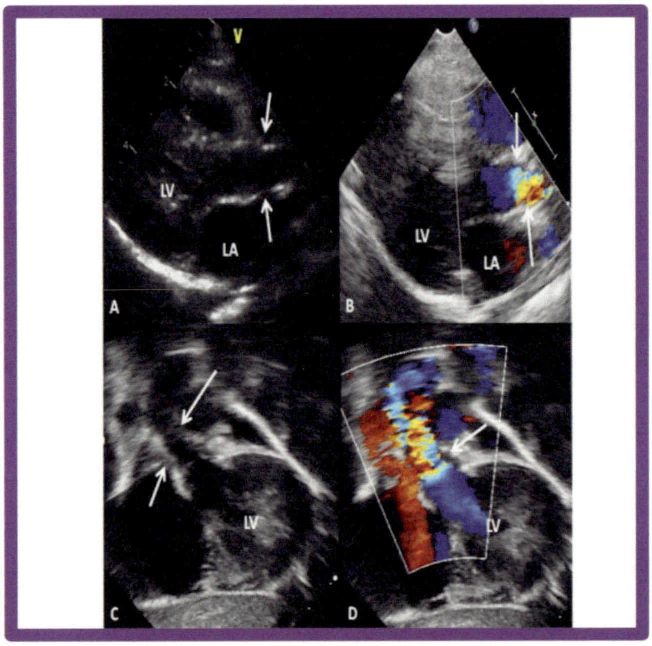

Figure 4.
Echo-Doppler studies in parasternal long axis (A and B) and subcostal (C and D) projections illustrating supra-valvar AS. Note that the stenosis is above the aortic valve as shown with arrows. Color flow imaging shows turbulence in Doppler flow signal as pointed out with arrows (B and D). An increased Doppler flow velocity was recorded superior to the aortic valve but is not illustrated in the above echo frames. LA, left atrium; LV, left ventricle. Reproduced from reference [18].

instantaneous gradient does not accurately reflect the true peak-to-peak systolic pressure gradient obtained in the cardiac catheterization laboratory because of the pressure recovery phenomenon [19]. Consequently, applicable corrections to account for pressure recovery should be made during the calculations of the pressure gradient. Turbulent flow is also demonstrated by color flow Doppler (**Figures 7D** and **8B**).

DOI: http://dx.doi.org/10.5772/intechopen.112887

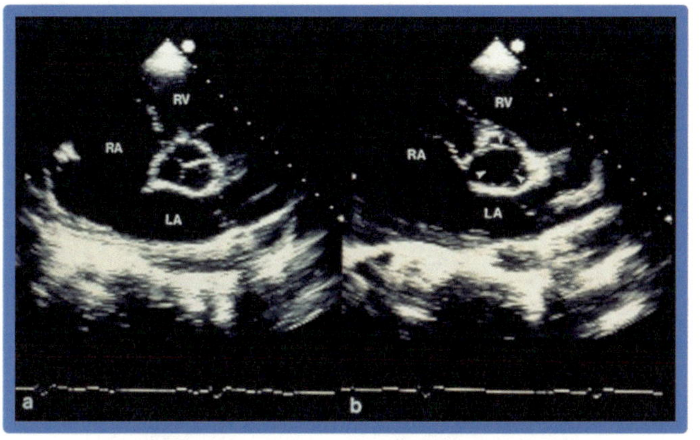

Figure 5.
Selected echo images in parasternal short axis view demonstrating normal tricuspid aortic valve in closed (A) and open (B) positions. LA, left atrium; RA, right atrium; RV, right ventricle.

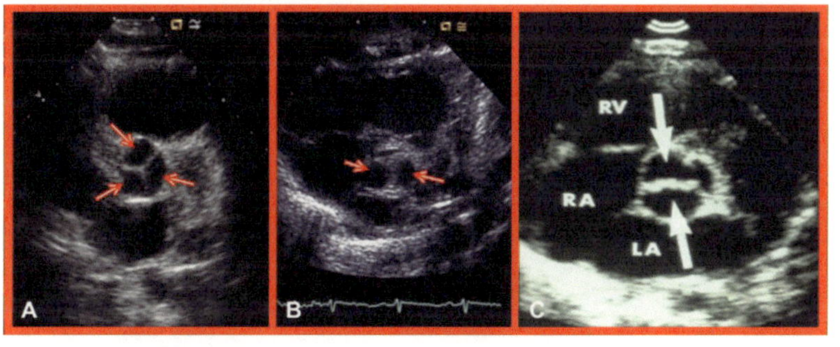

Figure 6.
Selected echo images in parasternal short axis view demonstrating normal tricuspid aortic valve (A), bicuspid aortic valve with vertical (B) and horizontal (C) commissures. The arrows point to the respective aortic valve leaflets.

The echo-Doppler studies in pediatric patients are sufficiently accurate such that there is generally no need for other imaging studies such as magnetic resonance imaging (MRI) and computed tomography (CT).

5.1.4 Other echocardiographic features

Annular hypoplasia and dysplasia of aortic valve leaflets have also been seen, mostly in neonates and young babies.

Left ventricular internal dimension (LVID) in diastole is usually normal for age. However, LVID may be increased in patients with long-standing and severe AS. Such left ventricular enlargements are more common in neonates with critical AS. Hypertrophy of the left ventricular musculature in a concentric manner is seen which is mostly proportionate to the severity of obstruction. The left ventricular shortening fraction may be increased, usually proportional to the degree of narrowing. However, in neonates with critical AS and patients with heart failure, it may be decreased. Post-stenotic dilatation of the aorta (Ao) is observed in most patients; the degree of such dilatation is not related to the degree of aortic valve obstruction [16–18].

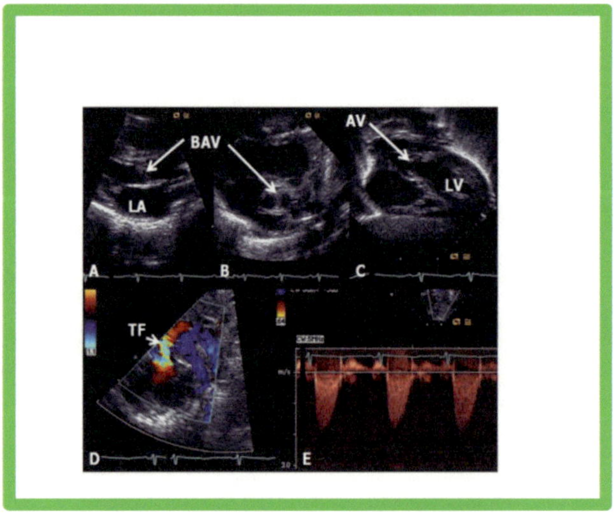

Figure 7.
Echo images illustrating a thick (A) and bicuspid (B) aortic valve (BAV) with doming of the aortic valve (AV) (C) pointed out by arrows. Color flow Doppler demonstrates turbulent flow (TF) at the aortic valve (arrow) (D). The Doppler velocity across the AV is low (<2 m/s) (E), suggesting trivial AS with a bicuspid aortic valve. LA, left atrium; LV, left ventricle. Reproduced from reference [18].

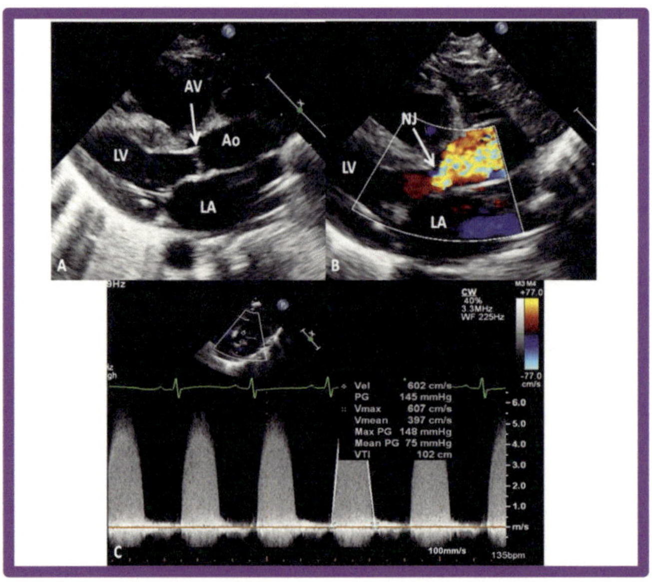

Figure 8.
Echo-Doppler studies of a patient with severe AS illustrating an aortic valve (AV) which is thick and domed (A). Color flow imaging demonstrates turbulent flow with a narrow jet (NJ) at the AV (arrow) (B). The Doppler velocity via the AV is high (>6 m/s) (C), suggesting very severe AS; the calculated peak instantaneous gradient is 148 mmHg with a mean of 75 mmHg. The patient has a bicuspid AV which is not demonstrated in these echo frames. Ao, ascending aorta; LA, left atrium; LV, left ventricle. Reproduced from reference [18].

5.2 Congenital AS in the young adults

The echo-Doppler studies in young adults with congenital AS are similar to those described in the preceding section, although an occasional patient with poor acoustic windows may require trans-esophageal echo evaluation or other imaging studies.

5.3 Calcific AS in the elderly

Like AS in the pediatric patient, echocardiographic studies are very useful in characterizing the aortic valve morphology, in quantitating the degree of obstruction, and in assessing left ventricular response to increased afterload. The aortic valve leaflets have increased echo density and decreased valve leaflet motion. It is frequently difficult to discern whether it is a tricuspid or bicuspid aortic valve. The Peak Doppler flow velocity is increased which is used to calculate the systolic pressure gradient across the aortic valve by a modified Bernoulli equation, as reviewed above in the section on “Congenital AS in the Pediatric Patient.” Other disease entities such as hypertrophic cardiomyopathy, mitral valve disease, and CHDs are excluded by echo studies. Left ventricular hypertrophy is usually detected by echo evaluation. Left ventricular ejection fraction can be quantitated; in most cases, it is preserved until late in the disease.

5.4 Aortic insufficiency

Echocardiographic, MRI, and CT features of AI were described in the chapter on “Transcatheter Therapies for Aortic Regurgitation – Where Are We in 2023?” by Shabbir and his associates and will not be repeated in this chapter.

6. Aortic valve surgery without valve replacement

Most chapters in this book deal with surgical or transcatheter replacement of the aortic valve. Other forms of surgery such as commissurotomy, plastic repair of aortic valve, and Ross procedure have not been addressed. These will be reviewed briefly.

6.1 Commissurotomy

Aortic valvotomy via aortotomy under cardiopulmonary bypass has been used with success [20]; however, most institutions currently use balloon aortic valvuloplasty as the initial treatment option.

6.2 Plastic repair of the aortic valve

Neocuspidization (plastic repair of aortic valve) either into a bicuspid or tricuspid aortic valve, as the case may be, with or without prosthetic material (patient’s native leaflet tissue, glutaraldehyde-treated autologous pericardium, non-treated autologous pericardium, expanded polytetrafluoroethylene (ePTFE) membrane, decellularized xenogenic tissue, glutaraldehyde-treated bovine pericardium, or untreated equine pericardium) and cusp augmentation to restore the aortic valve close to its normal structure and function has been used successfully [21–24].

6.3 Ross procedure

Aortic valve replacement with patient's own pulmonary valve and inserting a bioprosthetic valve in the pulmonary position [25, 26] has been used successfully to address severe AS cases both in neonates and older patients, although the risk of double valve disease exists [27].

Author details

P. Syamasundar Rao
Children's Heart Institute, Children's Memorial Hermann Hospital and McGovern Medical School, University of Texas Health Sciences Center at Houston, Houston, Texas, USA

*Address all correspondence to: p.syamasundar.rao@uth.tmc.edu

IntechOpen

© 2023 The Author(s). Licensee IntechOpen. This chapter is distributed under the terms of the Creative Commons Attribution License (http://creativecommons.org/licenses/by/3.0), which permits unrestricted use, distribution, and reproduction in any medium, provided the original work is properly cited.

References

[1] Angelini A, Ho SY, Anderson RH, et al. The morphology of the normal aortic valve as compared with the aortic valve having two leaflets. The Journal of Thoracic Cardiovasc Surgery. 1989;**98**:362-367

[2] McKay R, Smith A, Leung MP, Arnold R, Anderson RH. Morphology of the ventriculoaortic junction in critical aortic stenosis: Implications for hemodynamic function and clinical management. The Journal of Thoracic Cardiovasc Surgery. 1992;**104**:434-442

[3] Mitchell SC, Korones SB, Berendes HW. Congenital heart disease in 56,109 births. Incidence and natural history. Circulation. 1971;**43**:323-332. DOI: 10.1161/01.cir.43.3.323

[4] Hoffman JI, Kaplan S. The incidence of congenital heart disease. The Journal of the American College of Cardiology. 2002;**39**:1890-1900

[5] Braverman AC, Güven H, Beardslee MA, et al. The bicuspid aortic valve. Current Problems in Cardioldioloy. 2005;**30**:470-522

[6] Friedman T, Mani A, Elefteriades JA. Bicuspid aortic valve: Clinical approach and scientific review of a common clinical entity. Expert Review of Cardiovascular Therapy. 2008;**6**:235-248

[7] Movahed MR, Hepner AD, Ahmadi-Kashani M. Echocardiographic prevalence of bicuspid aortic valve in the population. Heart Lung Circulation. 2006;**15**:297-299. DOI: 10.1016/j.hlc.2006.06.001

[8] Stefani L, Galanti G, Toncelli L, Manetti P, Vono MC, Rizzo M, et al. Bicuspid aortic valve in competitive athletes. British Journal of Sports Medicine. 2008;**42**:31-35; discussion 35. DOI: 10.1136/bjsm.2006.033530

[9] Tutar E, Ekici F, Atalay S, Nacar N. The prevalence of bicuspid aortic valve in newborns by echocardiographic screening. The American Heart Journal. 2005;**150**:513-515. DOI: 10.1016/j.ahj.2004.10.036

[10] Jain R, Ammar KA, Kalvin L, Ignatowski D, Olet S, Tajik AJ, et al. Diagnostic accuracy of bicuspid aortic valve by echocardiography. Echocardiography. 2018;**35**:1932-1938. DOI: 10.1111/echo.14167

[11] Osnabrugge RL, Mylotte D, Head SJ, Van Mieghem NM, Nkomo VT, LeReun CM, et al. Aortic stenosis in the elderly: Disease prevalence and number of candidates for transcatheter aortic valve replacement: A meta-analysis and modeling study. Journal of the American College of Cardiology. 2013;**62**:1002-1012

[12] Coffey S, Roberts-Thomson R, Brown A, Carapetis J, Chen M, Enriquez-Sarano M, et al. Global epidemiology of valvular heart disease. Nature Reviews, Cardiology. 2021;**18**:853-864. DOI: 10.1038/s41569-021-00570-z

[13] Singh JP, Evans JC, Levy D, Larson MG, Freed LA, Fuller DL, et al. Prevalence and clinical determinants of mitral, tricuspid, and aortic regurgitation (the Framingham heart study). The American Journal of Cardiology. 1999;**83**:897-902. DOI: 10.1016/s0002-9149(98)01064-9 Erratum in: The American Journal of Cardiology. 1999;**84**:1143

[14] Gouveia e Melo R, Silva Duarte G, Lopes A, Alves M, Caldeira D, Fernandes

e Fernandes R, et al. Incidence and prevalence of thoracic aortic aneurysms: A systematic review and meta-analysis of population-based studies. Seminars in Thoracic Cardiovascular Surgery. 2022;**34**:1-16

[15] Rao PS. Diagnosis and management of acyanotic heart disease: Part I-obstructive lesions. The Indian Journal of Pediatrics. 2005;**72**:496-502

[16] Singh GK, Rao PS. Left heart outflow obstructions. In: Crawford MH, DiMarco JP, Paulus WJ, editors. Cardiology. 3rd ed. Edinburgh, UK: Mosby Elsevier; 2010. pp. 1507-1518. ISBN 978-0-7234-3485-6

[17] Rao PS. Congenital heart defects–A review. In. Rao PS, editor. Congenital Heart Disease-Selected Aspects. Rijeka, Croatia: InTech; 2012. pp. 3-44. ISBN: 978-953-307-472-6

[18] Rao PS. Echocardiographic evaluation of neonates with suspected heart disease. In: Rao PS, Vidyasagar D, editors. A Multidisciplinary Approach to Perinatal Cardiology. Vol. 1. New Castle upon Tyne, UK: Cambridge Scholars Publishing; 2021. pp. 314-408. ISBN-13: 978-1-5275-6722-1

[19] Singh GK, Mowers KL, Marino C, Balzer D, Rao PS. Effect of pressure recovery on pressure gradients in congenital stenotic outflow lesions in pediatric patients-clinical implications of lesion severity and geometry: A simultaneous Doppler echocardiography and cardiac catheter correlative study. The Journal of American Society of Echocardiography. 2020;**33**:207-217. DOI: 10.1016/j.echo.2019.09.001

[20] Alexiou C, Langley SM, Dalrymple-Hay MJ, Salmon AP, Keeton BR, Haw MP, et al. Open commissurotomy for critical isolated aortic stenosis in neonates. The Annals Thoracic Surgery. 2001;**71**:489-493. DOI: 10.1016/S0003-4975(00)02232-3

[21] El Khoury G, de Kerchove L. Principles of Aortic Valve Repair. Vol. 145. Amsterdam: Elsevier; 2013. pp. S26-S29. DOI: 10.1016/j.jtcvs.2012.11.071

[22] Poncelet AJ, El Khoury G, De Kerchove L, Sluysmans T, Moniotte S, Momeni M, et al. Aortic valve repair in the paediatric population: Insights from a 38-year single-centre experience. The European Journal Cardio-Thoracic Surgery. 2017;**51**:43-49. DOI: 10.1093/ejcts/ezw259

[23] Wiggins LM, Mimic B, Issitt R, Ilic S, Bonello B, Marek J, et al. The utility of aortic valve leaflet reconstruction techniques in children and young adults. The Journal of Thoracic and Cardiovascular Surgery. 2020;**159**:2369-2378. DOI: 10.1016/j.jtcvs.2019.09.176

[24] Wong SH, Nento D, Singh H, Agarwal A. Advances in the management of congenital malformations of the aortic valve. In: Rao PS, editor. Congenital Heart Defects–Recent Advances. London, UK, Rijeka, Croatia: IntechOpen; 2022. pp. 197-220

[25] Ross DN. Aortic root replacement with a pulmonary autograft--current trends. Journal of Heart Valve Disease. 1994;**3**:358-360

[26] Sharabiani MT, Dorobantu DM, Mahani AS, Turner M, Peter Tometzki AJ, Angelini GD, et al. Aortic valve replacement and the Ross operation in children and young adults. The Journal of American College of Cardiology. 2016;**67**:2858-2870. DOI: 10.1016/j.jacc.2016.04.021

[27] Etnel JR, Elmont LC, Ertekin E, Mokhles MM, Heuvelman HJ, Roos-Hesselink JW, et al. Outcome after aortic valve replacement in children: A systematic review and meta-analysis. The Journal of Thoracic and Cardiovascular Surgery. 2016;**151**(143-152):e3. DOI: 10.1016/j.jtcvs.2015.09.083

Section 2

Pathology of the Aortic Valve and Ascending Aorta

Chapter 2

Acquired Aortic Valve Diseases (Current Status of the Problem)

Abdumadjidov Khamidulla Amanullaevich and Urakov Shukhrat Tukhtaevich

Abstract

Acquired heart disease – the concept of "acquired heart disease" includes a variety of pathological conditions acquired during the life of the patient. The lion's share of these diseases are acquired heart defects. The significance of this problem is special for our region, since the incidence of rheumatic diseases and its complications in our Republic is still significant. However, in recent decades, statistical data on acquired defects, especially on aortic heart defects, have changed markedly. Thus, the prevalence of aortic heart disease among the elderly and senile is about 10.7%, significantly increasing for sclerotic lesions of the aortic valve – up to 25–48%. According to Euro Heart Survey on valvular heart disease, damage to the aortic valve was detected in 44.3% of patients with valvular heart disease (33.9% – aortic stenosis, 10.4% – aortic valve insufficiency. At the same time, aortic stenosis in 81.9% and insufficiency – in 50 .3% of patients were of degenerative origin. According to the statistics of our Republic, more than 400 patients with rheumatism per 100 thousand of the population are detected per year, of which, after an appropriate examination, in terms of the population of our Republic, more than 16,000 require surgical correction of acquired heart disease, which confirms the importance of discussing the problem for our healthcare.

Keywords: acquired heart defects, current data, research methods, treatment tactics, current of correction

1. Introduction

Aim of chapter. In connection with the foregoing, we think that the discussion of modern data on aortic malformation of acquired genesis, namely, the modern idea of changing the etiology, frequency of occurrence, clinical picture, as well as diagnostic issues, including new modern highly informative research methods, determining the tactics of surgical treatment with analysis indications and contraindications to a particular method of treatment, respectively, is of great scientific and practical importance. Therefore, we once again decided to discuss the above issues regarding aortic heart disease of acquired origin.

1.1 Actuality

The trend towards an increase in the general morbidity of the population with diseases of the circulatory system can be clearly seen [1, 2], both according to the results of world statistics, according to the results of the State Report on the state of health of the population of the Russian Federation (2002, 2003), and according to the Ministry of Health of Uzbekistan (2008). The number of open heart surgeries is increasing every year. Reconstructive operations on the aortic valve (AV) are in the center of attention of cardiac surgeons: in economically developed countries, this operation is already in second place in terms of frequency among all cardiac surgical interventions performed in the adult population. The reason for this is the changes that have taken place in the etiology of the formation of aortic valve disease and the change in the demographic structure of society itself. In developed countries, calcified aortic disease is the third most common nosological form after arterial hypertension and coronary heart disease [3].

Knowledge of the etiology of the process that led to aortic malformation can significantly influence both the surgical tactics and the protocol of postoperative treatment of patients and, as a result, the prognosis of the long-term period. Therefore, at all stages of treatment, one should strive to answer the question of the etiology of the primary process that caused valve dysfunction. Sometimes this answer can only be given by a surgeon who visually assesses the nature of the valve lesion already during the operation. In any case, elucidation of the etiology, even with a presumptive conclusion, is extremely important.

2. Etiology

Assessing our own experience, published data of colleagues from other countries and Russian clinics, it should be emphasized that even today aortic malformations of rheumatic etiology dominate in cardiac surgery hospitals, although not as clearly as in the statistics of half a century ago. This figure does not exceed 30–40%. However, if we take into account that only during the period from 1993 to 1998 in Russia the frequency of cardiac rheumatism increased by 7 times [1, 2], then in the future we should again expect an increase in the number of patients with rheumatic valvular defects.

The etiology of pathological changes in AK from the moment of the first operations has changed several times. If at the beginning rheumatic lesions, endocarditis, syphilis and atherosclerosis prevailed; then at present, atherosclerotic (degenerative) and congenital malformations (mainly bicuspid aortic valve) of the aortic valve come to the fore. Such changes in the etiology could not but affect the course of the disease itself, the clinic of the defect and, accordingly, the development of a specific tactic for the introduction of such patients.

The increase in surgical interventions on the aortic valve in the group of patients over 60 years of age has significantly increased the number of atherosclerotic "degenerative" (age-related) aortic valve defects. If the aortic defect is moderately pronounced and is combined with widespread atherosclerosis of the coronary arteries, the aorta and its branches, in combination with distinct specific disorders in lipid metabolism (total cholesterol, low density lipoproteins, triglycerides), then the atherosclerotic origin of the process on the valve is beyond doubt. This is a special and prognostically most severe group of patients. It is to this category of patients that the point of view of some authors extends that aortic stenosis is a special form of manifestation of atherosclerosis with risk factors identical to this systemic disease.

In a real clinical situation, no more than 50% of elderly patients with signs of aortic stenosis have changes in coronary vessels [4, 5]. Such patients have another dystrophic process in the valve with a reduced level of metabolic reactions due to age-related changes: atherosclerosis as such can only play the role of an accelerating factor, especially if accompanied by inflammatory changes in the aortic valve cusps specific for many atheromas due to Chlamydia invasion pneumoniae [6]. Age-related involutional calcium degeneration is, in our opinion, the most appropriate definition for such pathology of the aortic valve. As a special form, it often occurs in elderly patients and, as a rule, falls into the group of atherosclerotic malformations during analysis. The diagnostic line between these two groups of patients (atherosclerosis and age-related dystrophy) is very thin, but it is quite realistic to draw it with known experience. The practical significance of such a diagnosis can be expressed not only in a different prognosis, but also in the amount of drug therapy after surgery (the use of antiplatelet agents, lipid-lowering agents). The group of patients with congenital bicuspid aortic valve configuration adjoins the same type of "degenerative" defects with severe calcification. For us, this was unexpected, but the number of such patients increases as the number of operated elderly patients increases. Actually, the three main causes of aortic heart disease that we have already noted together account for at least 90% of the causes of aortic valve stenosis [4]. All these reasons lead to various pathomorphological, but the same type of functional changes in the aortic valve cusps, limiting their mobility. This process (fibrosis, thickening, formation of adhesions in the area of commissures, calcification) always takes a long time – years, or even decades. Other, rarer causes of aortic stenosis include previous and active infective endocarditis, systemic lupus erythematosus (Libman – Sachs verrucous aseptic endocarditis), hereditary metabolic disorders such as homozygous type II hyperlipoproteinemia and alkaptonuria (ochronosis), metastatic calcification of the aortic valve in patients with chronic renal failure [3].

Changes in the etiology of the disease over a fairly short period of time are associated primarily with the ongoing prevention of rheumatism and rheumatic heart disease. Secondly, such a restructuring in etiology is also associated with a change in the demographic structure of society in economically developed countries, where there is a constant increase in the population of elderly and senile age. Accordingly, this led to an increase in the number of elderly patients with acquired heart defects, where atherosclerotic and degenerative forms of AV malformation already prevail, which affected both the clinical picture of the disease and the age composition of operated patients. At present, either aortic stenosis or combined forms of defect occupy the main place in the structure of the forms of defect.

Statistics of detection of aortic heart disease in Uzbekistan by etiological factors:

1. Rheumatic lesion of aortic valve

2. Atherosclerotic (degenerative) lesion of aortic valve

3. Congenital lesion of aortic valve (bicuspid valve, etc.)

According to the recommendations of the European Society of Cardiology and the European Association of Cardiothoracic Surgeons, aortic valve disease should be surgically corrected in the presence of echocardiographic signs of severe stenosis (blood flow velocity on the valve is more than 400 cm/s, the average gradient on the valve is more than 40 mm.r.st., effective area orifice less than 1 cm^2, effective orifice area index less than 0.6 cm^2/m^2) and/or severe regurgitation (grade 3–4 insufficiency, central regurgitation over 65% of the area of the left ventricular cavity, vena contracta more than 0.6 cm, regurgitation volume more than 60 ml/contraction).

The indications for surgical correction of the defect were a severe degree of aortic valve stenosis (**Figure 1**), identified during clinical examination and confirmed by echocardiography data with an average transaortic pressure gradient of more than 40 mm Hg, the presence or absence of symptoms of heart failure, manifested at rest or during stress tests (decreased exercise tolerance), as well as in the presence of concomitant left ventricle systolic dysfunction (ejection fraction <50%).

Aortic valve insufficiency served as an indication for surgery in case of severe regurgitation in symptomatic patients, regardless of LV systolic function, in the absence of symptoms and the presence of LV systolic dysfunction (ejection fraction <50%). In addition, surgery has been indicated in the absence of symptoms and normal LV ejection fraction, but in the presence of LV dilatation (LV end-systolic dimension >50 mm). Performing neocuspidization according to the formulas is possible only in the absence of aortic root expansion (the diameter at the level of the sinotubular junction is not more than 35 mm and the diameter at the level of the fibrous ring is not more than 25 mm). Otherwise, it is necessary to perform neocuspidization in combination with aortic root replacement in the Moscow (Russian) conduit modification [7, 8].

Symptom complexes characteristic of a particular valvular defect determine modern treatment tactics to a much greater extent than the actual nature of the damage to the aortic cusps. Therefore, any attempt to identify the diagnosis of the condition, substantiate the indications for surgical intervention and surgical tactics only on the data of topical diagnostics (hole diameter, magnitude of leaflet prolapse, magnitude of the pressure drop across the valve, the presence or absence of signs of calcification, etc.)

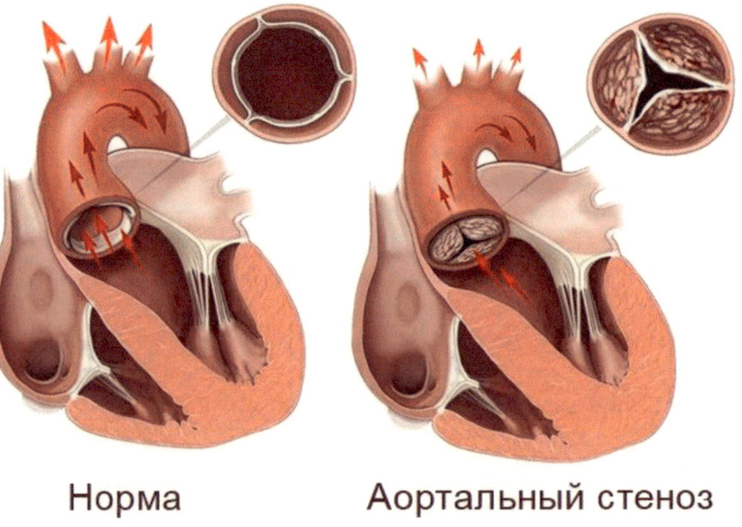

Figure 1.
Indications for surgical correction of aortic heart defects.

does not testify in favor of comprehensively a clinical analysis of the condition of a particular patient [9].

Cardiologists today reliably diagnose this pathology and promptly send such patients to cardiac surgeons. And yet, when deciding whether to operate on patients older than 70 years, we sometimes encounter some resistance from our fellow cardiologists [10]. Their doubts are based on both an objective factor – a higher risk of surgery, and a subjective one – the uncertainty of the individually "programmed" life expectancy of such elderly patients.

Therefore, in this publication, we specifically present the data of O'Keefe et al., [11], who managed to trace a group of 50 patients awaiting balloon dilatation of a stenotic aortic valve. The average age of patients exceeded 70 years, survival without surgery by the 3rd year of follow-up was only 25%. At the same time, in a randomized group of patients without aortic pathology, the survival rate was 77%. Considering that today the lethality of aortic grafting is minimal, these data should convincingly prove to cardiologists the need for an operative way of treating such patients [12].

In classical situations, the question "when to operate?" does not represent difficulties: digital radiography from the screen of the electro-optical converter, electrocardiography, echocardiography [10], MRI [13] with contrast are sufficient methods for making a topical diagnosis and assessing the state of the left ventricle of the heart. Performing a sounding of the heart cavities in patients with aortic defects in order to determine the pressure drop, regurgitation volume, end-diastolic pressure in the left ventricle or pulmonary capillary wedge pressure today can already be regarded as a diagnostic anachronism.

In practice, of course, we are especially wary of choosing a solution in patients with "minor" symptoms and, even more so, in patients with asymptomatic course. It is known that clinical manifestations and complaints may be absent even in severe severe aortic stenosis with an orifice area of less than 0.8 cm^3 and with a decrease in the ejection fraction to 25–30% [14].

An increase in the left ventricle of the heart up to 6 cm or more (in patients with aortic insufficiency), as well as hypertrophy with overload of the left ventricle (in patients with aortic stenosis), are sufficient instrumental criteria for the need for surgery in the presence of a topical diagnosis.

Doppler echocardiography allows you to set the magnitude of the pressure drop with almost the same accuracy as sounding the left ventricle. Understanding the conditionality and multifactorial dependence of this indicator, we consider its value to be 40–50 mm Hg. Art. a sufficient basis for a more detailed examination of the patient and the search for arguments in favor of the operation.

The calculation of the effective orifice is less dependent on the characteristics of blood flow through the area "left ventricle-aortic valve-ascending aorta", but this indicator is also quite arbitrary and "semi-quantitative". And yet, we always take into account the instructions of ultrasound diagnostics specialists to limit the opening of the valve leaflets to less than 1.5 cm, and with a hole size of less than 1 cm, the indications for surgery are almost absolute. An even more accurate expression of the degree of stenosis is the ratio of the size of the stenosis to the total body surface area – a value of less than 0.6 cm/m^2 is critical [3]. If at the same time there is information about valve calcification, then it is not worth postponing the operation, since the progression of the process is inevitable.

If the arguments in favor of the operation are not absolute, then with aortic stenosis we calculate the pressure loss on the valve (mm Hg/ml stroke volume) – the value is 1 mm Hg. Art./ml and more significant and weighty. If necessary, repeat these calculations under load. In aortic insufficiency, a decrease in the ejection fraction of less than 55% and its further decrease (or invariance) under stress test conditions also indicate the limit of compensatory reserves of the left ventricular myocardium and serve as a more than convincing criterion in favor of surgery.

In the presence of concomitant coronary pathology requiring surgical correction, or concomitant mitral valve defects, the criteria for revision and intervention on the aortic valve can be much more liberal and are often determined by the individual decision of the operating surgeon.

It should be remembered that aortic stenosis progresses regardless of any patterns. However, with degenerative defects, this process is faster than with rheumatic or in the presence of a bicuspid valve. With slow progression, the opening of the aortic valve narrows by 0.02 cm^2 per year, and with rapid progression, more than 0.3 cm^2 per year. When the peak velocity of blood flow through the valve reaches about 4 m/s, the two-year survival rate without surgery is only 21%. Thus, calcification, the rate of progression of stenosis during the year, and positive exercise tests (slight rise or even decrease in blood pressure during exercise) are real factors for deciding on surgery for asymptomatic aortic stenosis.

In asymptomatic aortic insufficiency, the prognosis is based on an assessment of left ventricular function and the degree of dilatation of the ascending aorta. Threatening signs are an increase in end-diastolic pressure of the left ventricle more than 70 mm, end-systolic pressure more than 50 mm (index more than 25 mm/m^2 of the patient's body surface), a decrease in the ejection fraction to 50%. If the ascending aorta is dilated more than 55 mm, surgery should be offered regardless of the degree of aortic regurgitation and left ventricular function. In patients with a bicuspid valve or with Marfan syndrome, the indications for surgery are even more stringent – the threshold for making a decision is the diameter of the ascending aorta is 50 mm.

Regular routine monitoring of the condition is necessary for all patients with symptoms of aortic valve disease and is mandatory every 12 months in order not to miss the time for possible surgical interventions.

3. Diagnostics of aortic heart defects

1. Clinical symptoms
2. Laboratory research
3. Electrocardiography's
4. X-ray examination
5. Doppler echocardiography
6. angiography, Aortography
7. MRI with contrast
8. Radioisotope research

3.1 X-ray examination and ECG in aortic disease

X-ray of the chest organs – evaluates the size and location of the heart, changes in the configuration of the heart (protrusion of the shadow of the heart in the projection of the aorta and left ventricle in aortic disease) (**Figures 2** and **3**).

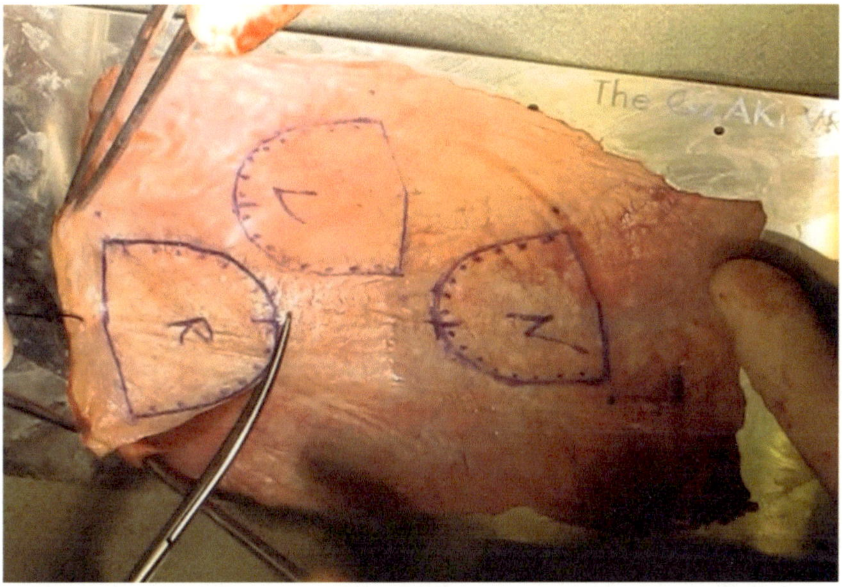

Figure 2.
ECG – Signs of left ventricular hypertrophy with overload.

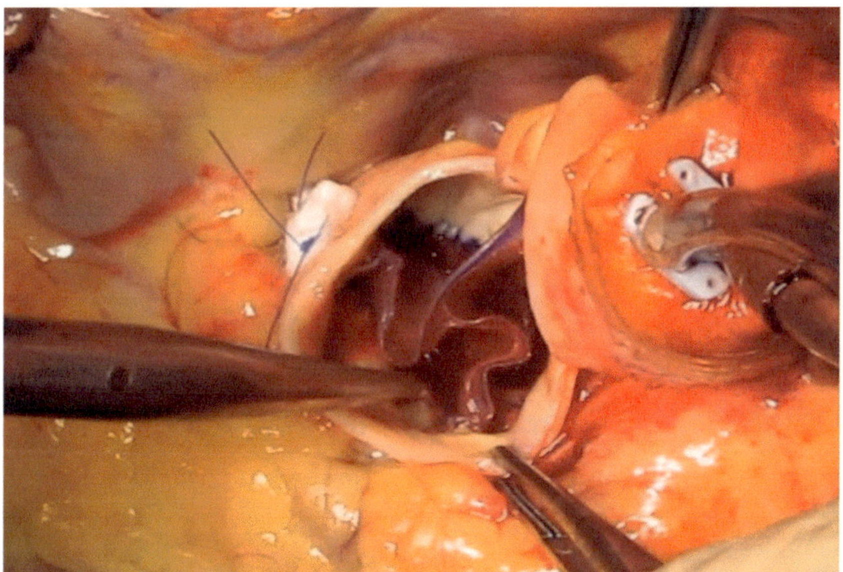

Figure 3.
Echocardiographic features of aortic stenosis.

Aortic stenosis thickening of the aortic valve cusps, decreased mobility.
Concentric LV hypertorphia.

Pressure gradient between aorta and LV
Assessment of the degree of calcification of the aortic valve and aortic root.
Assessment of the degree of left ventricular myocardial hypertrophy.
Assessment of the degree of dilatation of the cavities of the heart.
Doppler echocardiography.
Increased flow rate through the aortic valve into systole.
Calculation of the maximum and average systolic pressure gradient across the aortic valve.
Classification of the degree of aortic stenosis depending on the maximum and average transvalvular pressure gradient.
Calculate the area of the aortic orifice using the continuity equation:
positions and measurements, calculated parameters.
Calculation of the aortic orifice area index.

3.2 Echocardiographic signs of aortic insufficiency

The study of the size of the chambers of the heart, the mass of the myocardium of the left ventricle (**Figure 4**) [14].

The study of contractility of the left ventricle. The study of the volume, shape of the myocardium of the left ventricle.

Doppler echocardiography.

Pulse wave doppler.

Assessment of the degree of aortic regurgitation by the depth of the jet in the outflow tract of the left ventricle.

Continuous wave doppler also allows assessing the degree and significance of aortic regurgitation.

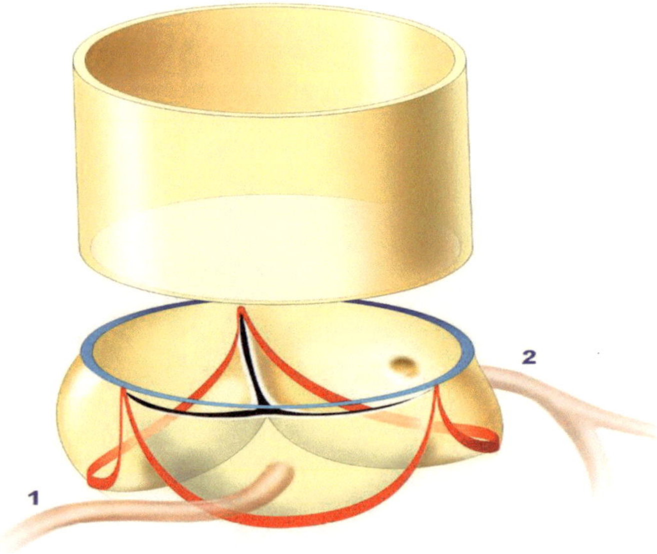

Figure 4.
Aortic insufficiency.

Ways to reliably assess the severity of aortic regurgitation:
Calculation of the half-decay time of the aortic pressure gradient regurgitation.
Calculation of the fraction of the regurgitant volume.

3.3 Invasive research methods for aortic stenosis

In order to measure the pressure gradient between the left ventricle and the aorta, probing of the heart cavities is performed. to which allows you to indirectly judge the degree of aortic stenosis. Ventriculography needed to detect concomitant mitral regurgitation. Aortography and coronary angiography are used for the differential diagnosis of aortic stenosis with an aneurysm of the ascending aorta and ischemic heart disease (**Figure 5**).

Magnetic resonance imaging (MRI) of the heart is a method of tomographic diagnostics, based on scanning the heart tissue with radio waves when the patient is in a powerful magnetic field. In the process of MRI, images of slices of the heart are obtained in different planes. High resolution characteristics of MRI make it possible to obtain detailed information about the structure of the cavities and valves of the heart, to conduct a study of the functional parameters of cardiac activity [8, 9, 13].

3.4 Invasive diagnostic methods for aortic insufficiency

Catheterization of the heart cavities with angiography in patients with aortic insufficiency is necessary to determine the magnitude of cardiac output, LV end-diastolic volume and regurgitation volume, as well as other necessary parameters.

3.5 Radionuclide studies of the myocardium in aortic disease

Radionuclide myocardial scintigraphy is used in evaluating the results of surgical correction of aortic heart defects.

With AS, LV wall tension occurs, which leads to coronary microcirculatory dysfunction. Scintigraphically after surgery, most patients show an improvement in myocardial perfusion.

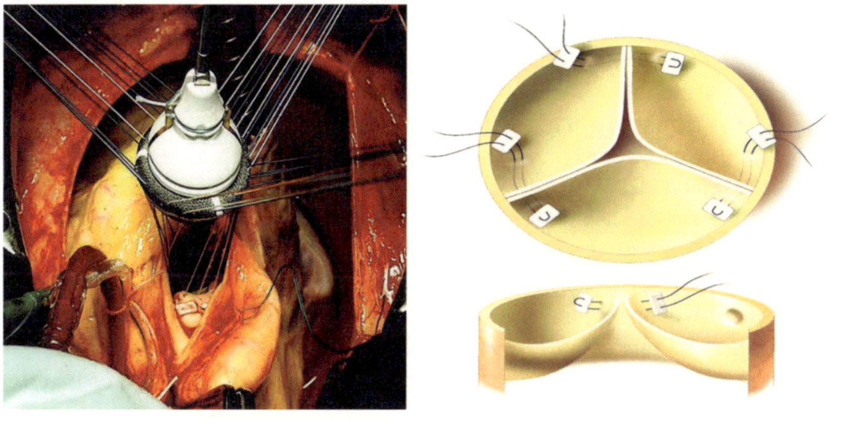

Figure 5.
Magnetic resonance imaging (MRI) of the heart.

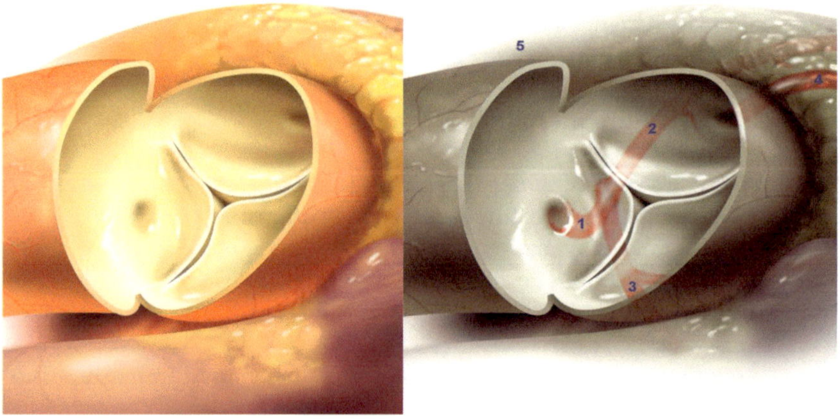

Figure 6.
Radionuclide myocardial scintigraphy of myocardium.

The above research methods (**Figure 6**) are performed in almost all specialized cardiology and cardiac surgery institutions, where they thoroughly deal with the problems of modern diagnostics and the solution of surgical tactics for the treatment of acquired aortic heart defects. We only considered it necessary to briefly dwell on the problems of diagnosing and determining the surgical tactics of acquired aortic valve defects, knowing that dynamically these issues are resolved individually, depending on the capabilities of clinics and specialists involved in "adult cardiac surgery" at the present stage.

3.6 Surgical methods for the treatment of aortic heart disease

The requirement of modern cardiac surgery is the widest possible use of valve-saving technologies in heart valve surgery, namely in the surgical treatment of aortic heart defects. However, as is known from the specialized literature, according to the leading authors of the post-Soviet period of development, the opinion remained that valve replacement operations were preferable in surgery for aortic heart defects, in view of the peculiarities of hemodynamics, the relationship of the left heart and the aortic valve. Therefore, the preferential performance of prosthetic aortic valves rather than plastic reconstructive interventions during these periods is explained. But, the trend towards the implementation of valve-saving technologies is especially noticeable in recent decades, when the development of a number of plastic interventions on aortic valves began [15–18]. It is appropriate to bring plastic surgeries, such as "Open valvuloplasty of the aortic valves" with stenosis, or preferential preservation of the structure of the valve, without gross morphological changes (calcification, gross fibrosis, etc.). Performing parietal resection of thickened leaflets with the addition of commissural sutures in case of fibrous change, stenosis or predominant stenosis of the aortic valves. It should be noted that they were performed with a normal tricuspid aortic valve structure. There are many attempts to perform plastic operations on the aortic valves. However, many of them did not have sufficiently stable good long-term results and required repeated valve replacement operations in a short period of postoperative follow-up. I think that among the many methods of plastic surgery on aortic valves, the following deserve attention:

1. There are several modifications of Operation Ozaki. The author's methods, the meaning of which is in the complete reconstruction of the aortic valve from the autopericardium or from the xenopericardium, differ in the types of meters and templates. So, for example, the Benaki operation uses gauges made from the flexible material nitinol, as opposed to the rigid Ozaki gauges. Due to the special properties of this material, gauges can be modeled, giving them the desired shape and allowing more convenient measurement of the distance between the commissures, then they are also used as templates for cutting the leaf. In addition to improved meters, Benaki's operation uses special "three-armed" forceps for the comfort of creating aortic valve neocusps [7]. Known special holding device for the formation and simultaneous plastics of the aortic valve leaflets (MAAZOUZI APS AORTIC PLASTY-SIZER). In the work of A.S. Nesmachny describes in detail the technique of using the device in clinical practice [7, 16, 19].

The positioning of future leaflets in the holding device before implantation allows quickly and accurately, in accordance with the diameter of the aortic annulus, to form a neovalve.

4. Stages of operation Ozaki

1. A known method of forming the leaflets of the aortic valve, cut after intraoperative measurement of intercommissural distances (**Figure 7**). The length of the

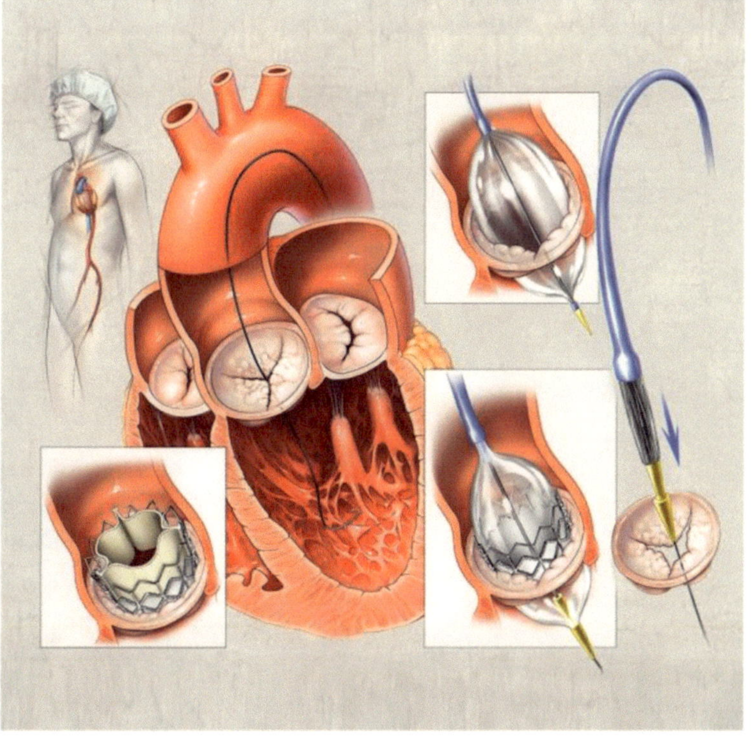

Figure 7.
Forming cusps from pericardium.

free edge of each nonvalve should be 20% greater than the intercommissural distance, the valve height is 0.866 of the intercommissural distance. The leaflets are fixed to the aortic ring with a continuous suture (**Figure 8**). The disadvantage of this method is the absence of the results of the application of this technique in clinical practice described in the literature.

2. It should be noted that in this case we are discussing the simplest, most effective methods of surgical correction of aortic defects, which are the fundamental methods of surgical treatment of this pathology.

3. Considering that in more complex variants of aortic malformations complicated by other changes in the aorta itself, its part, valvular or tubular apparatus, more complex, modified methods of surgical correction of aortic valve malformations are invariably performed [3, 17, 20]. An example is the performance of plastic surgeries on the aortic root, valvular apparatus, ascending (sometimes the arch, descending part) of the aorta, such as David-Jakub operations, Bental-DeBono's basic operation in various modifications, and others. We decided to note only the main points of plastic surgery on the aortic valve, using the Ozaki operation as an example.

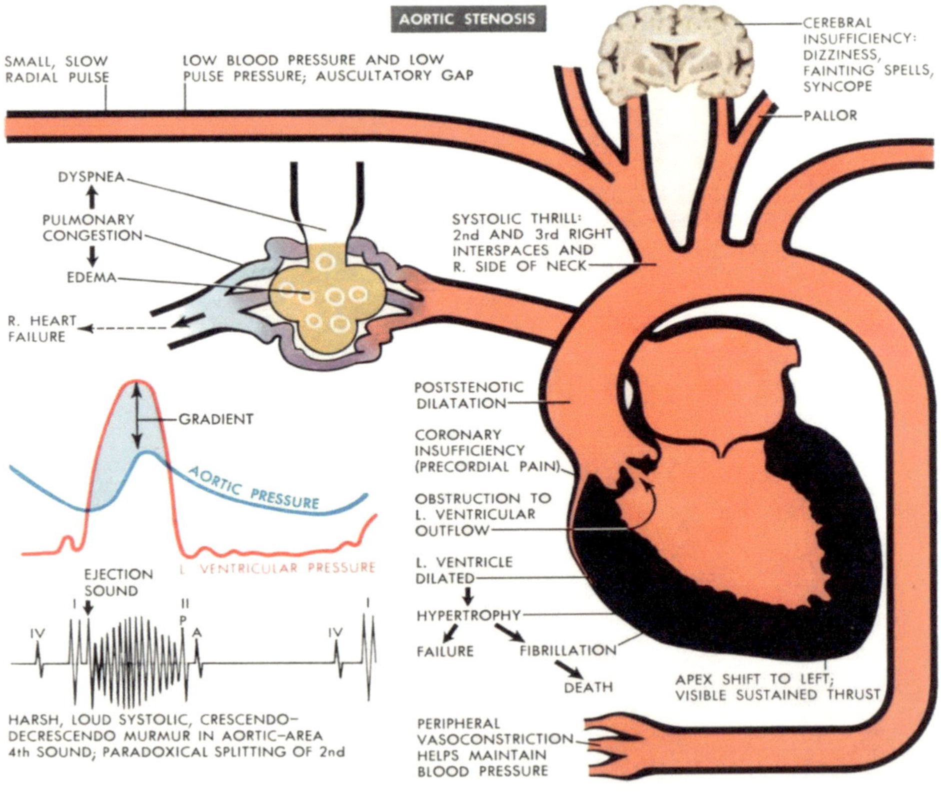

Figure 8.
Final view of the operation.

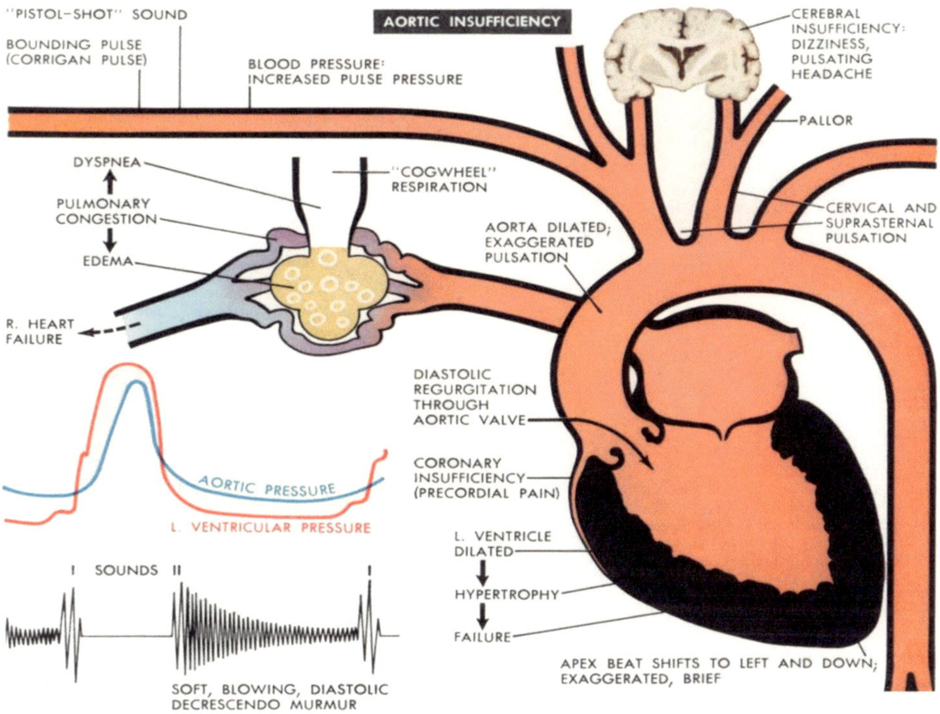

Figure 9.
Classic surgery: Aortic valve replacement and aortic valve leaflet plasty.

4. The classic operation – replacement of the aortic valve with artificial prostheses (**Figure 9**), is the most common method of surgical correction of aortic heart defects to date [21].

4.1 Endovascular aortic valve replacement

Here it is necessary to indicate the importance of choosing an aortic valve prosthesis, since the last decades have been marked by the rapid development of the production of biological valves, frameless, framed biological aortic valves, homografts, the use of biological valves for endovascular methods of aortic valve implantation, and many others [22–24].

But, I think our task is to determine the basics of the correct surgical tactics for the treatment of aortic heart defects, indicating the main methods for diagnosing these heart defects. To this end, we briefly want to acquaint the reader with the basics of the pathogenesis of the development of pathology, the anatomical and hemodynamic foundations of aortic heart defects [12, 25].

In recent decades, the technology of endovascular implantation of an artificial aortic valve has been developed (**Figure 10**).

The next high-tech operation is endovascular implantation of aortic valve prosthesis [22, 23, 26]:

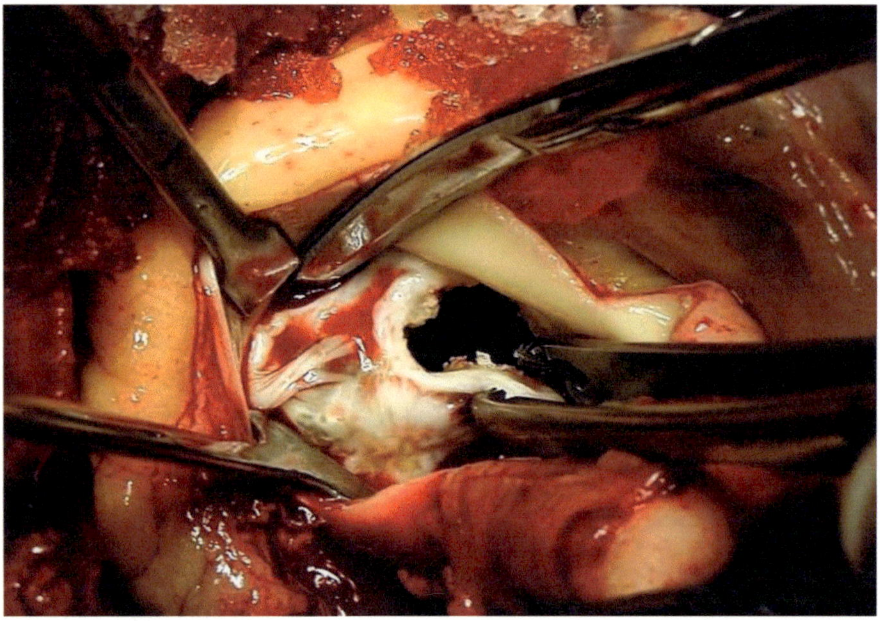

Figure 10.
Transcatheter aortic valve implantation.

5. Pathological anatomy (by the example of aortic stenosis)

The basis of pathological changes in aortic disease, in this case, aortic stenosis is rheumatic inflammation – valve valvulitis. Rheumatic valvulitis gradually leads to thickening and compaction of the aortic cusps. This is facilitated by the organization of fibrous overlays on the ventricular surface of the valve, as well as the growth of valve tissue due to mechanical irritation by blood flow. These factors underlie the soldering of the free edges of the leaflets, as a result of which the valve opening gradually decreases. In the area of commissures, fibrin plates form bridges that connect the valves between themselves and the aortic wall. Subsequently, the plates are organized into fibrous tissue. The narrowed valve opening has a triangular or slit-like shape and is usually located eccentrically. When the valves are wrinkled, one or another degree of aortic insufficiency is formed. In the altered valve, degenerative processes develop, followed by calcification. Calcification can move to structures adjacent to the aortic valve: the interventricular septum, the anterior leaflet of the mitral valve, the wall of the left ventricle. Bicuspid AV is often associated with a subvalvular membrane, sometimes with abnormal origin and course of the coronary arteries, the presence of three or even four coronary orifices, and in adulthood is complicated by calcification and/or endocarditis of the AV. Under the valvular membrane (Williams' disease) in the left ventricular outflow tract (LVOT) may or may not fuse with the AV leaflets, be circular or semilunar in shape in a limited area. Such patients have a characteristic "elf face" and lag behind in mental development. LVOT obstruction in hypertrophic cardiomyopathy (HCM) is often associated with anterior leaflet prolapse of the mitral valve (AMVP). Aortic stenosis causes significant morphological changes in the myocardium of the left ventricle (LV). Prolonged illness leads to progressive hypertrophy and the development of relative coronary insufficiency. Dystrophic changes develop in the heart muscle: protein and fatty degeneration of muscle fibers, and later diffuse and focal sclerosis [14].

6. Pathological physiology (by the example of aortic stenosis)

Hemodynamic manifestations of aortic stenosis develop with a decrease in the area of the aortic ostium less than 1 cm^2, which is usually combined with a pressure gradient between the LV and aorta of 50 mm Hg. Art. The "critical" area of the Aorta opening, corresponding to the picture of a sharp aortic stenosis, is 0.5–0.7 cm^2 with an aortic systolic gradient of 100–150 mm Hg. Art. To ensure adequate cardiac output, the LV during systole must develop a pressure of 200–250 mm Hg. Art. Possessing powerful compensatory capabilities, hypertrophied LV intensifies contractions and copes with the defect for a long time. Gradually, the amount of "residual" blood in the cavity of the left ventricle increases and diastolic filling increases. The cavity of the left ventricle expands, and tonogenic dilatation occurs. Additional mobilization of the myocardium occurs due to the activation of the Frank- Starling mechanism. When a further increase in the length of muscle fibers ceases to be accompanied by an increase in contraction, the so-called myogenic dilation occurs; LV decompensation gives rise to a phase of general heart failure. Long-term existence of AV stenosis and compensatory hyperfunction leads to the development of LV myocardial hypertrophy, the mass of which can reach 1200 g or more (at a rate of 250–300 g). The consequence of this is relative coronary insufficiency. In addition, in patients with aortic stenosis, there may be an absolute deterioration in coronary blood flow due to a sharp increase in intraventricular and intramyocardial pressure, as well as a drop in pressure at the base of the aorta (blood is ejected into the aorta in a thin and strong jet), making it difficult to fill the coronary arteries during diastole. For these reasons, in patients with aortic stenosis, angina pectoris occurs in 70% of cases, although only half of the patients have coronary atherosclerosis. Due to developing myocardial ischemia in this category of patients, the risk of sudden death is high [3, 27, 28]. When stenosis is combined with aortic valve insufficiency (more often with a bicuspid aortic valve), an increase in "preload" is added to the increased "afterload" of the LV, which leads to greater stress in the LV wall and a decrease in effective stroke volume.

7. Pathogenesis of development of aortic stenosis

Pathogenesis and changes in hemodynamics. The narrowing of the aortic orifice by more than 50% creates a significant obstruction to the flow of blood from the left ventricle to the systemic circulation. With its narrowing, the minute volume decreases by 75%, although the area of the hole, which is even 10–20% of the norm, is compatible with life [29]. To ensure more or less sufficient systolic ejection in aortic stenosis, a number of compensatory mechanisms are activated. One of them is the lengthening of the systole of the left ventricle and the increase in pressure in the cavity of the left ventricle. As a result, a large pressure gradient

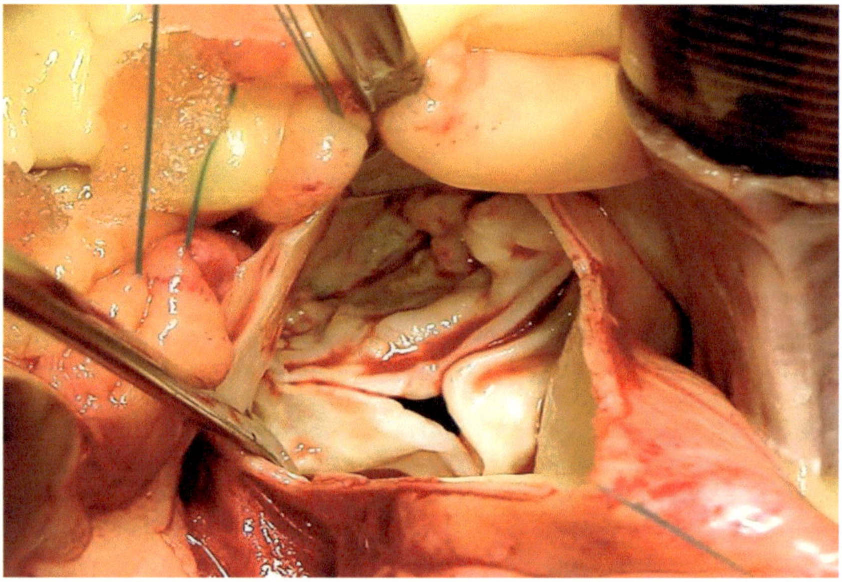

Figure 11.
Hemodynamic disturbances in aortic stenosis.

is created between the aorta and the left ventricle, the latter is sharply hypertrophied without a significant increase in the cavity. The narrowing of the mouth of the aorta, like no other defect, is characterized by severe hypertrophy of the left ventricle. The minute volume remains normal for a long time or slightly decreases, the defect remains compensated. With a pronounced degree of defect or a decrease in the contractility of the left ventricle, the minute volume decreases significantly. In the latter case, the left ventricle dilates, it increases the end-diastolic pressure. This further leads to a rise in pressure in the left atrium, and then retrograde in the pulmonary veins. There is passive (venous) pulmonary hypertension, which does not reach large values and usually does not lead to severe hypertrophy of the right ventricle. Over time, congestion may occur in the systemic circulation. Coronary blood flow in aortic stenosis is reduced, especially during systole, which is explained by the influence of high intraventricular pressure and increased resistance in the thickness of the myocardium to coronary inflow. The main cause of coronary insufficiency is considered to be a disproportion between the increased need for nutrition of a hypertrophied muscle and its relatively low blood supply [30]. Additional factors are slow filling of the aorta, a decrease in systolic and mean pressure in the aorta (especially in the circumference of the valves) (**Figure 11**).

8. Pathogenesis of the development of aortic valve insufficiency

As a result of incomplete closure of the aortic valve leaflets during diastole, there is a reverse flow of blood from the aorta to the left ventricle [31, 32]. From 6 to 50% or more of the systolic volume of blood can return to the left ventricle. As a result of increased blood supply (as well as normally from the atrium, and also additionally from the aorta), the left ventricle dilates, its function increases, since it must eject more blood during systole (ventricular systolic volume can reach 200–220 ml). As a result, the left ventricle is moderately hypertrophied due to the lack of resistance to the ejection of blood [32]. Dilatation of the same ventricle is compensatory, combined with the preservation of the contractile function of the left ventricle; it is called adaptive (tonogenic, primary), in contrast to the secondary (myogenic), which develops with a decrease in the contractile function of the myocardium. The defect is also compensated for by shortening the isometric contraction phase and lengthening the ejection phase, i.e., facilitating the expulsion of an increased amount of blood from the left ventricle. This is due to a more rapid increase (under the influence of additional blood volume coming from the aorta) pressure in the left ventricle to the level required to open the aortic valve, as well as a decrease in overall vascular resistance. With a large valvular defect and as decompensation develops, the diastolic pressure in the left ventricle increases, which results in isometric hyperfunction of the left atrium. The overload of the left atrium increases when, due to significant dilatation of the left atrium and left ventricle, the expansion of the left atrioventricular orifice, relative mitral valve insufficiency is formed. In the future, as decompensation progresses, congestion in the pulmonary circulation (passive pulmonary hypertension) may occur, pressure in the pulmonary artery rises, isometric hyperfunction and hypertrophy of the right ventricle develop, followed by right ventricular failure (**Figures 12–20**).

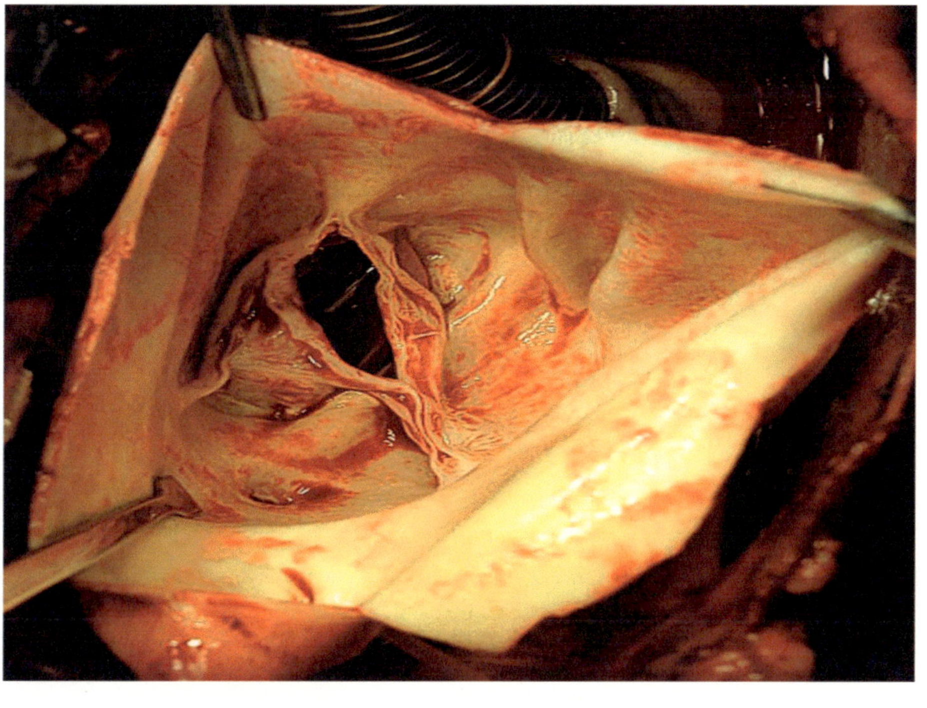

Figure 12.
Hemodinamic disorders in aortic insufficiency.

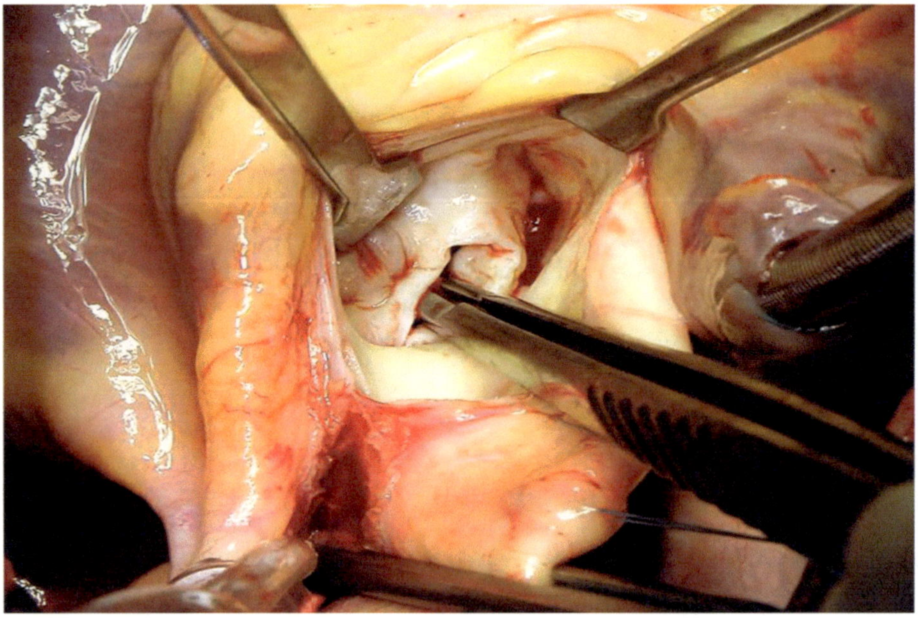

Figure 13.
Rheumatic lesions of the aortic valve.

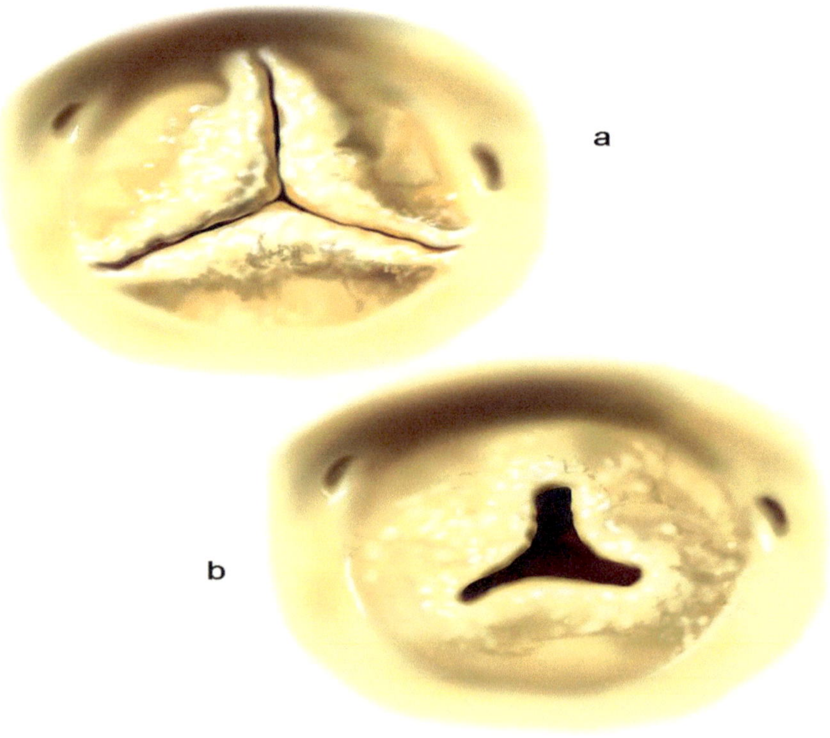

Figure 14.
Atherosclerotic degenerative changes of the aortic valve.

DOI: http://dx.doi.org/10.5772/intechopen.113014

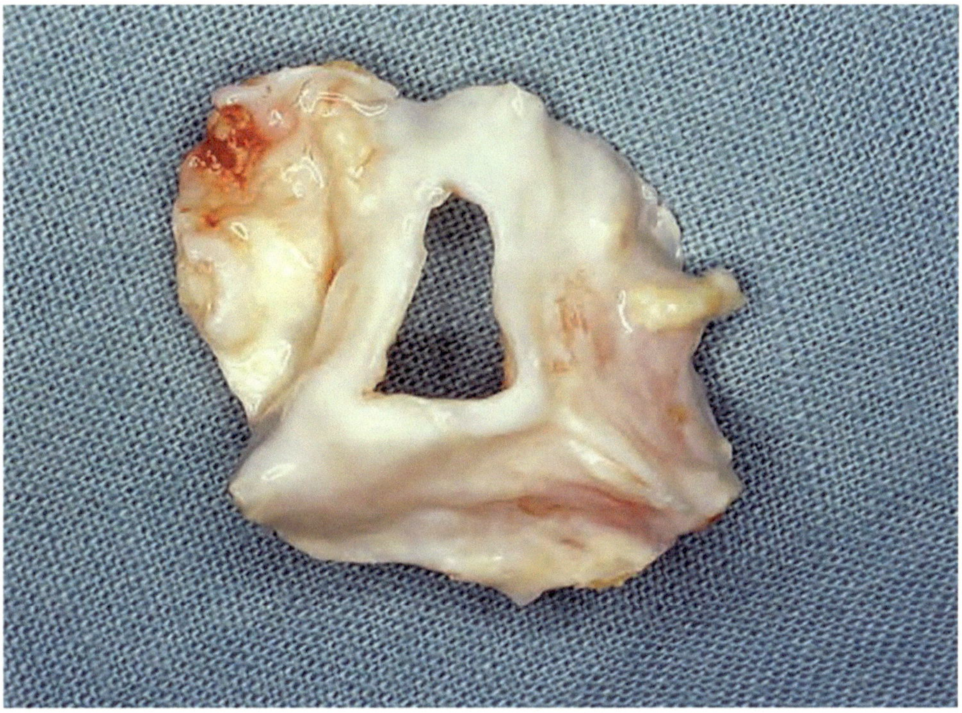

Figure 15.
Congenital aortic valve (bicuspid aortic valve) lesions.

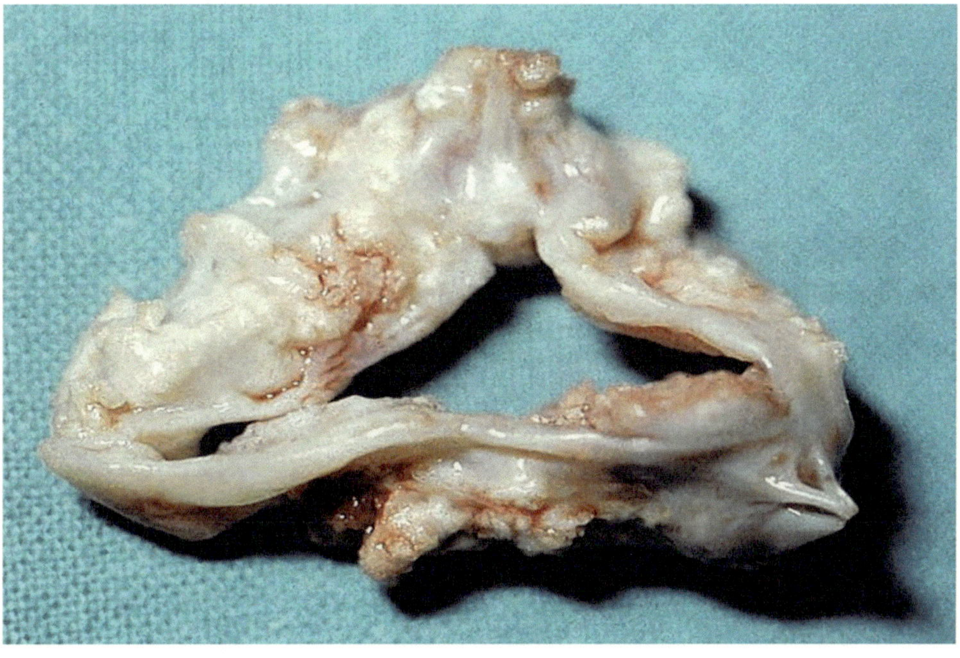

Figure 16.
Congenital aortic valve (bicuspid aortic valve) lesions.

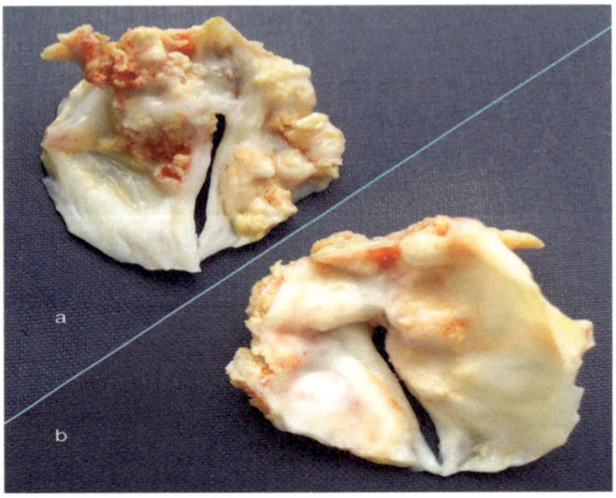

Figure 17.
Difference in calcinosis in rheumatic (a) and degenerative (b) lesions of the aortic valve.

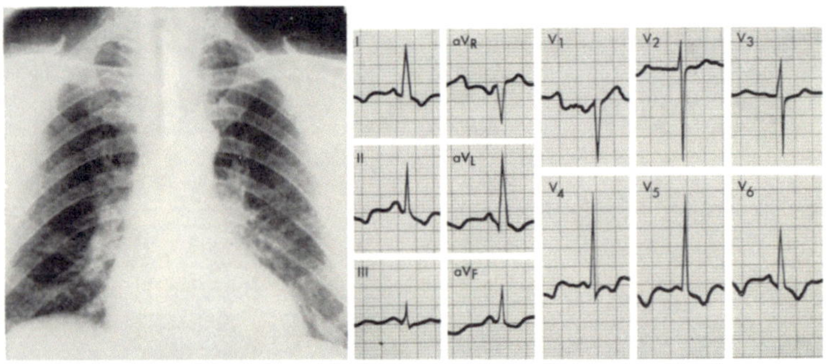

Figure 18.
Morphological picture of removed aortic valve (rheumatic lesions).

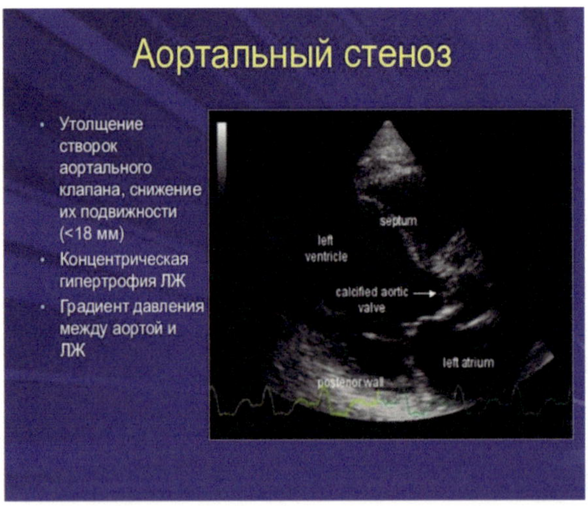

Figure 19.
Morphological picture of removed aortic valves (in degenerative lesion).

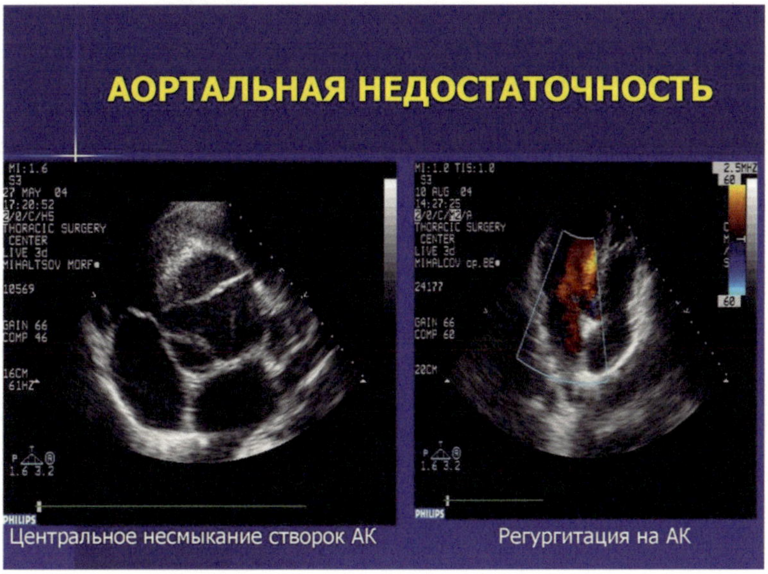

Figure 20.
Morphology of the valve in congenital defects of the aortic valve.

9. Conclusion

Thus, when discussing the above problem of cardiology and cardiac surgery, it should be noted that the statistics of detection of aortic malformations have indeed changed over the past decades, in terms of frequency, which come out on the third place after coronary heart disease and hypertension. A particularly large percentage refers to aortic stenosis. Another feature is the change in the etiological factors in the development of aortic heart defects. So, if earlier the rheumatic genesis of the development of aortic malformations prevailed all over the world, now the degenerative nature of the development of aortic malformations is clearly increasing.

The third feature is the change in the social structure of aortic heart disease, i.e. with a noticeable increase in the age of the population, the number of patients over 60 years of age who undergo open correction sharply prevails. It follows from the above that open corrections are also changed. It follows from the above that the principles of diagnosing aortic heart defects have also changed, non-invasive highly informative computer technologies are increasingly being used that help to accurately determine the surgical tactics of treatment and evaluate the results of corrections of aortic heart defects.

The combination of valvular pathology and atherosclerotic lesions of the coronary vessels and the aortic wall sharply increases. Accordingly, the number of simultaneous large reconstructive operations on the valves of the aorta and root, and coronary vessels and others is increasing. It follows from the above that the principles of diagnosing aortic heart defects have also changed, non-invasive highly informative computer technologies are increasingly being used that help to accurately determine the surgical tactics of treatment and evaluate the results of corrections of aortic heart defects. The combination of valvular pathology and atherosclerotic lesions of the coronary vessels and the aortic wall sharply increases.

Accordingly, the number of simultaneous large reconstructive operations on the valves of the aorta and root, and coronary vessels and others is increasing. Open corrections are made. Accordingly, there is a need to revise the approaches to studying the issues of etiology, clinic and diagnostics, determining the tactics of treatment, performing the stages of surgical correction and evaluating the results of the latter in patients with acquired aortic heart disease at the present stage of development of cardiology and cardiac surgery.

Author details

Abdumadjidov Khamidulla Amanullaevich[1,2]* and Urakov Shukhrat Tukhtaevich[1]

1 Department of Surgical Diseases, Bukhara State Medical Institute, Bukhara City, Republic of Uzbekistan

2 Bukhara State Medical Institute named after Ibn Sina, Bukhara City, Republic of Uzbekistan

*Address all correspondence to: hamidulla06@mail.ru

IntechOpen

© 2023 The Author(s). Licensee IntechOpen. This chapter is distributed under the terms of the Creative Commons Attribution License (http://creativecommons.org/licenses/by/3.0), which permits unrestricted use, distribution, and reproduction in any medium, provided the original work is properly cited.

References

[1] Semenov VY, Samorodskaya IV, Larina VN, et al. Mortality rates from acquired heart disease over a 15-year period in the Russian Federation and the United States of America. Creative Cardiology. 2017;**11**(3):235-246

[2] Rheumatic Heart Disease. Report of the WHO Secretariat. 141 Sessions. EB 141\4. Item 6.2 of the Provisional Agenda for May 1, 2017. Geneva: WHO; 2017

[3] Baumgartner H, Falk V, Bax JJ, et al. 2017 ESC/EACTS guidelines for the management of valvular heart disease. European Journal of Cardio-Thoracic Surgery. 2017;**52**(4):616-664

[4] Généreux P, Pibarot P, Redfors B, et al. Staging classification of aortic stenosis based on the extent of cardiac damage. European Heart Journal. 2017;**38**(45):3351-3358

[5] Iung B, Baron G, Butchart EG, et al. A prospective survey of patients with valvular heart disease in Europe: The euro heart survey on valvular heart disease. European Heart Journal. 2003;**24**(13):1231-1243

[6] Tabata N, Sinning JM, Kaikita K, et al. Current status and future perspective of structural heart disease intervention. Journal of Cardiology. 2019;**74**(1):1-12

[7] Komarov RN, Katkov AI, et al. Surgery of the aortic root and aortic valve: Past and present. Circulatory Pathology and Cardiac Surgery. 2019;**23**(4):9-25 (Ch. 23)

[8] Cawley PJ, Maki JH, Otto CM. Cardiovascular magnetic resonance imaging for valvular heart disease: Technique and validation. Circulation. 2009;**119**(3):468-478

[9] Ma L, Markl M, Chow K, et al. Aortic 4D flow MRI in 2 minutes using compressed sensing, respiratory controlled adaptive k-space reordering, and inline reconstruction. Magnetic Resonance in Medicine. 2019;**81**(6):3675-3690

[10] Lang RM, Badano V, et al. Recommendations for cardiac chamber quantification by echocardiography in adults: An update from the American Society of Echocardiography and the European Association of Cardiovascular Imaging. European Heart Journal-Cardiovascular Imaging. 2015;**16**(3):233-271

[11] De Kerchove L, el-Khoury G. Anatomy and pathophysiology of the ventriculo-aortic junction: Implication in aortic valve repair surgery. Annals of Cardiothoracic Surgery. 2013;**2**(1):57

[12] Pineda AM, Kiefer TL. Asymptomatic severe aortic valve stenosis—When to intervene: A review of the literature, current trials, and guidelines. Current Cardiology Reports. 2018;**20**(12):1-10

[13] Kocher N, Russe M, Kari F, et al. Visual, semi-quantitative analysis of blood flow distribution in aortic root aneurysms with different grades of aortic insufficiency using 4D flow MRI. In: European Congress of Radiology-ECR 2017. 2017

[14] Devereux RB, de Simone G, Arnett DK. Normal limits in relation to age, body size and gender of two-dimensional echocardiography aortic root dimensions in persons >15 years of age. The American Journal of Cardiology. 2012;**110**(8):1189-1194

[15] Akopov GA, Ivanov AS, et al. Long-term results of reconstructive operations on the aortic valve and ascending aorta. Bulletin of Transplantology and Artificial Organs. 2021;**XIII**(5):155-156 (Ch. 23)

[16] Ivanov AS, Akopov GA, et al. Reconstructive valve-preserving surgery of the aortic root. Bulletin of Transplantology and Artificial Organs. 2021;**23**(1):157-161 (Ch. 23)

[17] Carpentier A, Adams DH, Filsoufi F. Carpentier's Reconstructive Valve Surgery: From Valve Analysis to Valve Reconstruction. Philadelphia: Saunders; 2010. p. 268. ISBN: 9780721691688

[18] Glauber M, Miceli A. Minimally Invasive Aortic Valve Surgery. Cardiac Surgery. Cham: Springer; 2020. pp. 421-428

[19] Molchanov AN, Idov EM. Valve-preserving and plastic interventions on the aortic root and aortic valve (literature review). Bulletin of the Ural Medical Academic Science. 2017;**14**(1):75-85

[20] Adams DH, Filsoufi F. Carpentier's Reconstructive Valve Surgery: From Valve Analysis to Valve Reconstruction. Saunders/Elsevier; 2010

[21] Rajput FA, Zeltser R. Aortic Valve Replacement. 2019

[22] Maes F, Lerakis S, Ribeiro HB, et al. Outcomes from transcatheter aortic valve replacement in patients with low-flow, low-gradient aortic stenosis and left ventricular ejection fraction less than 30%: A substudy from the TOPAS-TAVI registry. JAMA Cardiology. 2019;**4**(1):64-70

[23] Osnabrugge RLJ, Mylotte D, Head SJ, et al. Aortic stenosis in the elderly: Disease prevalence and number of candidates for transcatheter aortic valve replacement: A meta-analysis and modeling study. Journal of the American College of Cardiology. 2013;**62**(11):1002-1012

[24] Siontis GCM, Praz F, Pilgrim T, et al. Transcatheter aortic valve implantation vs. surgical aortic valve replacement for treatment of severe aortic stenosis: A meta-analysis of randomized trials. European Heart Journal. 2016;**37**(47):3503-3512

[25] Rayner TA, Harrison S, Rival P, et al. Minimally invasive versus conventional surgery of the ascending aorta and root: A systematic review and meta-analysis. European Journal of Cardio-Thoracic Surgery. 2020;**57**(1):8-17

[26] Aalaei-Andabili SH, Bavry AA. Left ventricular diastolic dysfunction and transcatheter aortic valve replacement outcomes: A review. Cardiology and Therapy. 2019;**8**(1):21-28

[27] David TE, David CM, Ouzounian M, et al. A progress report on reimplantation of the aortic valve. The Journal of Thoracic and Cardiovascular Surgery. 2021;**161**(3):890-899

[28] Nishimura RA, O'Gara RT, Bavaria JE, Brindis RG, et al. 2019 AATS/ACC/ASE/SCAISTS expert consensus systems of care document. Cathether Cardiovascular Intervention. 2019;**94**(1):3-26

[29] Argulian E, Windecker S, Messerli FH. Misconceptions and facts about aortic stenosis. The American Journal of Medicine. 2017;**130**(24):398-402

[30] Campo J, Tsoris A, Kruse J, et al. Prognosis of severe asymptomatic aortic stenosis with and without surgery. The Annals of Thoracic Surgery. Jul

2019;**108**(1):74-79. DOI: 10.1016/j.athoracsur.2019.01.031. Epub 2019 Mar 21

[31] Akinseye OA, Pathak A, Ibebuogu UN. Aortic valve regurgitation: A comprehensive review. Current Problems in Cardiology. 2018;**43**(8):315-334

[32] Salem R, Zierer A, Karimian-Tabrizi A, et al. Aortic valve repair for aortic insufficiency or dilatation: Technical evolution and long-term outcomes. The Annals of Thoracic Surgery. 2020;**110**(6):1967-1973

Chapter 3

Ascending Aortic Aneurysm in Relation to Aortic Valve Phenotype

David Freiholtz, Per Eriksson and Hanna M. Björck

Abstract

Being born with a bicuspid aortic valve (BAV) is a significant risk factor for developing an ascending aortic aneurysm (AscAA). Research has uncovered different mechanisms influencing AscAA development in BAV-patients compared to those with normal tricuspid aortic valves (TAV). BAV-associated AscAA may result from intrinsic hemodynamic or genetic alterations, possibly even embryonic origins. During embryonic development, neural crest cells and the second heart field contribute to the ascending aorta's formation, with defective signaling potentially increasing susceptibility to aneurysm development. BAV can manifest with different phenotypes, impacting clinical outcomes. The degenerative AscAA in TAV-patients differs from BAV-associated AscAA, marked by fibrosis, smooth muscle cell loss, and inflammation. AscAA in TAV-patients rarely appears in those with aortic stenosis, suggesting a link between aortic valve disease and degenerative AscAA. This chapter aims to describe suggested molecular mechanisms driving aneurysm formation in BAV- and TAV-patients.

Keywords: ascending aortic aneurysm, bicuspid aortic valve, embryology, valvulogenesis, vascular inflammation, aortic stenosis, aortic regurgitation

1. Introduction

Ascending aortic aneurysm (AscAA), defined as a dilatation of the ascending aorta 1.5 times the expected diameter [1], is a silent, potentially fatal disease with regrettably little known of its underlying pathomechanisms. The condition is most often discovered incidentally during radiological examinations, and no screening for the disease is performed. AscAA in general has a reported incidence of 5 per 100,000 patient-years [2]. The most significant risk factor for developing AscAA, with 80 times increased risk compared to the general population [3], is the common congenital heart malformation, the bicuspid aortic valve (BAV) [4–6]. The embryonic development of the aortic valve and ascending aorta are spatiotemporally associated, and implications of this, aortic flow disturbances and/or genetics have been proposed for the cooccurrence of BAV and AscAA [7–9]. Notably, the ascending aortic media is structurally well preserved in patients with concomitant aneurysm and BAV [10] (**Figure 1A**). Contrastingly, an aneurysm of the ascending aorta in patients with normal tricuspid aortic valves (TAV) is characterized by marked degenerative insults and immune cell infiltration [11] and almost exclusively occurs in association with aortic

IntechOpen

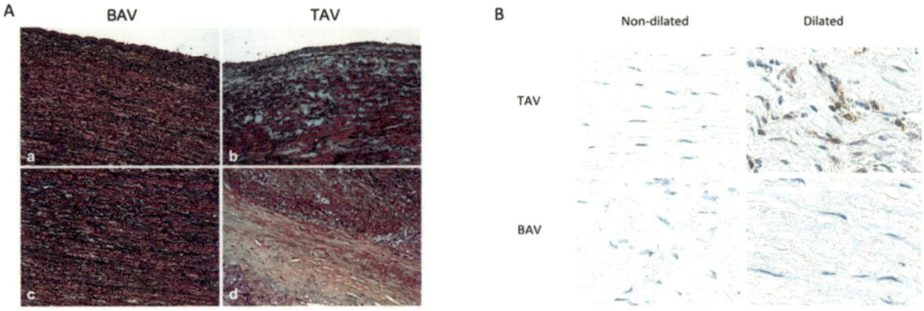

Figure 1.
(A) Movat pentachrome stainings of dilated aortas from patients with BAV (a, c) and TAV (b, d). In TAV-associated aneurysm, clear signs of degeneration, fibrosis, smooth muscle cell loss, and extracellular matrix component deposition can be seen. Magnification x20. Adapted from Freiholtz et al. [10].
(B) Immunohistochemical stainings of CD4+ cells in ascending aortic tissue of BAV- and TAV-patients, magnification x40. Adapted from Folkersen et al. [11].

valve regurgitation, not aortic valve stenosis [12]. In this chapter, we will describe the potential effects of aortic valve cuspidity and aortic valve disease on ascending aortic aneurysm formation and development.

2. A spatiotemporal embryonic association of the aorta and aortic valve

Valvulogenesis involves the initial formation of endocardial cushions in the atrioventricular canal and outflow tract via a process known as endocardial-to-mesenchymal transition. Specifically, delamination, endocardial cell migration, and remodeling events give rise to mesenchymal cells, subsequently forming the atrioventricular canal leaflets (mitral and tricuspid) and semilunar valves (aortic and pulmonary) [13]. However, lineage tracing studies in various animal models have demonstrated that the formation of semilunar valves is a more complex process involving other cell lineages, including cardiac neural crest cells as well as second heart field [14]. Interestingly, cardiac neural crest cells are crucial for arteriopulmonary septation and also give rise to vascular smooth muscle cells (VSMCs) of the ascending aorta and the aortic arch [15]. In the aortic root, the adluminal media is derived from neural crest cells, while the outer media/adventitia originates from second heart field [16, 17].

Evidently, there is a direct embryonic relationship of the adult ascending aorta and the aortic valve. During embryogenesis, various signaling pathways, such as Wnt/β-catenin, NOTCH, and transforming growth factor β (TGFβ), play a crucial role in regulating cell migration, proliferation, and extracellular matrix (ECM) deposition in the developing valves and ascending aortic wall [13, 18–22]. Defects in these signaling pathways may indeed lead to dysfunctional valvulogenesis and the formation of a BAV [15].

3. Embryonic origin of the bicuspid aortic valve: Impact on clinical manifestations of AscAA

BAV is the most common congenital malformation of the heart, with a prevalence of 1–2% in the general population [23]. It is characterized by the occurrence of two, as opposed to the normal three, aortic valvular cusps, and its morphotype may be classified by the number of raphe – a fusion of the lanulae valvarum of the left-coronary (L), the right-coronary (R) or the noncoronary cusp (N) [24]. A fusion of two cusps, confers a type-I BAV where the most common variant is fusion of the R and L cusps, followed by R–N and L–N. A type II BAV entails fusion of two raphe, and type 0 BAV represents a BAV with only two valvular sinus. Interestlingly, studies investigating the involvement of cardiac progenitor cells in the development of different BAV phenotypes have suggested that the type 1 BAV fusions R–L and R–N (i.e., the most common BAV phenotypes) have separate developmental aberrations. In particular, the R–L fusion was shown to be associated with abnormal behavior of neural crest cells [15], whereas an eNOS mutation has been proposed as a cause for the R–N fusion and a predisposition to aortic dilatation and dissection [25, 26]. The latter finding may suggest a role of second heart field in the development of type 1 R–N BAV as eNOS is expressed by endocardial cells, cardiomyocytes, and VSMCs, all of which are derived from the second heart field [27].

A possible consequence of different cardiac progenitor cells conferring different BAV phenotypes could be that specific regions of the ascending aorta are affected depending on the individual's phenotype. Indeed, we and others have shown an association between BAV phenotype and different clinical manifestations [27, 28]. Furthermore, the R–L phenotype was associated with larger aortic root dimensions, which has been well-documented in echocardiography cohorts [29–32]. Additionally, patients with type 0 BAV tended to present clinically at an earlier age than those with other phenotypes, and a similar trend was observed in men in this study [28]. Interestingly there are trends showing that R–L and type 0 phenotypes are associated with a higher prevalence of ascending aortic dilatation at any segment compared with the R–N phenotype, which relation to aortopathy has historically been conflictingly [28]. For instance, a large study on a surgical cohort reported a lack of ascending aortic root dilatation in combination with R–N phenotype [33].

4. Characteristics of BAV-associated ascending aortopathy

As described above, an association between impaired embryonic signaling between different cardiac progenitor cells and the formation of a BAV has been suggested, likely contributing to aortopathogenesis. The cardiac progenitor cells involved in valvulogenesis migrate and populate the ascending aortic media [18]. The literature has as such focused on the aortic media as causative of aortopathy. The adult ascending aortic media is laminarly structured with VSMCs sandwiched between load-bearing elastin and collagen [34]. Albeit BAV has been known as a risk factor for disease since 1844 [35], it was first during 1984, in necropsy studies by Larson et al., that structural differences between BAV-associated aortopathy and degenerative ascending aortic aneurysm were proposed in light of vastly different rates of acute aortic syndromes [36]. Histologically, one can observe very small differences in the ascending aorta of BAV patients with or without aneurysm, i.e., the elastin is intact, there is VSMC apoptosis, although notably without mucoid extracellular matrix accumulation (MEMA), and the aortic intima-media exhibits few signs of inflammation [10]. Still, the nondilated aorta of individuals with BAV displays a seemingly thinner intima [37].

In past years, researchers have focused on the aortic media in BAV-associated aortopathy with findings of differential VSMC phenotypes in BAV and TAV aortopathies

[11, 38]. Not only have these cells been found to undergo apoptosis [39] without apparent MEMA [10], but BAV VSMCs also exhibit distinct morphology. In BAV patients, VSMCs are less differentiated, indicating a defect in the phenotypic switch process, leading to significantly lower expression of differentiated, contractile VSMC markers, such as smoothelin, calponin, and SM22alpha [40, 41]. Additionally, VSMC dissociated from aneurysmal tissue exhibit differences in proliferation and migration comparing BAV and TAV VSMC. Specifically, in an ORIS migration assay, TAV VSMCs showed a faster migration and a higher proliferation rate than BAV VSMCs [10]. Although these cells exhibit such characteristics and behavior in aneurysmal tissue, the less differentiated and immature VSMCs are observed in both nondilated and dilated BAV populations [40], leading the mind to wonder if this VSMC phenotype might itself not be driving aneurysm development.

Interestingly, we and others have observed a mesenchymal-like state of endothelial cells in the ascending aorta of BAV patients, even prior to aortic dilatation [7, 42, 43]. Moreover, the expression of the endothelial-specific marker CD31 is decreased in nondilated BAV aorta, indicating a less differentiated endothelial phenotype [10]. Also, there are signs of a compromised basal membrane, with decreased expression of laminin gamma 1 [10], the main monomer in laminin trimers of large artery basal membranes [44]. This, together with reports of alterations in endothelial junction protein expression in nondilated BAV, such as increased protein turnover of CDH5, decreased expression of CLDN5, and increased mRNA expression of *CDH2* with dilatation compared to TAV patients [45], indeed implicates dysfunctional endothelium in BAV. Electron microscopy further strengthens this observation with signs of junctional degradation and a less intact endothelium in nondilated BAV individuals compared with TAV [45]. The genetic variants and missense mutations of ROBO4 found to associate with BAV aortopathy further strengthen the role of the endothelium in the AscAA development of BAV patients [46], as ROBO4 is an arbiter of vascular integrity and endothelial barrier function [47, 48]. The study by Gould et al. demonstrates the endothelial barrier impairment by infiltration of albumin into the ascending aortic wall [46], but we, too, have observed this to be a general characteristic of BAV ascending aortas, no matter if they are dilated or not [10].

Thus, the endothelium, too, has a seemingly important role in the distinct aortic wall phenotype observed in BAV patients. This is further supported by numerous animal models with endothelial-specific mutations producing offspring with a higher prevalence of BAVs. Most notably, in regards to endothelial function, mice lacking eNOS result in 40% BAV progeny [25]. Mice with $GATA5^{-/-}$ (with 25% BAV progeny) indicate that dysfunctional endothelial phenotype, as they also display lower expression of endothelial-specific markers – CDH5, TIE2, and eNOS, is related to BAV [49]. However, a drawback of these studies is that the prevalence of, or propensity to develop, aortopathy was not investigated. Nonetheless, the endothelial-specificity of eNOS, and the fact that GATA5 is mostly restricted to the endocardium, disappearing at mid-gestation and is required for early differentiation of cardiac progenitors into endothelial/endocardial cells, suggests a connection between the BAV phenotype and disturbed endothelial function.

An observed consequence of impaired endothelial function related to BAV is increased permeability. Ascending aortas of nondilated and dilated BAV patients exhibit greater infiltration of albumin in the aortic intima-media compared to TAV patients, which in nondilated state have a normal functional endothelium [10, 46]. The infiltration of plasma proteins into the aortic wall of BAV patients and potential consequences to VSMC phenotype thereof has to our knowledge, not been investigated. It is, however, a promising line of research in search of circulating biomarkers influencing the cellular phenotype of ascending aortas in BAV patients. One might speculate that such a biomarker might guide practices of surveillance and indications of ascending aortic surgery.

5. Genetics and hemodynamics in BAV aortopathy

Analyses of the genetic contribution to BAV and its associate aortopathy in a large family-based study suggested that genetics and the presence of BAV independently influence ascending aortic diameter [50]. These investigations highlight the first and oldest hypothesis of BAV-associated AscAA development, namely the hemodynamic hypothesis [51]. Indeed, several studies have suggested a contribution of BAV-associated impaired flow to aneurysm development [52, 53]. A plethora of radiological tools, such as low-sensitive cardiac magnetic resonance imaging with full volumetric coverage of the ascending aorta, have allowed multiple flow-specific investigations on BAV aortopathy in the previous decade. As such, it is clear that hemodynamic alterations are intrinsic to BAV, even in the absence of severe valve disease, by virtue of its anatomy. Hemodynamic alterations in the presence of a BAV include flow jets, eccentric helical flow, and increased ascending aortic wall-shear stress. Observations of increased wall-shear stress and intramural stresses underpin the hypothesis that these hemodynamic alterations indeed participate in AscAA development and progression [54]. Not only are disturbances in ascending aortic flow pathognomic of BAV, but signs of flow-dependent cellular and histological changes have also been observed. Grewal et al. have published data suggesting a jet-associated phenotypic switch of the inner ascending aortic media by virtue of hemodynamic alterations [55]. Similarly, in support of a hemodynamic component in ascending aortopathy is a spatial differential expression of matrix proteins and smooth muscle cell depletion compared to a more circumferentially homogenous Marfan-or TAV-associated aorta [56, 57]. Furthermore, aortic endothelial cells isolated from BAV patients exhibit differential expression of flow-related *KLF2, KLF4, PECAM1,* and *CDH5* compared with TAV ECs [58]. Still, as explored by Gauer et al., the expression of eNOS synthase does not differ between different ascending aortic regions in BAV, despite being subject to different hemodynamic forces and wall-shear stress [59]. Another topic obscuring the influence of hemodynamics on BAV aortopathy is the remedy of BAV through aortic valve repair and the possible progression of ascending aortic dilatation. There are conflicting reports on the pace at which the BAV aorta continues to dilate following aortic valve repair, showing both a faster growth and a normal rate of dilatation [60, 61]. There are still no investigations on transcatheter aortic valve replacement in BAV patients and the continued dilatation of the ascending aorta.

The second hypothesis of BAV development, i.e., the genetic hypothesis, is gaining more favor, and indeed genome-wide association studies are finding noncoding variants of genes like *GATA4* associating with BAV [62] Albeit GATA4 deletion hampers endothelial-to-mesenchymal transition in transfected cells, and are through this mechanism believed to influence BAV-development [62]. GATA4-variants and mutations, while not functionally investigated, are further implicated in BAV development by a well-described association with congenital heart defects [63–65]. While GATA4 is associated with the presence of a BAV, genetic variants of ROBO4 – a gene associated with endothelial cell performance and function [47, 48], are also implicated in both BAV development and its associated aortopathy [46]. Even still, variants of SMAD6 are associated with BAV-associated aortopathy [66].

Of note, exploration of genetic causes of nonfamilial BAV aortopathy cannot be disentangled from the concomitant hemodynamic alterations, and as such, both genetic and an altered hemodynamic are likely to contribute to disease development. This way, the current state of the literature warrants an integration of genetic and molecular factors being investigated in association with hemodynamic factors.

6. Degenerative ascending aortic aneurysm

While degenerative AscAA manifests with the same clinical manifestation as the BAV-associated AscAA, i.e., a dilated aorta, it is histomorphologically vastly different [67]. A comprehensive global gene expression analysis was conducted on ascending aortic intima-media obtained from both nondilated and dilated ascending aortas of 131 patients with BAV and TAV (i.e., degenerative AscAA), showing significant molecular disparities in the underlying pathophysiology between BAV and TAV- aortopathy [11]. The degenerative form of AscAA is marked by fibrotic, inflammatory, and degenerative changes [7, 68]. The histopathology of degenerative AscAA was first described by Erdheim in 1929 as idiopathic cystic medial necrosis [69]. Although this descriptor of the changes has been abandoned by contemporary science, the changes describe the loss of VSMCs with the subsequent accumulation of ECM components. Cystic medial necrosis is, by the current histopathological consensus on degenerative thoracic aortic disease [70], instead described as MEMA, whereby dead VSMCs deposit primarily collagens and proteoglycans to the site of injury [71]. Furthermore, one of the main load-bearing proteins, elastin [72], which, together with the VSMCs, make up the lamellar units of the vascular media, appear fragmented and thinned out with disease progression [70]. Furthermore, there are multiple reports of low-grade inflammation and infiltrated leukocytes into the aortic intima-media of degenerative AscAA [11].

Although the main histopathological characteristics of degenerative AscAA are described in the pathological consensus, structured histopathological studies reveal a degree of heterogeneity in AscAA tissue from patients undergoing ascending aortic repair. The degree of inflammatory activity and location of infiltrated leukocytes, i.e., subintimal or mid-media, varies without known associations to patient characteristics [11]. Noteworthy is also the reported experience of surgeons treating aortic diseases, where degenerative AscAA differ significantly from descending aortic aneurysm or abdominal aortic aneurysms (AAA), in particular with respect to the absence of mural thrombi or macroscopic signs of atherosclerosis [73]. Taken together, this indicates, in our minds, that the degenerative changes described in the pathological consensus apply to most AscAA patients despite some reports of heterogeneity as pronounced inflammation or microscopic atherosclerotic lesions.

AscAA in patients with tricuspid aortic valves can manifest as part of monogenic syndromes, where inherited genetic mutations play a significant role in the development of aortopathy. Mutations in genes encoding ECM proteins, such as FBN1 in Marfan syndrome, COL3A1 in vascular Ehlers–Danlos syndrome, and TGFBR1 and TGFBR2 in Loeys–Dietz syndrome, disrupt the structural integrity of the aortic wall [74]. These mutations lead to abnormal ECM synthesis, impaired collagen and elastin assembly, and risk of ascending aortic dilatation.

In the absence of monogenic diseases, molecular drivers of degenerative AscAA development may be matrix metalloproteinsases (MMP), TGFβ signaling pathway disruptions, and inflammation [11, 75]. MMPs are a family of enzymes involved in the breakdown of ECM components. Excessive MMP activity has been observed in AscAA, particularly MMP-2 [76], −3 [77], −9 [78], −14, and − 19 [79]. Increased MMP expression and degraded ECM structures, such as elastin, induce VSMC death, weakening the aortic wall and promoting aneurysm formation [80]. Dysregulated TGFβ signaling is central in AscAA in monogenic conditions like Marfan syndrome and Loeys–Dietz syndrome [81, 82] but may too contribute to disease progression in polygenic contexts. The disruption of TGFβ signaling results in increased production of TGFβ ligands, which, paradoxically, can lead to defective TGFβ signaling and impaired ECM maintenance and turnover [83]. Altered TGF-β signaling disrupts the balance between ECM synthesis and degradation, consequently leading to aneurysm development. Inflammatory processes also play a role in degenerative AscAA pathogenesis. Macrophages and T lymphocytes infiltrate the aortic wall, releasing pro-inflammatory cytokines and chemokines with reports of upregulated inflammatory genes [84]. This immune system activation contributes to chronic inflammation, subsequent oxidative stress, and ECM remodeling, thereby exacerbating degenerative characteristics and aneurysm growth [85–88].

The clear difference between degenerative and BAV-associated AscAA strengthens the idea that these diseases are indeed separate. Instead, degenerative AscAA appears more similar to AAA at a molecular level, although genetic analyses have demonstrated a limited overlap [74, 89].

Atherosclerotic processes are often implicated in AAA, with accumulation of lipids, immune cells, and ECM components within the abdominal aortic wall [90]. Lipid deposition and macrophage infiltration contributes to the release of pro-inflammatory cytokines and the production of reactive oxygen species, resulting in chronic inflammation, endothelial dysfunction, and vascular degeneration [91, 92]. Oxidative stress further promotes inflammation, ECM degradation, and apoptosis of vascular cells, exacerbating AAA progression [93]. Moreover, proteolytic enzymes, such as MMPs (in particular MMP-1, −2, −3, −9, −12, and − 13) and elastases, are secreted by immune and vascular SMCs leading to increased degradation of ECM components and weakening the abdominal aortic wall [80, 94]. Of note, in the context of differential mechanisms driving aneurysm development, the abdominal aorta is subject to different hemodynamic forces than the ascending aorta, including flow disturbances, pulsatile flow, and increased wall-shear stress. These hemodynamic forces induce endothelial dysfunction, inflammation, and arterial wall remodeling, contributing to AAA formation [95]. Of note, intracranial aneurysms (IAs) are also influenced by hemodynamic forces, specifically in the context of formation and rupture [96]. Regions of disturbed flow, such as bifurcations and curvatures, are particularly vulnerable [96]. Also, similarly to AscAA and AAA, proteolytic enzymes (e.g., MMP-2 and -9) are involved in the pathogenesis of IA [97].

Genetic predisposition also plays a significant role in IA development. Mutations in genes encoding components of the ECM, such as collagen type IV alpha-1 and alpha-2, have been identified in familial cases of IA [98, 99]. These mutations hamper the structural integrity of the intracranial arterial wall, causing a propensity to IA formation. Inflammation and immune responses also contribute to IA pathogenesis. Inflammatory cells infiltrate the arterial wall, releasing cytokines and promoting oxidative stress [100–102]. This leads to ECM degradation, smooth muscle cell apoptosis, and arterial wall remodeling, ultimately contributing to aneurysm formation and growth (**Figure 2**).

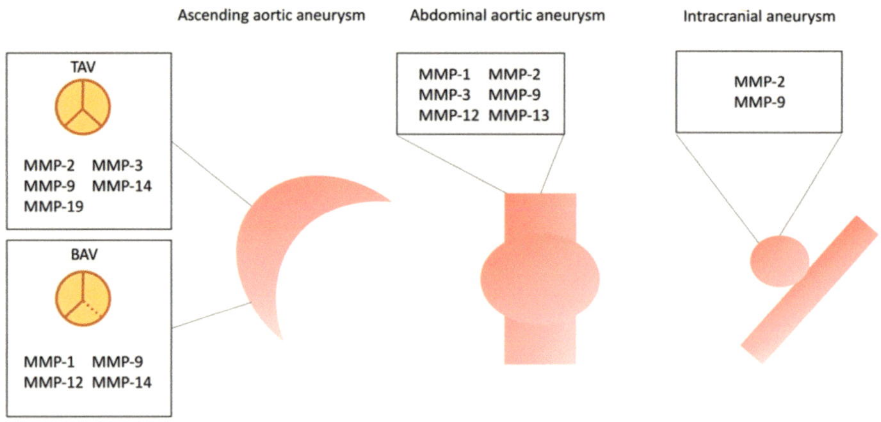

Figure 2.
Matrix metalloproteinases associated with degenerative aneurysmal disease.

It is important to note that while there are similarities in the molecular drivers between AscAA, IA, and AAA, there are also distinct differences. AscAA is often associated with monogenic connective tissue disorders or proteolytic enzyme degenerative effects, whereas IAs are more often influenced by polygenic genetic factors, hemodynamic forces, and inflammation [103]. AAA is influenced by atherosclerotic processes, proteolytic enzyme activity, oxidative stress, hemodynamic forces, inflammation, and ECM remodeling [74, 98]. It is important to note that while these molecular drivers are often associated with AscAA, IA, and AAA, there can be considerable heterogeneity in the underlying mechanisms between individual patients. Moreover, there may be overlapping molecular pathways and interactions, requiring further studies. Understanding the molecular drivers of aneurysmal disease is crucial for developing targeted therapies and interventions to prevent its progression and improve patient outcomes.

7. Implications of aortic valve disease on degenerative ascending aortic aneurysm

There are signs that degenerative AscAA is also associated with aortic valve disease when examining the surgical ASAP-cohort (described in detail elsewhere [12]); BAV-associated aortopathy has an equal prevalence of aortic stenosis (AS) and aortic regurgitation (AI). Contrastingly TAV-associated (degenerative) AscAA often associates with AI but very seldomly AS. This may imply that AS has protective effects on AscAA development, or the inverse, that AscAA patients are protected from AS.

The association of AI with degenerative AscAA may in part represent secondary causes of AI, i.e., disease of surrounding structures [104]. However, AI, combined with degenerative AscAA, was also prevalent in the absence of aortic root dilatation, as seen in the ASAP cohort, pointing toward a primary cause of AI to AscAA formation. Notably, AI is a well-known prognostic factor in clinical outcomes of patients undergoing ascending aortic repair [105]. A worse surgical outcome for AscAA/AI repair is reported in both BAV and TAV individuals [106].

Interestingly, further strengthening the association of AI to AscAA formation is the fact that degenerative changes are noted in ascending aortas of patients with normal aortic diamters and AI. Specifically, elastin fragmentation, thinning and MEMA (indicative of VSMC death) have been observed in patients with AI but not AS [105, 107]. One apparent line of investigation not yet explored is whether this association can be observed in individuals with BAV without dilatation but with respective aortic valve disease [37]. Neither have implications of AI-associated ascending aortic degeneration been investigated as a possible player in AscAA formation.

8. Summary

In summary, the impact of aortic valve cuspidity on ascending aortic aneurysm is well-established. Specifically, BAV aortopathy has been associated with endothelial instability and endothelial-to-mesenchymal transition, possibly of embryonic origin. Moreover, different BAV fusion types may impose different mechanisms of aortopathy, with different aortic segments being affected. TAV-associated degenerative aneurysms, on the other hand, are molecularly more similar to AAA with clear medial degeneration and inflammation. Also, aortic valve disease may play a role in degenerative aneurysm formation, with aortic dilatation occurring almost exclusively in combination with aortic regurgitation. This is further supported by histopathological evidence.

As the aortic valve and ascending aorta are not only anatomically proximate but also embryonically associated and physiologically interacting, the impact of aortic valve cuspidity and disease on ascending aortopathy is warranted further research specifically to explore more patient-specific molecular mechanisms. An elucidation of the molecular underpinnings of AscAA development in different conditions of the aortic valve will help guide novel diagnosis and treatment strategies.

Conflict of interest

The authors declare no conflict of interest.

Author details

David Freiholtz*, Per Eriksson and Hanna M. Björck
Karolinska Institutet, Stockholm, Sweden

*Address all correspondence to: david.freiholtz@ki.se

IntechOpen

© 2023 The Author(s). Licensee IntechOpen. This chapter is distributed under the terms of the Creative Commons Attribution License (http://creativecommons.org/licenses/by/3.0), which permits unrestricted use, distribution, and reproduction in any medium, provided the original work is properly cited.

References

[1] Isselbacher EM, Preventza O, Black JH, Augoustides JG, Beck AW, Bolen MA, et al. 2022 ACC/AHA guideline for the diagnosis and Management of Aortic Disease: A report of the American Heart Association/American College of Cardiology Joint Committee on clinical practice guidelines. Circulation. 2022;**146**(24):E334-E482

[2] Gouveia e Melo R, Silva Duarte G, Lopes A, Alves M, Caldeira D, e Fernandes RF, et al. Incidence and prevalence of thoracic aortic aneurysms: A systematic review and meta-analysis of population-based studies. Seminars in Thoracic and Cardiovascular Surgery. 2022;**34**(1):1-16

[3] Michelena HI, Khanna AD, Mahoney D, Margaryan E, Topilsky Y, Suri RM, et al. Incidence of aortic complications in patients with bicuspid aortic valves. Journal of the American Medical Association. 2011;**306**(10):1104-1112

[4] Sillesen AS, Vøgg O, Pihl C, Raja AA, Sundberg K, Vedel C, et al. Prevalence of bicuspid aortic valve and associated Aortopathy in Newborns in Copenhagen, Denmark. JAMA - Journal of the American Medical Association. 2021;**325**(6):561-567

[5] Masri A, Kalahasti V, Alkharabsheh S, Svensson LG, Sabik JF, Roselli EE, et al. Characteristics and long-term outcomes of contemporary patients with bicuspid aortic valves. Journal of Thoracic and Cardiovascular Surgery. 2016;**151**(6):1650-1659

[6] Masri A, Svensson LG, Griffin BP, Desai MY. Contemporary natural history of bicuspid aortic valve disease: A systematic review. Vol. 103. Heart. 2017;**103**(17):1323-1330

[7] Grewal N, Gittenberger-De Groot AC, von der Thusen J, Wisse LJ, Bartelings MM, Deruiter MC, et al. The development of the ascending aortic wall in tricuspid and bicuspid aortic valve: A process from maturation to degeneration. Journal of Clinical Medicine. 2020;**9**(4):908

[8] Stock S, Mohamed SA, Sievers HH. Bicuspid aortic valve related aortopathy. General Thoracic and Cardiovascular Surgery. 2019;**67**(1):93-101

[9] Abdulkareem N, Smelt J, Jahangiri M. Bicuspid aortic valve aortopathy: Genetics, pathophysiology and medical therapy. Interactive Cardiovascular and Thoracic Surgery. 2013;**17**(3):554-559

[10] Freiholtz D, Bergman O, Lång K, Poujade FA, Paloschi V, Granath C, et al. Bicuspid aortic valve aortopathy is characterized by embryonic epithelial to mesenchymal transition and endothelial instability. Journal of Molecular Medicine. 2023;**1**:1-11

[11] Folkersen L, Wågsäter D, Paloschi V, Jackson V, Petrini J, Kurtovic S, et al. Unraveling divergent gene expression profiles in bicuspid and tricuspid aortic valve patients with thoracic aortic dilatation: The ASAP study. Molecular Medicine. 2011;**17**(11-12):1365-1373

[12] Jackson V, Petrini J, Caidahl K, Eriksson MJ, Liska J, Eriksson P, et al. Bicuspid aortic valve leaflet morphology in relation to aortic root morphology: A study of 300 patients undergoing open-heart surgery. European Journal of Cardio-thoracic Surgery. 2011;**40**(3):e118-e124

[13] Hinton RB, Lincoln J, Deutsch GH, Osinska H, Manning PB, Benson DW, et al. Extracellular matrix remodeling and organization in developing and diseased aortic valves. Circulation Research. 2006;**98**(11):1431-1438

[14] Stefanovic S, Etchevers HC, Zaffran S. Outflow tract formation—Embryonic origins of Conotruncal congenital heart disease. Journal of Cardiovascular Development and Disease. 2021;**8**(4):42

[15] Grewal N, Lindeman JH, Klautz A, Driessen A, Klautz RJM, Poelmann RE. Normal and abnormal development of the aortic valve and ascending aortic wall: A comprehensive overview of the embryology and pathology of the bicuspid aortic valve. Annals of Cardiothoracic Surgery. 2022;**11**(4):380-388

[16] Phillips HM, Mahendran P, Singh E, Anderson RH, Chaudhry B, Henderson DJ. Neural crest cells are required for correct positioning of the developing outflow cushions and pattern the arterial valve leaflets. Cardiovascular Research. 2013;**99**(3):452-460

[17] Soto-Navarrete MT, López-Unzu MÁ, Durán AC, Fernández B. Embryonic development of bicuspid aortic valves. Progress in Cardiovascular Diseases. 2020;**63**(4):407-418

[18] Armstrong EJ, Bischoff J. Heart Valve Development. Circulation Research. 2004;**95**(5):459-470

[19] De la Pompa JL, Epstein JA. Coordinating tissue interactions: Notch Signaling in cardiac development and disease. Developmental Cell. 2012;**22**(2):244-254

[20] Thiery JP, Acloque H, Huang RYJ, Nieto MA. Epithelial-mesenchymal transitions in development and disease. Cell. 2009;**139**(5):871-890

[21] Wang Y, Fang Y, Lu P, Wu B, Zhou B. NOTCH Signaling in aortic valve development and calcific aortic valve disease. Frontiers in Cardiovascular Medicine. 2021;**8**:682298

[22] High FA, Zhang M, Proweller A, Tu LL, Parmacek MS, Pear WS, et al. An essential role for Notch in neural crest during cardiovascular development and smooth muscle differentiation. Journal of Clinical Investigation. 2007;**117**(2):353-363

[23] Tutar E, Ekici F, Atalay S, Nacar N. The prevalence of bicuspid aortic valve in newborns by echocardiographic screening. American Heart Journal. 2005;**150**(3):513-515

[24] Sievers HH, Schmidtke C. A classification system for the bicuspid aortic valve from 304 surgical specimens. Journal of Thoracic and Cardiovascular Surgery. 2007;**133**(5):1226-1233

[25] Peterson JC, Wisse LJ, Wirokromo V, van Herwaarden T, Smits AM, Gittenberger-De Groot AC, et al. Disturbed nitric oxide signalling gives rise to congenital bicuspid aortic valve and aortopathy. DMM Disease Models and Mechanisms. 2020;**13**(9):dmm044990

[26] Aicher D, Urbich C, Zeiher A, Dimmeler S, Schäfers HJ. Endothelial nitric oxide synthase in bicuspid aortic valve disease. Annals of Thoracic Surgery. 2007;**83**(4):1290-1294

[27] Sawada H, Rateri DL, Moorleghen JJ, Majesky MW, Daugherty A. Smooth muscle cells derived from second heart field and cardiac neural crest reside in spatially distinct domains in the Media of the Ascending Aorta—Brief Report.

Arteriosclerosis, Thrombosis, and Vascular Biology. 2017;**37**(9):1722-1726

[28] Granath C, Mohamed SA, Olsson C, Grattan M, Mertens L, Franco-Cereceda A, et al. Valve disease and aortopathy associations of bicuspid aortic valve phenotypes differ between men and women. Open Heart. 2021;**8**(2):e001857

[29] Habchi KM, Ashikhmina E, Vieira VM, Shahram JT, Isselbacher EM, Sundt TM, et al. Association between bicuspid aortic valve morphotype and regional dilatation of the aortic root and trunk. The International Journal of Cardiovascular Imaging. 2017;**33**(3):341-349

[30] Evangelista A, Gallego P, Calvo-Iglesias F, Bermejo J, Robledo-Carmona J, Sánchez V, et al. Anatomical and clinical predictors of valve dysfunction and aortic dilation in bicuspid aortic valve disease. Heart. 2018;**104**(7):566-573

[31] Della CA, Bancone C, Dialetto G, Covino EFE, Manduca S, Montibello VMV, et al. The ascending aorta with bicuspid aortic valve: A phenotypic classification with potential prognostic significance. European Journal of Cardio-Thoracic Surgery. 2014;**46**(2):240-247

[32] Roman MJ, Pugh NL, Devereux RB, Eagle KA, Holmes K, LeMaire SA, et al. Aortic dilatation associated with bicuspid aortic valve: Relation to sex, Hemodynamics, and valve morphology (the National Heart Lung and blood institute-sponsored National Registry of genetically triggered thoracic aortic aneurysms and cardiovascular conditions). The American Journal of Cardiology. 2017;**120**(7):1171-1175

[33] Jackson V, Olsson C, Eriksson P, Franco-Cereceda A. Aortic dimensions in patients with bicuspid and tricuspid aortic valves. Journal of Thoracic and Cardiovascular Surgery. 2013;**146**(3):605-610

[34] Kusner JJ, Brown JY, Gleason TG, Edelman ER. The natural history of bicuspid aortic valve disease. Structure Heart. 2022;**7**(2):100119

[35] Braverman AC, Güven H, Beardslee MA, Makan M, Kates AM, Moon MR. The bicuspid aortic valve 470 Curr Probl Cardiol, September 2005. Current Problems in Cardiology. 2005;**30**:470-522

[36] Larson EW, Edwards WD. Risk factors for aortic dissection: A necropsy study of 161 cases. The American Journal of Cardiology. 1984;**53**(6):849-855

[37] Grewal N, Girdauskas E, Idhrees M, Velayudhan B, Klautz R, Driessen A, et al. Structural abnormalities in the non-dilated ascending aortic wall of bicuspid aortic valve patients. Cardiovascular Pathology. 2023;**62**:107478

[38] Maleki S, Björck HM, Paloschi V, Kjellqvist S, Folkersen L, Jackson V, et al. Aneurysm development in patients with bicuspid aortic valve (BAV): Possible connection to repair deficiency? Aorta (Stamford). 2013;**1**(1):13-22

[39] Balint B, Yin H, Nong Z, Arpino JM, O'Neil C, Rogers SR, et al. Seno-destructive smooth muscle cells in the ascending aorta of patients with bicuspid aortic valve disease. eBioMedicine. 2019;**43**:54-66

[40] Ignatieva E, Kostina D, Irtyuga O, Uspensky V, Golovkin A, Gavriliuk N, et al. Mechanisms of smooth muscle cell differentiation are distinctly altered in thoracic aortic aneurysms associated with bicuspid or tricuspid aortic valves. Frontiers in Physiology. 2017;**8**:536

[41] Ailawadi G, Moehle CW, Pei H, Walton SP, Yang Z, Kron IL, et al. Smooth muscle phenotypic modulation is an early event in aortic aneurysms. Journal of Thoracic and Cardiovascular Surgery. 2009;**138**(6):1392-1399

[42] Maleki S, Poujade FA, Bergman O, Gådin JR, Simon N, Lång K, et al. Endothelial/epithelial mesenchymal transition in ascending aortas of patients with bicuspid aortic valve. Frontiers in Cardiovascular Medicine. 2019;**6**:182

[43] Björck HM, Du L, Pulignani S, Paloschi V, Lundströmer K, Kostina AS, et al. Altered DNA methylation indicates an oscillatory flow mediated epithelial-to-mesenchymal transition signature in ascending aorta of patients with bicuspid aortic valve. Scientific Reports. 2018;**8**(1):2777

[44] Di Russo J, Hannocks MJ, Luik AL, Song J, Zhang X, Yousif L, et al. Vascular laminins in physiology and pathology. Matrix Biology. 2017;**57-58**:140-148

[45] Maleki S, Kjellqvist S, Paloschi V, Magné J, Branca RMM, Du L, et al. Mesenchymal state of intimal cells may explain higher propensity to ascending aortic aneurysm in bicuspid aortic valves. Scientific Reports. 2016;**6**(June):1-16

[46] Gould RA, Aziz H, Woods CE, Seman-Senderos MA, Sparks E, Preuss C, et al. ROBO4 variants predispose individuals to bicuspid aortic valve and thoracic aortic aneurysm. Vol. 51. Nature Genetics. 2019;**51**(1):42-50

[47] Park KW, Morrison CM, Sorensen LK, Jones CA, Rao Y, Bin CC, et al. Robo4 is a vascular-specific receptor that inhibits endothelial migration. Developmental Biology. 2003;**261**(1):251-267

[48] Okada Y, Yano K, Jin E, Funahashi N, Kitayama M, Doi T, et al. A three-kilobase fragment of the human Robo4 promoter directs cell type-specific expression in endothelium. Circulation Research. 2007;**100**(12):1712-1722

[49] Laforest B, Andelfinger G, Nemer M. Loss of Gata5 in mice leads to bicuspid aortic valve. Journal of Clinical Investigation. 2011;**121**(7):2876-2887

[50] Martin LJ, Hinton RB, Zhang X, Cripe LH, Benson DW. Aorta measurements are heritable and influenced by bicuspid aortic valve. Frontiers in Genetics. 2011;**2**:61. DOI: 10.3389

[51] Girdauskas E, Borger MA, Secknus MA, Girdauskas G, Kuntze T. Is aortopathy in bicuspid aortic valve disease a congenital defect or a result of abnormal hemodynamics? A critical reappraisal of a one-sided argument. European Journal of Cardio-Thoracic Surgery. 2011;**39**(6):809-814

[52] den Reijer PM, Sallee D 3rd, van der Velden P, Zaaijer ER, Parks WJ, Ramamurthy S, et al. Hemodynamic predictors of aortic dilatation in bicuspid aortic valve by velocity-encoded cardiovascular magnetic resonance. Journal of Cardiovascular Magnetic Resonance: Official Journal of the Society for Cardiovascular Magnetic Resonance. 2010;**12**(1):4. DOI: 10.1186/1532-429X-12-4

[53] Hope MD, Hope TA, Meadows AK, Ordovas KG, Urbania TH, Alley MT, et al. Bicuspid aortic valve: Four-dimensional MR evaluation of ascending aortic systolic flow patterns. Radiology. 2010;**255**(1):53-61

[54] Pasta S, Gentile G, Raffa GM, Bellavia D, Chiarello G, Liotta R, et al. In Silico shear and intramural stresses are linked to aortic valve morphology

in dilated ascending aorta. European Journal of Vascular and Endovascular Surgery. 2017;**54**(2):254-263

[55] Grewal N, Girdauskas E, DeRuiter M, Goumans MJ, Lindeman JH, Disha K, et al. The role of hemodynamics in bicuspid aortopathy: A histopathologic study. Cardiovascular Pathology. 2019;**41**:29-37

[56] Cotrufo M, Della Corte A, De Santo LS, Quarto C, De Feo M, Romano G, et al. Different patterns of extracellular matrix protein expression in the convexity and the concavity of the dilated aorta with bicuspid aortic valve: Preliminary results. The Journal of Thoracic and Cardiovascular Surgery. 2005;**130**(2):504-511

[57] Della Corte A, Quarto C, Bancone C, Castaldo C, Di Meglio F, Nurzynska D, et al. Spatiotemporal patterns of smooth muscle cell changes in ascending aortic dilatation with bicuspid and tricuspid aortic valve stenosis: Focus on cell-matrix signaling. Journal of Thoracic and Cardiovascular Surgery. 2008;**135**(1):8-18

[58] Maleki S, Björck HM, Folkersen L, Nilsson R, Renner J, Caidahl K, et al. Identification of a novel flow-mediated gene expression signature in patients with bicuspid aortic valve. Journal of Molecular Medicine. 2013;**91**(1):129-139

[59] Gauer S, Balint B, Kollmann C, Federspiel JM, Henn D, Bandner-Risch D, et al. Dysregulation of endothelial nitric oxide synthase does not depend on hemodynamic alterations in bicuspid aortic valve aortopathy. Journal of the American Heart Association. 2020;**9**(18):e016471

[60] Regeer MV, Versteegh MIM, Klautz RJM, Schalij MJ, Bax JJ, Marsan NA, et al. Effect of aortic valve replacement on aortic root dilatation rate in patients with bicuspid and tricuspid aortic valves. Annals of Thoracic Surgery. 2016;**102**(6):1981-1987

[61] Yoshioka Y, Yajima S, Sakaniwa R, Tadokoro N, Kainuma S, Kawamoto N, et al. Does the residual aorta dilate after replacement of the bicuspid aortic valve and ascending aorta? Journal of Thoracic Disease. 2023;**15**(3):994-1008

[62] Yang B, Zhou W, Jiao J, Nielsen JB, Mathis MR, Heydarpour M, et al. Protein-altering and regulatory genetic variants near GATA4 implicated in bicuspid aortic valve. Nature Communications. 2017;**8**:15481

[63] Abbasi S, Mohsen-Pour N, Naderi N, Rahimi S, Maleki M, Kalayinia S. In silico analysis of GATA4 variants demonstrates main contribution to congenital heart disease. Journal of Cardiovascular and Thoracic Research. 2021;**13**(4):336-354

[64] Behiry EG, Al-Azzouny MA, Sabry D, Behairy OG, Salem NE. Association of NKX2-5, GATA4, and TBX5 polymorphisms with congenital heart disease in Egyptian children. Molecular Genetics & Genomic Medicine. 2019;**7**(5):e612

[65] Garg V, Kathiriya IS, Barnes R, Schluterman MK, King IN, Butler CA, et al. GATA4 mutations cause human congenital heart defects and reveal an interaction with TBX5. Nature. 2003;**424**(6947):443-447. DOI: 10.1038/nature01827

[66] Gillis E, Kumar AA, Luyckx I, Preuss C, Cannaerts E, van de Beek G, et al. Candidate gene resequencing in a large bicuspid aortic valve-associated thoracic aortic aneurysm cohort: SMAD6 as an important contributor. Frontiers in Physiology. 2017;**8**:400

[67] Heng E, Stone JR, Kim JB, Lee H, MacGillivray TE, Sundt TM. Comparative histology of aortic dilatation associated with bileaflet versus trileaflet aortic valves. Annals of Thoracic Surgery. 2015;**100**(6):2095-2101

[68] Federspiel JM, Schnabel PA, Tschernig T, Balint B, Schwab T, Laschke MW, et al. Aortic aneurysms with tricuspid aortic valve have more degeneration than unicuspid aortic valve aneurysms. European Journal of Cardio-thoracic Surgery. 2021;**60**(2):333-340

[69] Erdheim J. Medionecrosis aortae idiopathica. Virchows Archiv für Pathologische Anatomie und Physiologie und für Klinische Medizin. 1929;**273**(2):454-479

[70] Halushka MK, Angelini A, Bartoloni G, Basso C, Batoroeva L, Bruneval P, et al. Consensus statement on surgical pathology of the aorta from the Society for Cardiovascular Pathology and the association for European cardio-vascular pathology: II. Noninflammatory Degenerative Diseases-Nomenclature and Diagnostic Criteria Cardiovascular Pathology. 2016;**25**(3):247-257

[71] Leone O, Pacini D, Foà A, Corsini A, Agostini V, Corti B, et al. Redefining the histopathologic profile of acute aortic syndromes: Clinical and prognostic implications. The Journal of Thoracic and Cardiovascular Surgery. 2018;**156**(5):1776-1785

[72] Wagenseil JE, Mecham RP. Elastin in large artery stiffness and hypertension. Journal of Cardiovascular Translational Research. 2012;**5**(3):264-273

[73] Weininger G, Ostberg N, Shang M, Zafar M, Ziganshin BA, Liu S, et al. Lipid profiles help to explain protection from systemic atherosclerosis in patients with ascending aortic aneurysm. Journal of Thoracic and Cardiovascular Surgery. 2022;**163**(2):e129-e132

[74] Pinard A, Jones GT, Milewicz DM. Genetics of thoracic and abdominal aortic diseases. Circulation Research. 2019;**124**(4):588-606

[75] Ikonomidis JS, Ruddy JM, Benton SM, Arroyo J, Brinsa TA, Stroud RE, et al. Aortic dilatation with bicuspid aortic valves: Cusp fusion correlates to matrix metalloproteinases and inhibitors. Annals of Thoracic Surgery. 2012;**93**(2):457-463

[76] Rabkin SW. Differential expression of MMP-2, MMP-9 and TIMP proteins in thoracic aortic aneurysm - comparison with and without bicuspid aortic valve: A meta-analysis. VASA. 2014;**43**(6):433-442

[77] Matusiewicz M et al. Upregulated sulfatase and downregulated MMP-3 in thoracic aortic aneurysm. Advances in Clinical and Experimental Medicine. 2020;**29**(5):565-572

[78] Lemaire SA, Wang X, Wilks JA, Carter SA, Wen S, Won T, et al. Matrix metalloproteinases in ascending aortic aneurysms: Bicuspid versus trileaflet aortic valves1. Journal of Surgical Research. 2005;**123**(1):40-48

[79] Jackson V, Olsson T, Kurtovic S, Folkersen L, Paloschi V, Wågsäter D, et al. Matrix metalloproteinase 14 and 19 expression is associated with thoracic aortic aneurysms. The Journal of Thoracic and Cardiovascular Surgery. 2012;**144**(2):459-466

[80] Rabkin SW. The role matrix Metalloproteinases in the production of aortic aneurysm. Progress in Molecular

Biology and Translational Science. 2017;**147**:239-265

[81] Velchev JD, Van Laer L, Luyckx I, Dietz H, Loeys B. Loeys-Dietz Syndrome. Advances in Experimental Medicine and Biology. 2021;**1348**:251-264

[82] Zeigler SM, Sloan B, Jones JA. Pathophysiology and pathogenesis of Marfan syndrome. Advances in Experimental Medicine and Biology. 2021;**1348**:185-206

[83] Isselbacher EM, Cardenas CLL, Lindsay ME. Hereditary influence in thoracic aortic aneurysm and dissection. Circulation. 2016;**133**(24):2516-2528

[84] Li Y, Ren P, Dawson A, Vasquez HG, Ageedi W, Zhang C, et al. Single-cell transcriptome analysis reveals dynamic cell populations and differential gene expression patterns in control and aneurysmal human aortic tissue. Circulation. 2020;**142**(14):1374-1388

[85] Kuzmik GA, Sang AX, Elefteriades JA. Natural history of thoracic aortic aneurysms. Journal of Vascular Surgery. 2012;**56**(2):565-571

[86] Pannu H, Tran-Fadulu V, Milewicz DM. Genetic basis of thoracic aortic aneurysms and aortic dissections. American Journal of Medical Genetics. Part C, Seminars in Medical Genetics. 2005;**139C**(1):10-16

[87] Saeyeldin A, Velasquez C, Mahmood S, Brownstein A, Zafar M, Ziganshin B, et al. Thoracic aortic aneurysm: Unlocking the "silent killer" secrets. General Thoracic and Cardiovascular Surgery. 2019;**67**(1):1-11

[88] He R, Guo DC, Sun W, Papke CL, Duraisamy S, Estrera AL, et al. Characterization of the inflammatory cells in ascending thoracic aortic aneurysms in patients with Marfan syndrome, familial thoracic aortic aneurysms, and sporadic aneurysms. Journal of Thoracic and Cardiovascular Surgery. 2008;**136**(4):922-929

[89] Gyftopoulos A, Ziganshin BA, Elefteriades JA, Ochoa Chaar CI. Comparison of genes associated with thoracic and abdominal aortic aneurysms. Aorta (Stamford, Conn.). 2023;**11**(3):125-134. DOI: 10.1055/s-0043-57266

[90] Sakalihasan N, Limet R, Defawe OD. Abdominal aortic aneurysm. Vol. 365. Lancet. 2005;**365**(9470):1577-1589

[91] Golledge J. Abdominal aortic aneurysm: Update on pathogenesis and medical treatments. Nature Reviews. Cardiology. 2019;**16**(4):225-242

[92] Deroo E, Stranz A, Yang H, Hsieh M, Se C, Zhou T. Endothelial dysfunction in the pathogenesis of abdominal aortic aneurysm. Biomolecules. 2022;**12**(4):509

[93] Wiernicki I, Parafiniuk M, Kolasa-Wolosiuk A, Gutowska I, Kazimierczak A, Clark J, et al. Relationship between aortic wall oxidative stress/proteolytic enzyme expression and intraluminal thrombus thickness indicates a novel pathomechanism in the progression of human abdominal aortic aneurysm. The FASEB Journal. 2019;**33**(1):885-895

[94] Jacob MP. Extracellular matrix remodeling and matrix metalloproteinases in the vascular wall during aging and in pathological conditions. Biomedicine and Pharmacotherapy. 2003;**57**(5-6):195-202

[95] Gao JP, Guo W. Mechanisms of abdominal aortic aneurysm progression: A review. Vascular Medicine. 2022;**27**(1):88-96

[96] Brown RD, Broderick JP. Unruptured intracranial aneurysms: Epidemiology, natural history, management options, and familial screening. Lancet Neurology. 2014;**13**(4):393-404

[97] Laurent D, Small C, Lucke-Wold B, Dodd WS, Chalouhi N, Hu YC, et al. Understanding the genetics of intracranial aneurysms: A primer. Clinical Neurology and Neurosurgery. 2022;**212**:107060. DOI: 10.1016/j.clineuro.2021.107060

[98] Bakker MK, Ruigrok YM. Genetics of intracranial aneurysms. Stroke. 2021;**52**(9):3004-3012

[99] Ruigrok YM, Rinkel GJE, Wijmenga C. Genetics of intracranial aneurysms. Lancet Neurology. 2005;**4**(3):179-189

[100] Zhang Z, Fang Y, Lenahan C, Chen S. The role of immune inflammation in aneurysmal subarachnoid hemorrhage. Experimental Neurology. 2021;**336**:113535. DOI: 10.1016/j.expneurol.2020.113535

[101] Jin J, Duan J, Du L, Xing W, Peng X, Zhao Q. Inflammation and immune cell abnormalities in intracranial aneurysm subarachnoid hemorrhage (SAH): Relevant signaling pathways and therapeutic strategies. Frontiers in Immunology. 2022;**13**:1027756

[102] Okada T, Suzuki H. Toll-like receptor 4 as a possible therapeutic target for delayed brain injuries after aneurysmal subarachnoid hemorrhage. Neural Regeneration Research. 2017;**12**(2):193-196

[103] Samuel N, Radovanovic I. Genetic basis of intracranial aneurysm formation and rupture: Clinical implications in the postgenomic era. Neurosurgical Focus. 2019;**47**(1):E10

[104] Akinseye OA, Pathak A, Ibebuogu UN. Aortic valve regurgitation: A comprehensive review. Current Problems in Cardiology. 2018;**43**(8):315-334

[105] Benedik J, Pilarzcyk K, Wendt D, Price V, Tsagakis K, Perrey M, et al. Is there any difference in aortic wall quality between patients with aortic stenosis and those with regurgitation? European Journal of Cardio-Thoracic Surgery: Official Journal of the European Association for Cardio-Thoracic Surgery. 2013;**44**(4):754-759. DOI: 10.1093/ejcts/ezt123

[106] Balint B, Federspiel JM, Schwab T, Ehrlich T, Ramsthaler F, Schäfers HJ. Aortic regurgitation is associated with ascending aortic Remodeling in the nondilated aorta. Arteriosclerosis, Thrombosis, and Vascular Biology. 2021;**41**(3):1179-1190

[107] Sequeira Gross TM, Lindner D, Ojeda FM, Neumann J, Grewal N, Kuntze T, et al. Comparison of microstructural alterations in the proximal aorta between aortic stenosis and regurgitation. Journal of Thoracic and Cardiovascular Surgery. 2021;**162**(6):1684-1695

Section 3

Technique of Transcatheter Aortic Valve Replacement

Chapter 4

Transcatheter Aortic Valve Replacement Technique and Current Approaches

Ali Yasar Kilinc and Mustafa Ucar

Abstract

Aortic stenosis (AS) is a chronic, progressive disease. The most common cause of aortic stenosis etiology in advanced age is calcific, degenerative aortic stenosis. Once patients become symptomatic, the disease progresses rapidly. Treatment is surgical aortic replacement. Advanced age and the presence of comorbid conditions increase the risk of surgery. Therefore, a significant number of patients cannot be treated. For this purpose, transcatheter aortic valve interventions were developed and started to be used all over the world. In this article, we discussed the technical features of the transcatheter aortic valve replacement (TAVR) procedure, the types of valves used and the complications of the procedure. Clinical results of the procedure and comparisons with other treatment methods will not be included in our article.

Keywords: aortic stenosis, balloon expandable, cusp overlap, self-expandable, transcatheter, heart valve

1. Introduction

Aortic stenosis (AS) is the most common type of valvular heart disease in developed countries. Incidence of AS increases due to the prolongation of life expectancy. Until the 2000s, surgical aortic valve replacement (SAVR) was the unique treatment for symptomatic AS. In 2002, Cribier et al. [1] performed a transcatheter aortic valve replacement (TAVR) procedure with a balloon-expandable valve in an inoperable patient and a new era began.

First, TAVR was approved for patients with high surgical risk but currently as more data gleaned, the focus expanded to the intermediate- and low-risk patients as well [2]. All the available transcatheter heart valves belong to one of the following categories: balloon-expandable valves (BEVs) or self-expandable valves (SEVs). BEV expands using the radial strength of the balloon, in contrast, SEV is deployed until it faces the resistance of the annular wall, adapting to anatomy of aortic annulus [3]. Another classification is according to leaflets mounted within the stented frame to native aortic annulus. Based on this grouping, valves can be classified as supra-annular and intra-annular. Supra-annular valves are designed to avoid interaction with native annulus. This prevents blood flow obstruction. Also, supra-annular valves lead to lower transvalvular gradients and higher effective orifice area [4]. On the other hand, intra-annular valves lead to less interaction with coronary ostia, thereby minimizing the risk of obstruction [5].

2. Transcatheter aortic valve types

2.1 Self-expandable valves

Self-expandable valve family includes Evolut R, Evolut Pro, Evolut Pro+, *Evolut FX (Medtronic, Minneapolis, MN, USA), Portico, Navitor (Abbott Vascular, Santa Clara, CA, USA), Acurate Neo (Boston Scientific, Marlborough MA, USA), Allegra (Biosensors, Singapore, Singapore, and New Valve Technology, Hechingen, Germany) and Biovalve (Biotronik, Buelach, Switzerland).

2.1.1 CoreValve/evolut family

First, the SEV 'CoreValve' was initially presented by Medtronic. In CoreValve US Pivotal Trial, TAVR showed higher survival rates compared to SAVR at 1 year [6]. The main disadvantages of this system were large size of delivery system, increased postprocedure permanent pacing rate, increased rate of paravalvular leak (PVL) and relatively increased stroke rates [7–10]. After the CoreValve system, Evolut R, Pro and Pro+ were designed by Medtronic (**Figure 1**). All models contain tri-leaflet porcine pericardial tissue on a Nitinol frame and work in a supra-annular position. Evolut R system has favorable outcomes compared to the CoreValve system, especially on paravalvular leak. Evolut Pro kept all features of Evolut R, is recapturable and repositionable to assist in optimal deployment. Also, this system has an extra porcine pericardial wrap over first 1.5 cells to reduce PVL [11, 12]. Evolut Pro+ platform can treat an even larger annulus range up to 30 mm diameter. Evolut FX valve was recently developed with enhanced visualization capabilities [13]. Platforms use transvascular ways. Evolut R and Evolut Pro+ have four annular diameter sizes. The size of 23 mm is suitable for 18–20 mm aortic valve annuli, 26 mm for annuli 20–23 mm, 29 mm for annuli 23–26 mm and 34 mm for annuli 26–29 mm. Evolut R platform uses 14 French (Fr) equivalent sheath. But 34 mm Evolut R and Evolut Pro platform use 16 Fr sheath. Evolut Pro+ platform uses 14 Fr sheath (18 Fr sheath is necessary for a 34 mm valve). Generally before implantation, predilatation is recommended. Usually rapid pacing is

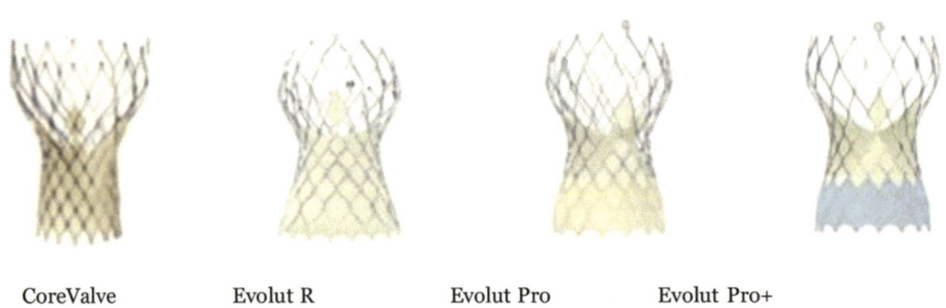

Figure 1.
CoreValve/evolut valve design.

DOI: http://dx.doi.org/10.5772/intechopen.111904

	Evolut r	Evolut pro	Portico	Acurate neo
Approval	FDA, CE	FDA, CE	CE	CE
Leaflet position	Supra-annular	Supra-annular	Intra-annular	Supra-annular
Leaflet structure	Porcine	Porcine	Bovine	Porcine
Valve sizes	23,26,29,34	23,26,29 (pro+34 also)	23,25,27,29	23,25,27
Resheathability	Yes	Yes	Yes	No
Self-positioning	No	No	No	Yes

Table 1.
Comparison of self-expandable valves' basic features.

not necessary but in aortic regurgitation and high annuli diameter, controlled pacing (90–130 rates/min) can be used (**Table 1**).

2.1.2 Portico and Navitor

Portico is the first resheathable and repositionable SEV. Its intra-annular design provides early valve function and reduces hemodynamic interaction during the procedure. Portico has large frame cells that enhance coronary access. Available sizes are 23 mm, 25 mm, 27 mm and 29 mm. Both platforms use transvascular ways. The 14 Fr sheath is suitable for 23–25 mm valves and the 15 Fr sheath is suitable for 27–29 mm valves [14, 15]. Navitor is a new generation of Portico valves (**Figure 2**). It has an external cuff to reduce PVL. Abbott published 30-day results. All-cause mortality 0%, permanent pacemaker 15%, major vascular complications 0.8% and mean gradient 7.4 mmHg, higher than minimal PVL 0%, were observed. Highlighted potential risk is associated with increased rates of permanent pacemaker implantation [16].

2.1.3 Acurate TA and Acurate NEO

Acurate TA is used for transapical access and Acurate Neo is used for transvascular access. Unlike other SEVs, Acurate cannot be repositioned. It has a supra-annular design with three stabilization arches that help bioprosthetic valve alignment. Implantation has two steps from 'up to down'. First aortic side releases then subannular side releases. Because of this unique opening style, the platform protects

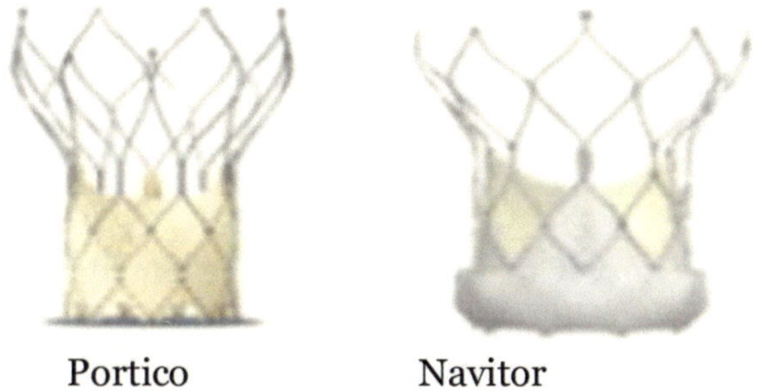

Figure 2.
Portico/Navitor valve design.

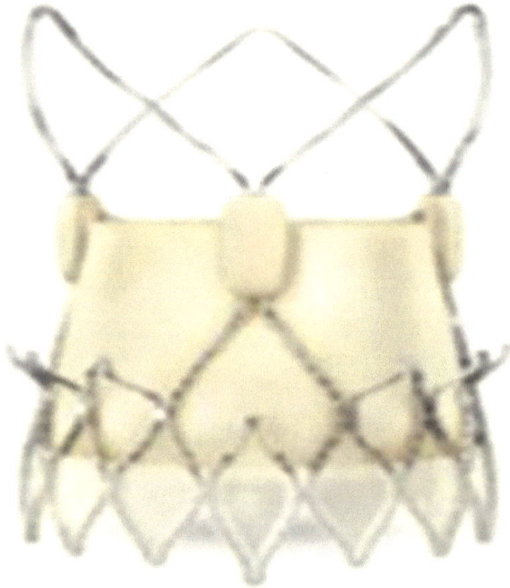

Figure 3.
Acurate neo design.

hemodynamics, allows blood flow and decreases embolization risk. Acurate Neo is especially suitable for low coronary distances and horizontal aorta (**Figure 3**). Acurate Neo has the lowest permanent pace ratio in all SEVs. This is a consequence of lower radial force. Due to lower radial force, conduction system trauma reduces. But this low radial force makes necessary predilatation and postdilatation. Acurate Neo has three sizes (23 mm, 25 mm and 27 mm) [17].

2.1.4 Allegra valve

Allegra (Biosensors, Singapore, Singapore, and New Valve Technology, Hechingen, Germany) has a tri-leaflet Nitinol stent roof made of bovine pericardium in the supra-annular position (**Figure 4**). The access way is transvascular. The delivery system includes three-stage release technology for implantation. Unlike other valves, the delivery system and valve are first placed toward the left ventricle. Then the valve starts to open from the middle part (Permaflow position). Because of low radial force, predilatation is recommended. In 2016 after the first results of the Allegra valve were positive, it received European Conformity, i.e., Conformité Européene (CE) approval in March 2017 [18, 19].

2.1.5 Biovalve

Biovalve (Biotronic, Buelach, Switzerland) is a new-generation valve with supra-annular structure, consisting of a skirt on a Nitinol roof and three leaflets made from porcine pericardium. This platform presents a large orifice area. The delivery system has a diameter of 18 Fr, suitable for transfemoral access, 360 degree flexible structure and ergonomic design. The valve can be resheathed up to 80% of implantation [20].

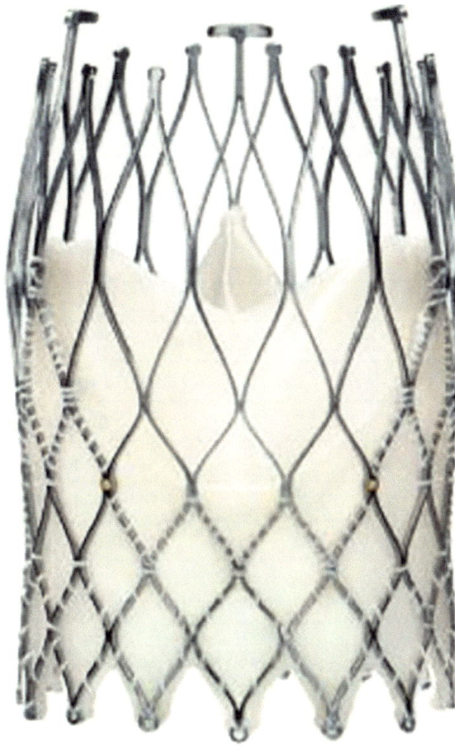

Figure 4.
Allegra valve design.

2.2 Balloon-expandable valves

Implantation of a transcatheter heart valve (THV) via a balloon-expandable system played an important role in the early stages of TAVR. The first clinical experience started with the Cribier-Edwards valve. After the technological developments, new-generation devices are made available. BEVs are Saphien family (Edwards Lifesciences Corporation, Irvine, CA, USA), Myval (Meril Life Sciences Pvt. Ltd., Vapi, Gujarat, India), Inovare (Braile Biomedical, São José do Rio Preto, Brazil) and Colibri (Colibri Heart Valve, Broomfield, USA). All BEVs are placed in an intra-annular position.

2.2.1 Saphien BEV family

Saphien is the first BEV. This family includes Saphien XT, Saphien 3 and Saphien 3 Ultra. The valves are made of tri-leaflet bovine pericardium mounted on a cobalt-chromium stent frame (**Figure 5**). Saphien XT valves are available in 20, 23, 26 and 29 mm sizes. This platform uses a 16 F sheath for 20 and 23 mm valves, 18 F sheath for a 26 mm valve and 20 F sheath for a 29 mm valve. Saphien 3 platform is compatible with the 14 F sheath for the 20 mm, 23 mm, and 26 mm valves and with the 16 F sheath for the 29 mm valve. All these sheaths are expandable and called 'eSheath'. Sapien 3 and Sapien 3 Ultra valves are suitable for transfemoral processing up to 5.5 mm femoral artery diameter. The major improvement in Sapien 3 is polyethylene

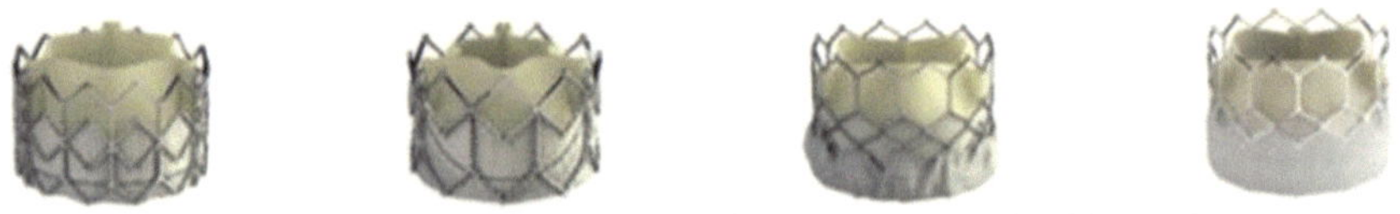

Figure 5.
Saphien BEV family.

Special condition	First choice
Small annulus (<23 mm)	Evolut R/Pro
Large annulus (>27 mm)	Evolut R/Pro
Low coronary distance	Acurate Neo
Small vascular diameter	Evolut R/Pro, Portico
Valve in valve	Evolut R/Pro, Acurate Neo
Concomitant coronary artery disease	Acurate Neo, Portico
Easy to use	Acurate Neo, Portico

Table 2.
Recommendations for [all conditions].

terephthalate (PET) outer skirt to reduce PVL and an open cell upper frame geometry to avoid obstruction and allow access to coronary arteries [21]. The last generation of Saphien family is Saphien 3 Ultra. This valve is based on Saphien 3 platform but has 40% taller skirt design to avoid PVL better. The 20, 23 and 26 mm valves feature a new skirt design, while the 29 mm valve remains in the existing Saphien 3 platform [22].

Saphien 3 and Saphien 3 Ultra have some unique indications for use. The Food Drug and Administration (FDA) has approved them for mitral and pulmonary procedures. But this issue is beyond the scope of this article (**Table 2**).

2.2.2 Myval BEV

Myval's design is created with hexagons. Its special design has large open cells toward the aortic end, while it has closed cells toward ventricular end to maintain higher radial force (**Figure 6**). Unlike other valves, Myval has a large number of sizes, such as conventional (20, 23, 26 and 29 mm), medium (21.5, 24.5 and 27.5 mm) and extra large (30.5 and 32 mm). Myval THV of size 32 mm got CDSCO (Central Drugs Standard Control Organization, India) approval and 30.5 mm is pending CDSCO approval. Medium sizes are for avoiding a serious complication of BEV, annular rupture. The platform uses 14 F delivery system [23].

2.2.3 Inovare BEV

Inovare BEV consists of tri-leaflet bovine pericardial valves mounted in a cobalt-chromium stent frame and is available in four sizes of 20, 22, 24 and 26 mm (**Figure 7**). The valve is implanted using the transapical and transaortic approach [24].

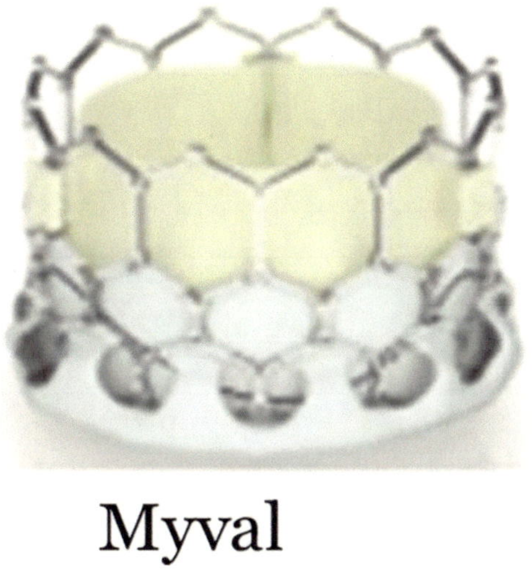

Figure 6.
Myval design.

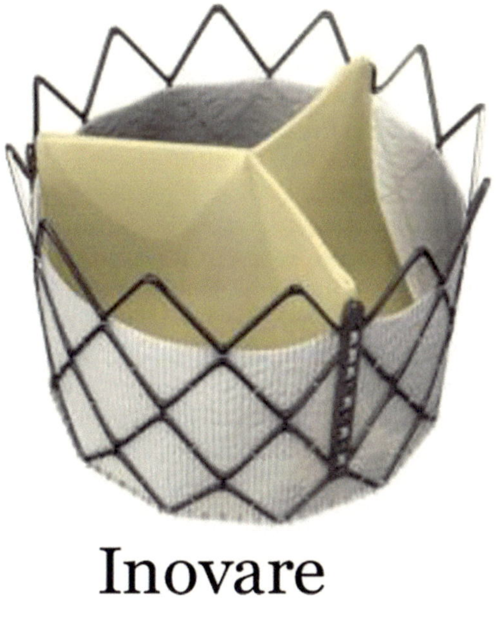

Figure 7.
Inovare design.

2.2.4 Colibri BEV

There are limited clinical data and Colbri BEV is a prefabricated TAVR system. The valve has a unique folding technique and is made of three independent porcine pericardium pieces. The first implantation was performed in November 2012 [24].

Scenario	Favor BEV	Favor SEV
Severely calcified annulus		+
Small annulus		+
Large annulus	+	
Bicuspid aortic valve	+	+
Small femoral arteries		+
Concomitant coronary artery disease	+	
Preexisting conduction abnormalities	+	
Reduced ejection fraction		+

Table 3.
General recommendations for choosing a proper valve.

Table 3 summarizes general recommendations for choosing a proper valve; however, the most important recommendation is to use the platform that the operator is experienced to handle.

3. Accesses in TAVR procedure

Over the past 20 years, TAVR has become an alternative treatment for severe aortic stenosis. For this treatment, operators need a suitable access. According to the current guidelines, femoral approach is the first choice [25, 26].

3.1 Transfemoral approach

Transfemoral access is the first choice in TAVR procedures. This is because operators are experienced in handling femoral access and possible complications can be managed easily. Despite technical improvement in vascular sheath diameters, 10–20% of all patients are not suitable for undergoing transfemoral access due to advanced peripheral arterial disease [27]. So for these unsuitable patients, alternative access sites have been searched. TAVR can be performed alternatively via transapical, transaortic, transsubclavian/transaxillary, transcarotid, transcaval and suprasternal approaches. But before searching for an alternative site, it is very important to evaluate iliofemoral anatomy. First of all starting from the carotid arteries, subclavian-axillary arteries, aorta and iliofemoral arteries are evaluated with multidetector computed tomography (CT). Minimal lumen diameter is determined. It is very important to evaluate iliofemoral arteries and aortic tortuosity and calcification. Circumferential calcifications, calcification protruding into the vessel lumen and anteriorly located calcifications mostly interfere with femoral access. If problems can be solved, femoral access should be used. Balloon angioplasty and lithotripsy, e.g., can be used to modify calcification and/or stenosis. Such Lunderquist and Back-up Mayer guidewires can be used to handle iliofemoral and aorta tortuosity. The plaques in aortic arch, porcelain aorta and thoracoabdominal aneurysms should be evaluated. After all if femoral access is not suitable, alternative sites should be detected. The most important criterion is operator's experience.

3.2 Transapical approach

The first transapical TAVR implantation was performed in 2005 [28]. During first years of TAVR, transapical approach was considered as the first alternative if femoral approach were not feasible. Transapical approach is more invasive than other concepts. Only BEVs are suitable for a transapical approach. Compared to the transfemoral approach, the advantages of the transapical approach are that valve alignment is easier, there are no vascular complications, less fluoroscopy time is required, and less contrast is used. Receiving general anesthesia, postoperative pain and bleeding from left ventricle (results in tamponade) are important limitations.

3.3 Transaortic approach

Transaortic approach is a highly invasive procedure compared to other vascular approaches. Transaortic intervention is performed through a right anterior mini-thoracotomy through an incision in the second intercostal space or mini-sternotomy puncture into the ascending aorta. BE and SE valves are suitable for this approach. Major advantages of this concept are less vascular complications, no necessity for left ventricular puncture and good contractility of valve. Major limitations are the need for general anesthesia, previous cardiac surgery (especially beware of left internal mammary artery (LIMA) and bypass grafts) and porcelain aorta. The distance from cannulation to annulus should be ideally 6–8 cm.

3.4 Subclavian/axillary approach

Subclavian/axillary approach is a useful alternative when transfemoral approach is not feasible. The procedure can be performed under general anesthesia or sedation and local anesthesia. Transsubclavian access is mainly via surgical approach but percutaneous access is possible too [29]. Right subclavian/axillary artery is rarely used for TAVR because of anatomical limitations. The main disadvantage of subclavian access is vascular complications. This artery is frailer than femoral artery. Because of subclavian anatomy, a manual compression might not be feasible. In subclavian access, calcification, stenosis, tortuosity, mammarian and vertebral artery relationship and during surgical cut-down brachial plexus should be evaluated carefully. Minimal subclavian artery diameter should be 5.5 cm. If there is a patent LIMA graft, subclavian access is relatively contraindicated [30].

Transaxillary approach was previously performed by surgical cut-down, nowadays this approach is done completely percutaneously. So that makes this approach first choice alternative way when transfemoral access is not feasible. Axillary artery is outside of thorax so manual compression is possible. The most ideal vascular entry point is between the medial of the pectoralis minor muscle and the outer side of the first rib, and puncture can be performed more easily when the arm is opened to the side [31]. Left axillary is generally preferred because of similarity between femoral artery exit angle. The ideal puncture site is the deltopectoral sulcus. Laterally puncture can cause brachial plexus injury, medially puncture can cause hemo−/pneumothorax and difficulty in compression. Major limitations are nearly same as transsubclavian approach but manual compression and completely percutaneous intervention are advantages.

3.5 Transcarotid approach

The first successful transcarotid approach was performed by Modine et al. in 2010 [32]. The procedure can be performed by a surgical cut-down or percutaneously. It is a safe procedure but we need to be aware of some special conditions. Carotid artery system should be carefully examined. Stenosis >50% or atheromatous plaques have higher risks for embolization. Contralateral carotid artery, vertebral arteries and posterior cerebral circulation, status of communicant arteries should be examined. Both carotid arteries can be used but the left carotid approach should be preferred because of its angulation with aorta. While performing the procedure, operators should be aware of vagus nerve, laryngeal nerve and respiratory tract.

One of the most important concerns of this procedure is periprocedural stroke. According to a study, comparing transfemoral approach with transcarotid/transsubclavian TAVR, after propensity-score matching, no significant differences in early and long-term outcomes were observed [33].

3.6 Suprasternal approach

Brachiocephalic artery is a new alternative site for TAVR when transfemoral approach is not feasible. The first suprasternal TAVI procedure was performed in 2015 [34]. This approach does not require sternotomy. Advantage of this access is short distance improving catheter stability. Tortuosity, vessel size, calcification and cervical neck anatomy should be evaluated carefully. Eudailey et al. presented a retrospective study from three centers in the USA of those patients who underwent suprasternal TAVR. A total of 84 patients were included in the study. Thirty-day survival was 98.8% and 0% transischemic attack or stroke was observed [35].

3.7 Transcaval approach

Because of increased stroke risk during carotid and subclavian approach and alternative sites are not feasible, a new intervention site should be searched. After understanding that caval-aortic truck physiology and detection of retroperitoneal pressure are always higher than those of vena cava inferior, in 2014 Greenbaum et al. performed the first transcaval TAVR [36]. This procedure, is extraordinary as it contains coronary, peripheral, congenital techniques and instruments. Before starting the procedure, aorta, vena cava inferior and adjacent structures should be evaluated carefully. The procedure starts with femoral vein puncture. After arriving at the suitable site, an aortacaval fistula is created with chronic total occlusion guidewire (e.g., Conquest or Astato). After passing the aorta valve, the delivery system is advanced via fistula. After the valve is deployed, fistula is closed with an Amplatzer device. In some cases, adjunctive aortic balloon inflations or covered stent implantation might be necessary. Follow-up CT angiography should be obtained at first and twelfth month after the procedure. This procedure is completely percutaneous and can be used when femoral approach is not feasible.

In conclusion, access for TAVR is a crucial step in patient management. Transfemoral approach is the first choice but, if not feasible, alternative access sites should be discussed in a heart team.

4. Techniques of procedure

After vascular access, a venous access (generally femoral vein) is obtained for pacing during procedure. Nowadays, pacing over the wire technique, which consists of left ventricle (LV) stimulation through the stiff guidewire, is being used. Two arterial accesses are obtained. The main site is for the delivery system and second site is for pigtail. Pigtail is used for reference and aortography. For passing through the calcified aortic valve, generally an Amplatz left 1 (AL1) catheter is used with a soft straight guide wire. When AL1 catheter fails, Amplatz left 2 (AL-2), Judkins right 4 (JR-4) or Amplatz right 1 (AR-1) catheters can be tried in accordance with the anatomy of the ascending aorta and aortic annulus. Using the left anterior oblique (LAO) projection can be useful. After passing the valve, the catheter is advanced to the ventricle and a 300 cm J-tip guidewire is exchanged. A pigtail is advanced over this guidewire. J-tip guidewire is changed to a stiffer guidewire while pigtail is in left ventricle. Safari and Confida are first choices but according to tortuosity stiffer wires, such as Amplatz Super Stiff, Lunderquist Extra Stiff or Backup Maier, can be used. Operators should be aware that the stiff side of the wire must be away from ventricle wall and the position of the wire must be maintained during all manipulations. Patients have severe calcifications and for those who can tolerate rapid pacing, predilatation should be performed with a suitable balloon. The balloon size should not exceed minimal annulus diameter. During full balloon inflation, contrast application via a pigtail catheter can help estimate suitable valve size, interaction with coronaries and probable PVL. In case of severe aortic regurgitation and hemodynamic instability, the valve prosthesis should be ready for insertion before the balloon procedure is completed. Next is valve insertion. Platform should advance, beware of aortic wall interaction. Because of high stent frames, future coronary interventions can be challenging in SEV. With the developing technology, commissural alignment can be achieved using different markers [37]. These markers are different for each valve platform. Fluoroscopic imaging should be followed from the groin to the aortic root. In severe tortuosity and calcific anatomy, detachment may occur in the capsule where the valve is loaded. In such a case, a stiffer wire should be used.

The angle in which the aortic cusps are in the same plane on fluoroscopic imaging is called the coplanar angle (golden angle). Nowadays, a new term is created called the 'Cusp overlap angle'. In this fluoroscopic image, the right and left cusps are superposed and the noncoronary cusp is separated. Compared to other angles, the cusp overlap angle shows more distance between basal annular plane and conduction system. Coplanar angle is the standard plane for many platforms. But SEV platforms use cusp overlap angle because of a high implantation plane for avoiding the need for a permanent pacemaker. According to the noncoronary cusp, >5 mm depth is related to the need for a permanent pacemaker and < 1 mm depth is related to migration. In these situations, SEV platforms allow resheathing.

At the end of the procedure after pulling back the platform, vascular closure is crucial. This is because access site complications are one of the most important mortality and morbidity causes during and postprocedure phase. Dedicated closure devices are used for these issues. But using these devices needs an expert. When closure is done, the patient is taken to the intensive care unit (ICU) for observation.

5. Summary and conclusions

Transcatheter aortic valve replacement (TAVR) is a minimally invasive treatment for those patients with severe aortic stenosis who cannot be treated surgically due to surgical risk. The first human experience was demonstrated in 2002 and after this date, it started to be performed all over the world. As the experience on this subject increases, TAVR has been brought to the agenda in patients with intermediate and low surgical risk, and studies on this subject are continuing. The procedure is generally performed by femoral approach. Different approaches (transapical, transaortic, subclavian/axillary, transcarotid, suprasternal and transcaval) can be used in patients who are not anatomically suitable for the femoral approach. Venous access was also obtained with two arterial access. A temporary pacemaker is placed via the venous route. Main arterial site is for delivery system and second site is for pigtail. Two types of valves can be used in the TAVR process: self-expandable (SE) and balloon-expandable (BE). In this chapter, we discuss valve types, which valve type will be preferred in which patient, the technical parts of different accesses and the specific complications of the procedures, and the points to be considered during the procedure.

Author details

Ali Yasar Kilinc[1]* and Mustafa Ucar[2]

1 Cardiology Department, Arnavutkoy State Hospital, İstanbul, Turkey

2 Cardiology Department, Celal Bayar University, Manisa, Turkey

*Address all correspondence to: aliyasar_kilinc@hotmail.com

IntechOpen

© 2023 The Author(s). Licensee IntechOpen. This chapter is distributed under the terms of the Creative Commons Attribution License (http://creativecommons.org/licenses/by/3.0), which permits unrestricted use, distribution, and reproduction in any medium, provided the original work is properly cited.

References

[1] Cribier A, Eltchaninoff H, Bash A, Borenstein N, Tron C, Bauer F, et al. Percutaneous transcatheter implantation of an aortic valve prosthesis for calcific aortic stenosis: First human case description. Circulation. 2002;**106**(24):3006-3008

[2] Petrou P. The economics of TAVI: A systematic review. International Journal of Cardiology. Heart & Vasculature. 2023;**44**:101173. DOI: 10.1016/j.ijcha.2023.101173

[3] Rotman OM, Bianchi M, Ghosh RP, Kovarovic B, Bluestein D. Principles of TAVR valve design, modelling, and testing. Expert Review of Medical Devices. 2018;**15**:771-791

[4] Hahn RT, Leipsic J, Douglas PS, Jaber WA, Weissman NJ, Pibarot P, et al. Comprehensive echocardiographic assessment of Normal transcatheter valve function. JACC: Cardiovascular Imaging. 2019;**12**:25-34

[5] Pellegrini C, Rheude T, Michel J, Alvarez-Covarrubias HA, Wünsch S, Mayr NP, et al. Comparison of latest generation supra-annular and intra-annular self-expanding transcatheter heart valves. Journal of Thoracic Disease. 2020;**12**:6769-6779

[6] Adams DH, Popma JJ, Reardon MJ, Yakubov SJ, Coselli JS, Deeb GM, et al. Transcatheter aortic-valve replacement with a self-expanding prosthesis. The New England Journal of Medicine. 2014;**370**:1790-1798

[7] Mieghem NMV, Nuis RJ, Piazza N, Apostolos T, Ligthart J, et al. Vascular complications with transcatheter aortic valve implantation using the 18 Fr Medtronic CoreValve system: The Rotterdam experience. EuroIntervention. 2010;**5**:673-679

[8] Van der Boon RM, Nuis R-J, Van Mieghem NM, Jordaens L, Rodés-Cabau J, van Domburg RT, et al. New conduction abnormalities after TAVI–frequency and Causes. Nature Reviews. Cardiology. 2012;**9**:454-463

[9] Sherif MA, Abdel-Wahab M, Stöcker B, Geist V, Richardt D, Tölg R, et al. Anatomic and procedural predictors of paravalvular aortic regurgitation after implantation of the Medtronic CoreValve bioprosthesis. Journal of the American College of Cardiology. 2010;**56**:1623-1629

[10] Eggebrecht H, Schmermund A, Voigtländer T, Kahlert P, Erbel R, Mehta RH. Risk of stroke after transcatheter aortic valve implantation (TAVI): A meta-analysis of 10,037 published patients. EuroIntervention. 2012;**8**:129-138

[11] Forrest JK, Mangi AA, Popma JJ, Khabbaz K, Reardon MJ, Kleiman NS, et al. Early outcomes with the Evolut PRO repositionable self-expanding transcatheter aortic valve with pericardial wrap. Journal of the American College of Cardiology. Cardiovascular Interventions. 2018;**11**:160-168

[12] Jilaihawi H, Zhao Z, Du R, Staniloae C, Saric M, Neuburger PJ, et al. Minimizing permanent pacemaker following repositionable self-expanding transcatheter aortic valve replacement. Journal of the American College of Cardiology. Cardiovascular Interventions. 2019;**12**:1796-1807

[13] Panagides V, Mesnier J, Nuche J, Delarochellière R, Paradis J-M,

Kalavrouziotis D, et al. From the Evolut pro to the Evolut FX self-expanding transcatheter aortic valve replacement systems: Current status and future perspectives. Expert Review of Medical Devices. 2022;**19**:561-569

[14] Willson AB, Rodès-Cabau J, Wood DA, Leipsic J, Cheung A, Toggweiler S, et al. Transcatheter aortic valve replacement with the St. Jude Medical Portico valve: First-in-human experience. Journal of the American College of Cardiology. 2012;**60**(7):581-586. DOI: 10.1016/j.jacc.2012.02.045

[15] Sgroi C, Tamburino CI, Patanè M. Transcatheter aortic valve implantation: Abbott portico. In: Tamburino C, Barbanti M, Capodanno D, editors. Percutaneous Treatment of Left Side Cardiac Valves. 3rd ed. Cham: Springer; 2018. pp. 431-442

[16] Navitor TM. TAvI system. In: Copyright © 2021 Abbott. Abbott Park, Illinois, U.S.A. Abbott data on file CL1014440. Available from: https://www.structuralheartsolutions.com/structural-heart-products-solutions/aortic-valve-navitor/clinical-data/ [Accessed: December 24, 2021]

[17] Hamm K, Reents W, Zacher M, Kerber S, Diegeler A, Schieffer B, et al. Transcatheter aortic valve implantation using the ACURATE TA and ACURATE neo valves: A four-year single-Centre experience. EuroIntervention. 2017;**13**(1):53-59. DOI: 10.4244/EIJ-D-16-00898

[18] Wolfrum M, Moccetti F, Piuhola J, Lehtola H, Baz JA, Iñiguez A, et al. The Allegra transcatheter heart valve: Short term results from a multi-center registry. Catheterization and Cardiovascular Interventions. 2021;**98**(6):1204-1209. DOI: 10.1002/ccd.29833

[19] Wenaweser P, Stortecky S, Schütz T, Praz F, Gloekler S, Windecker S, et al. Transcatheter aortic valve implantation with the NVT Allegra transcatheter heart valve system: First-in-human experience with a novel self-expanding transcatheter heart valve. EuroIntervention. 2016;**12**(1):71-77. DOI: 10.4244/EIJv12I1A13

[20] Schäfer U, Kempfert J, Verheye S, Maisano F, Thiele H, Landt M, et al. Safety and performance outcomes of a self-expanding transcatheter aortic heart valve: The BIovALvE Trials. JACC. Cardiovascular Interventions. 2020;**13**(2):157-166. DOI: 10.1016/j.jcin.2019.07.058

[21] Herrmann HC, Thourani VH, Kodali SK, Makkar RR, Szeto WY, Anwaruddin S, et al. One-year clinical outcomes with SAPIEN 3 transcatheter aortic valve replacement in high-risk and inoperable patients with severe aortic stenosis. Circulation. 2016;**134**:130-140

[22] Barbanti M, Costa G. SAPIEN 3 ultra transcatheter aortic valve device. Journal of the American College of Cardiology. Cardiovascular Interventions. 2020;**13**:2639-2641

[23] Kawashima H, Soliman O, Wang R, Ono M, Hara H, Gao C, et al. Rationale and design of a randomized clinical trial comparing safety and efficacy of Myval transcatheter heart valve versus contemporary transcatheter heart valves in patients with severe symptomatic aortic valve stenosis: The LANDMARK trial. American Heart Journal. 2021;**232**:23-38

[24] Ribeiro HB, Urena M, Allende R, Amat-Santos IJ, Rodés-Cabau J. Balloon-expandable prostheses for transcatheter aortic valve replacement. Progress in Cardiovascular Diseases. 2014;**56**(6):583-595. DOI: 10.1016/j.pcad.2014.02.001

[25] Vahania A, Beyersdorf F, Praz F, Milojevic M, Baldus S, et al. 2021 ESC/EACTS guidelines for the management of valvular heart disease. European Heart Journal. 2022;**43**(7):561-632

[26] 2020 ACC/AHA Guideline for the Management of Patients With Valvular Heart Disease. Journal of the American College of Cardiology. 2021;**77**(4):e25-e197. DOI: 10.1016/j.jacc.2020.11.018

[27] Auffret V, Lefevre T, Van Belle E, Eltchaninoff H, Iung B, Koning R, et al. FRANCE TAVı ınvestigators. Temporal trends in transcatheter aortic valve replacement in FRANCE: FRANCE 2 to FRANCE TAVı. Journal of the American College of Cardiology. 2017;**70**(1):42-55. DOI: 10.1016/j.jacc.2017.04.053

[28] Ye J, Cheung A, Lichtenstein S, et al. Transapical aortic valve implantation in humans. The Journal of Thoracic and Cardiovascular Surgery. 2006;**131**:1194-1196

[29] Schafer U, Deuschl F, Schofer N, et al. Safety and efficacy of the percutaneous transaxillary access for transcatheter aortic valve implantation using various transcatheter heart valves in 100 consecutive patients. International Journal of Cardiology. 2017;**232**:247-254

[30] Bruschi G, Fratto P, de Marco F, et al. The transsubclavian retrograde approach for transcatheter aortic valve replacement: Single-center experience. The Journal of Thoracic and Cardiovascular Surgery. 2010;**140**:911-915

[31] Overtchouk P, Modine T. Alternate access for TAVı: Stay clear of the chest. Interventional Cardiology. 2018;**13**(3):145-150. DOI: 10.15420/icr.2018.22.1

[32] Modine T, Lemesle G, Azzaoui R, et al. Aortic valve implantation with the CoreValve ReValving System via left carotid artery access: First case report. The Journal of Thoracic and Cardiovascular Surgery. 2010;**140**:928-929

[33] Villecourt A, Faroux L, Muneaux A, et al. Comparison of clinical outcomes after transcarotid and transsubclavian versus transfemoral transcatheter aortic valve implantation: A propensity-matched analysis. Archives of Cardiovascular Diseases. 2020;**113**:189-198

[34] Kiser AC, O'Neill WW, de Marchena E, et al. Suprasternal direct aortic approach transcatheter aortic valve replacement avoids sternotomy and thoracotomy: First-in-man experience. European Journal of Cardio-Thoracic Surgery. 2015;**48**:778-783

[35] Eudailey KW, Olds A, Lewis CT, et al. Contemporary suprasternal transcatheter aortic valve replacement: A multicenter experience using a simple, reliable alternative access approach. Catheterization and Cardiovascular Interventions. 2020;**95**:1178-1183

[36] Greenbaum AB, O'Neill WW, Paone G, Guerrero ME, Wyman JF, Rl C, et al. Caval-aortic access to allow transcatheter aortic valve replacement in otherwise ineligible patients: Initial human experience. Journal of the American College of Cardiology. 2014;**63**(25 pt A):2795-2804. DOI: 10.1016/j.jacc.2014.04.015

[37] Buono A, Morello A, Pero G, Corcione N, Bettari L, Saccocci M, et al. Commissural alignment with new-generation self-expanding transcatheter heart valves during aortic replacement. Cardiovascular Revascularization Medicine. 2021;**S1553-8389**(21):00563-00567. DOI: 10.1016/j.car-rev. 2021.07.027

Section 4

Management of Aortic Stenosis

Chapter 5

Perspective Chapter: Transcatheter Interventions in the Management of Aortic Valve Stenosis

P. Syamasundar Rao

Abstract

Transcatheter interventions that are useful in the management of valvar aortic stenosis will be reviewed. This chapter focuses on congenital aortic valve stenosis. The procedure of balloon aortic valvuloplasty (BAV) and the results were reviewed; BAV offers good relief of aortic valve obstruction and serves as substitute to surgery and is considered a favored option in the management of aortic stenosis in all age groups. However, BAV in elderly patients with calcific aortic stenosis offers only a temporary relief of aortic valve obstruction and BAV is not recommended for this subgroup of patients. Except for neonates, most patients are discharged home within 24-hours after BAV. While there is conclusive data for provision of pressure gradient relief both acutely and at follow-up as well as deferral of any surgery after BAV, the development of aortic insufficiency (AI) at long-term follow-up is a most important drawback. In neonates, severe AI may develop necessitating surgical intervention. Notwithstanding these drawbacks, BAV is presently believed to be a therapeutic procedure of option in the treatment of valvar aortic stenosis in pediatric and young adult patients. Methodical follow-up to identify reappearance of aortic obstruction and development of substantial AI is suggested.

Keywords: aortic stenosis, balloon aortic valvuloplasty, aortic insufficiency, aortic valve re-stenosis, long-term results

1. Introduction

The author (PSR) has had interest in the diagnosis and management of aortic stenosis over the years and contributed several original papers, editorials, reviews, letters to the editor, and book chapters [1–29] on this subject. The purpose of this chapter is to provide an updated review of transcatheter management of congenital aortic valve stenosis.

Aortic stenosis (AS) is a relatively common congenital heart defect (CHD); mostly seen as an isolated defect though it may be found along with other CHDs such as Shone's syndrome and aortic coarctation. The incidence of valvar AS is 5–6% of all CHDs. Its occurrence is more frequent in males than in females. The pathology of AS varies from one patient to the next; commissural fusion of bicuspid aortic valve leaflets is the most common pathology. Fusion of tricuspid aortic valve leaflets resulting in AS is seen less frequently. Aortic valve with a single cusp (unicuspid) is observed mostly in the

IntechOpen

newborn with critical obstruction. Quadricuspid aortic valve is extremely rare. There is concentric hypertrophy of the left ventricle (LV); this is proportional to the degree of obstruction caused by fusion of the aortic valve leaflets. Dilatation of the ascending aorta is also seen; however, the extent of aortic dilatation is independent of the degree of aortic valve obstruction [5, 6, 30, 31]. Clinical features and diagnostic studies used in the assessment of the degree of aortic valve stenosis were previously reviewed elsewhere [5, 14, 16, 19, 22, 27, 30, 31] and will not be discussed in this chapter.

Initially, surgical methodologies were utilized to provide relief of aortic valve obstruction; these include, commissurotomy of the fused aortic valve leaflets via aortotomy [32], plastic repair of aortic valve (neocuspidization) with or without the use of prosthetic material [33–36], and aortic valve replacement with mechanical [37, 38], bioprosthetic [39, 40] or patient's own pulmonary valve (Ross procedure) [41, 42], all procedures performed under cardio-pulmonary bypass. Following the use by Kan and her associates of the techniques of Dotter [43] and Gruntzig [44] to open the pulmonary valve [45], Lababidi et al. [46, 47] employed this technique to open the aortic valve. Subsequently, balloon aortic valvuloplasty has become first-line therapy to address AS at most institutions [5, 10, 21, 22]. In this chapter, catheter interventional procedures used in the management of congenital aortic valve stenosis will be reviewed.

2. Indications for balloon aortic valvuloplasty

The indication for transcatheter intervention including AS should be similar to that utilized for surgical therapy. Indications for intervention are largely based on the degree of aortic valve obstruction, as assessed by pressure gradients across the aortic valve immediately preceding balloon aortic valvuloplasty (BAV). A peak-to-peak systolic pressure gradient across the aortic valve greater than 50 mmHg with either symptomatology or ST-T wave changes in the electrocardiogram (ECG) indicative of myocardial ischemia or a peak-to-peak systolic pressure gradient of more than 70 mmHg regardless of symptomatology or ECG abnormalities [2, 5, 7, 10] are indications for BAV. While these criteria are generally agreed upon, it should be noted that catheter interventions in children are commonly performed under general anesthesia at most institutions at the present time and therefore, the trans valvar gradient measurement secured under conscious sedation protocol are not applicable. Consequently, pre-procedure trans valvar gradients measured by Doppler technique are used for determining criteria for BAV. The same 50/70 mmHg gradient criteria alluded to above may be used, but one must ensure that: (1) Doppler recordings from multiple sites in a calm, resting patient should be secured; and (2) correction for pressure recovery phenomenon [27] should be applied.

In neonates with severe/critical AS, the pressure gradients across the aortic valve may not be high if left ventricular function is poor and therefore, the pressure gradient criteria set forth above are not applicable. If clinical signs of congestive heart failure (CHF) are detected; ductal-dependent systemic circulation, requiring administration of prostaglandin E_1 (PGE_1) is present; or poor left ventricular function on echocardiogram is recorded; the described gradient criteria are not necessary for going ahead with BAV [18, 24].

Adolescent and adult AS patients with the above-described trans valvar pressure gradient criteria should also undergo BAV. Because of the enthusiasm expressed by several centers for transcatheter aortic valve replacement (TAVR) [48–50], it should be pointed out that the TAVR should only be used for calcific AS in the elderly patients and the non-calcific AS in adolescents and adults should be treated with the less aggressive BAV [25].

Patients with recurrent AS following prior BAV or surgical aortic valvotomy are also candidates for BAV subject to meeting pressure gradient criteria listed above. Trivial or mild aortic insufficiency (AI) is not a contraindication, but moderate to severe AI is a contraindication for BAV because of the concern for further increasing AI [3, 5, 10, 22].

3. Technique of balloon aortic valvuloplasty

The most commonly used method of accomplishing BAV is percutaneous femoral arterial route for most children, adolescents and adults and will be described first. Then, other methods used in different age groups will be reviewed.

Cardiac catheterization is performed to confirm clinical and echocardiographic diagnosis of AS after obtaining informed consent as per institutional norms. Most pediatric interventions are performed under general anesthesia at the present time while conscious sedation is used in adult subjects. After securing venous and arterial access, 100 units/kg of heparin (maximum 3000 units) is intravenously administered and activated clotting times checked periodically and kept above 200 s by administering additional doses of heparin as needed.

A #4- to #7-F multipurpose or right coronary artery catheter is positioned in the ascending aorta and advanced into the left ventricle (LV) via the stenotic aortic valve with the assistance of a floppy-tipped coronary guide wire (in infants), a 0.035-inch straight Benston guide wire (Cook) or a similar guide wire. Other types of catheters and guide wires may be utilized, at the discretion of the cardiologist if there is difficulty in crossing the aortic valve. Peak to peak systolic pressure gradient is recorded by pressure pullback across the aortic valve (**Figures 1** and **2**). If possible, concurrent pressures recording from both the LV and aorta are also documented (**Figure 3**). But, if there is

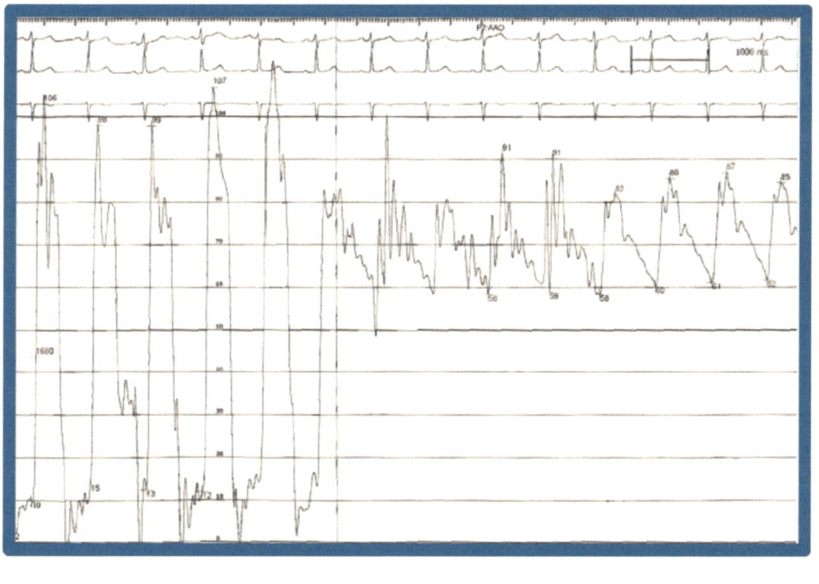

Figure 1.
Pressure pullback tracing from the left ventricle (LV) to the aorta (Ao) demonstrating a peak-to-peak gradient of 21 mmHg across the aortic valve; this would suggest that the aortic stenosis is mild, provided the cardiac index is within normal range. (Reproduced from reference [22]).

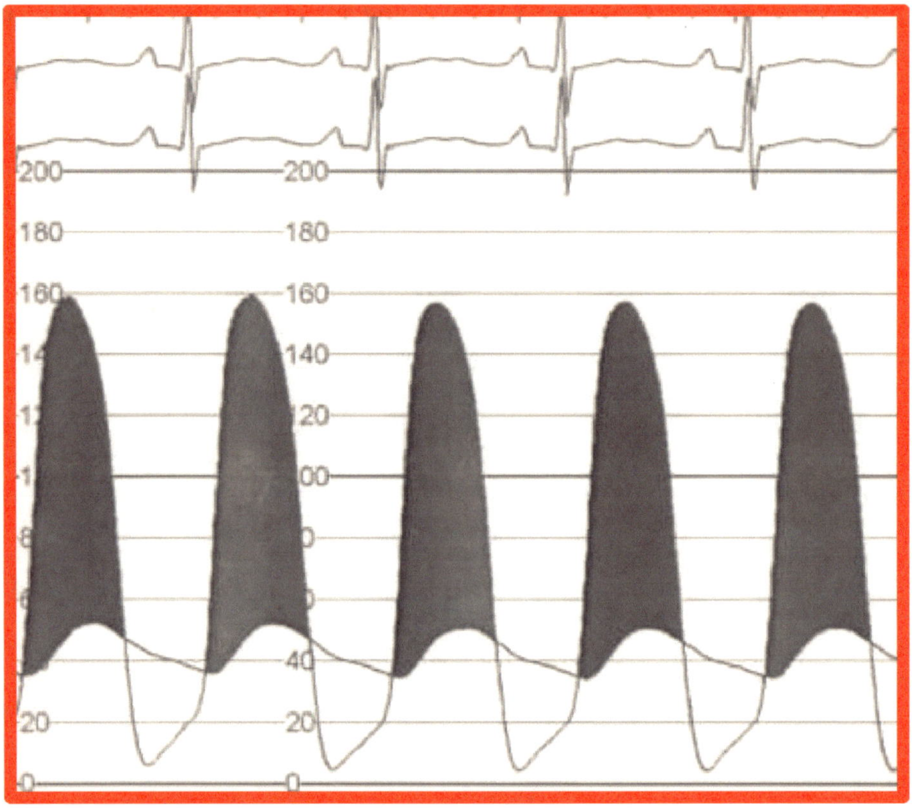

Figure 2.
Simultaneous pressure recordings from the left ventricle (LV) and the aorta (Ao) demonstrating a peak-to-peak gradient of 110 mmHg across the aortic valve suggesting that the aortic stenosis is very severe. (Reproduced from reference [22]).

significant difficulty in crossing the aortic valve, no pressure pullback should be made; in its place, prior recording of the aortic pressure is utilized to calculate the peak-to-peak systolic pressure gradient across the aortic valve (**Figure 3**).

Angiograms from the aorta and LV (**Figure 4**) are secured and the diagnosis is confirmed. Most common cine-angiographic projections used are left anterior oblique and right anterior oblique; these views are likely to highlight the features of AS and associated subvalvar and supravalvar anomalies.

Once the diagnostic data confirm the indications for BAV, an extra-stiff J-tipped Amplatz guide wire (Cook, Bloomington, IN) or an apex guide wire (Cook) in older children and adults is placed in the LV apex, via the catheter already in place. A balloon valvuloplasty catheter with a balloon diameter that is 80–100% of the annulus of the aortic valve is threaded over the guidewire already in place. The balloon diameter should not go above the annulus of the aortic valve. The aortic valve annulus measurements secured by the echocardiogram prior to the procedure and by the left ventricular angiogram during the procedure are used for the purpose balloon diameter selection. The length of the balloon to be used is largely based on the age and size of the patient. In young babies and neonates, a 2 cm long balloon is used. In older infants and young children, a 3 cm long balloon is preferred. In older children, adolescents and adults, a 4–5.5 cm long balloon is selected. Balloon inflation (**Figure 5**) with diluted contrast

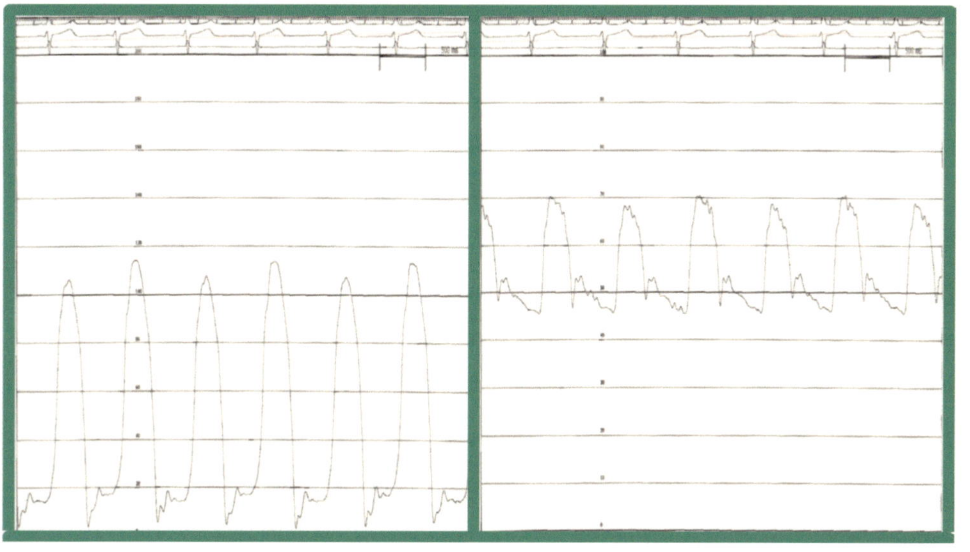

Figure 3.
Left ventricular (LV) and ascending aortic (AAo) pressures recorded separately showing a peak-to-peak gradient of 55 mmHg across the aortic valve. Pressure pullback was not recorded because of the difficulty in crossing the aortic valve initially. (Reproduced from reference [22]).

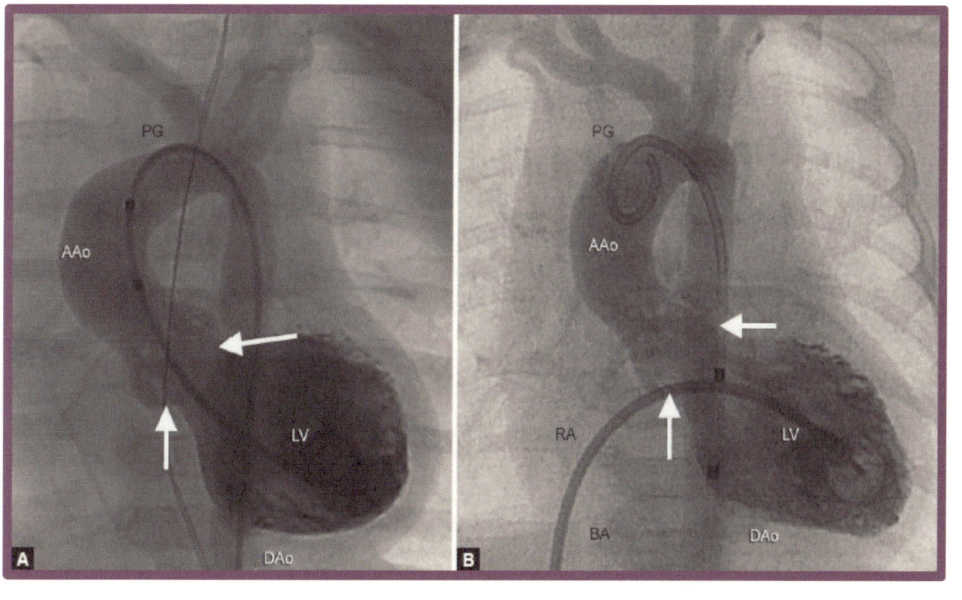

Figure 4.
Selected cine frames from left ventricular (LV) cine angiograms in posterior-anterior view in two neonates with severe aortic stenosis: (A) a pigtail (PG) catheter was introduced into the LV retrogradely; (B) a Berman angiographic (BA) catheter was advanced from the right atrium (RA), across a patent foramen ovale (not marked) into the left atrium (not marked) and from there into the LV. These angiograms demonstrate the aortic valve annulus (arrows in A and B). Note the domed and thickened aortic valve leaflets. (Reproduced from reference [24]).

material (1 in 4) to a pressure not to exceed the burst pressure quoted by the manufacturer of the balloon catheter is undertaken. The landmarks of the scout film (**Figure 4**) at the same camera angulations are used during balloon inflation. I usually perform two to three more balloon inflations, each for a duration of 5 s, 5 minutes in-between.

If the aortic valve annulus is too big to dilate with a single balloon, a double-balloon method may be used. In this procedure, two balloon catheters are concurrently positioned across the aortic valve (**Figures 6** and 7). The effective balloon diameter may be computed by using the formula shown below [51]; this also should not go above the diameter of the aortic valve annulus.

$$\frac{D_1 + D_2 + \pi\left(\frac{D_1}{2} + \frac{D_2}{2}\right)}{\pi} \tag{1}$$

Where D_1 and D_2 indicate diameters of the balloons utilized.

This formulation was made simpler by Narang et al. [52]: Effective balloon diameter = $0.82\ (D_1 + D_2)$.

A propensity to eject the dilating balloon while inflating the balloon exists. Consequently, we utilize stiff guidewires and long balloons. Other interventionists recommend adenosine-induced transient cardiac standstill [53] or fast right ventricular pacing [54] to attain steady position of the balloon while performing BAV. In the author's

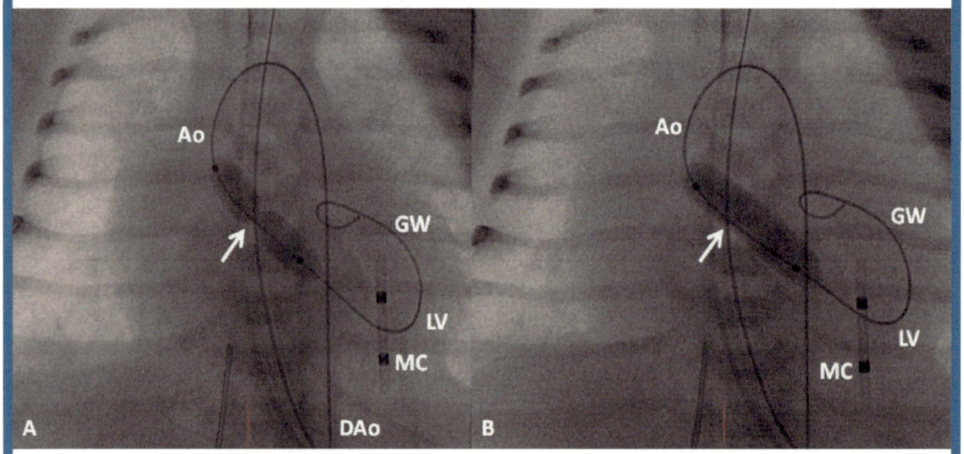

Figure 5.
Selected cine frames in posterior-anterior projections illustrating a balloon dilatation catheter across the stenosed aortic valve. Waisting of the balloon (arrow) was seen during the early phases of inflation of the balloon (A) which was completely abolished on further inflation of the balloon (B). Ao, aorta; DAo, descending aorta; GW, guide wire; LV, left ventricle; MC, marker catheter. (Reproduced from reference [22]).

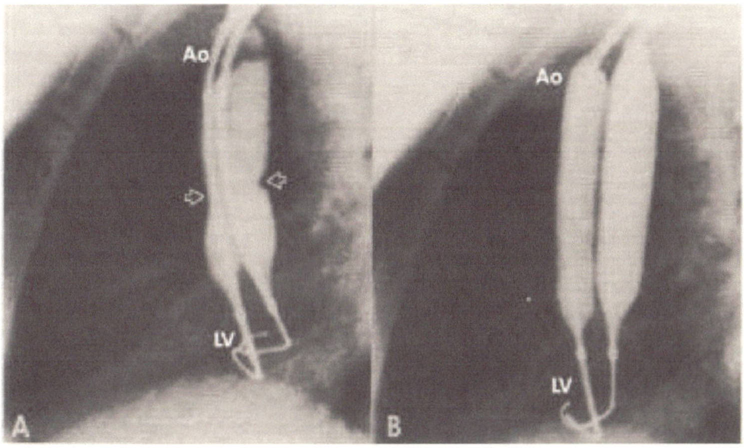

Figure 6.
Selected cineradiographic frames in straight lateral projection demonstrating two balloons placed across the aortic valve; the balloons were positioned retrogradely via both the femoral arteries. Balloon waisting (arrows) during the initial phases of balloon inflation (A) was completely abolished on further inflation of the balloons (B). Ao; aorta; LV, left ventricle. (Reproduced from reference [5]).

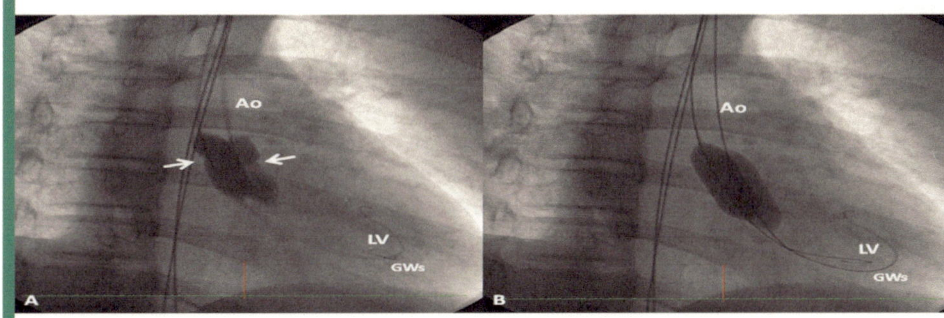

Figure 7.
Selected cineradiographic frames in right anterior oblique projection demonstrating two balloons placed across the aortic valve; the balloons were positioned retrogradely via both the femoral arteries. Balloon waisting (arrows) during the initial phases of balloon inflation (A) was completely abolished on further inflation of the balloons (B). Ao; aorta; GWs, guide wires; LV, left ventricle. (Reproduced from reference [22]).

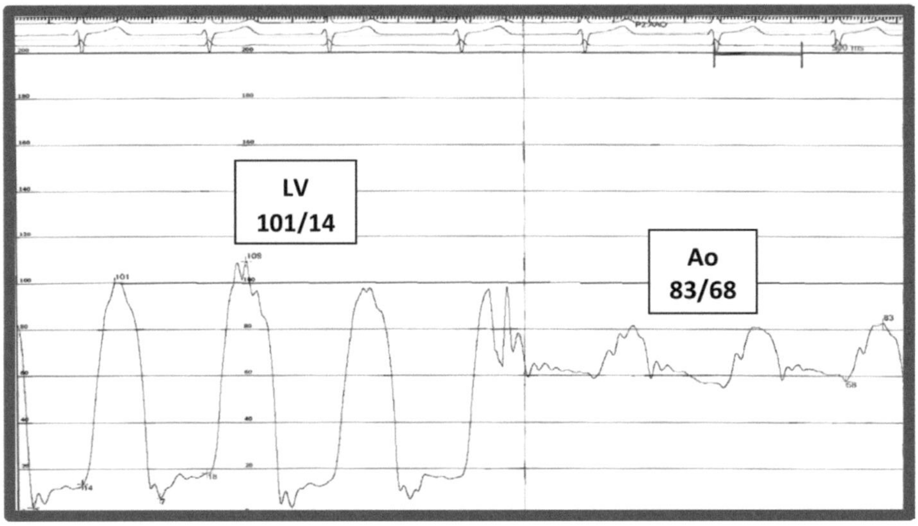

Figure 8.
Pressure pullback tracing across the aortic valve following balloon aortic valvuloplasty, demonstrating a residual peak-to-peak gradient of 18 mmHg, indicating good result of the procedure. Ao, aorta; LV, left ventricle. (Reproduced from reference [22]).

personal experience, use of stiff guide wires and long balloons was found to be satisfactory [1, 3, 5, 7, 10] to successfully accomplish BAV. Nucleus balloons (NuMed) with a "barbell" configuration and hourglass shaped V8 aortic valvuloplasty balloons (Venus Medtech) have a theoretical advantage of keeping the balloon within the aortic valve [29]. While this seems attractive, the bulky nature of these balloon catheters is problematic.

Following the completion of BAV, pressure pullback recording across the aortic valve (**Figure 8**) is performed and angiograms from the LV and/or aortic root are secured 15 minutes following BAV. The catheters and sheaths are withdrawn, and the procedure concluded. Vascular occlusion devices such as Angio-Seal (St Jude Medical) and others occlusion systems [55, 56] may be used if large balloon catheters are utilized for BAV.

3.1 Balloon aortic valvuloplasty in neonates

Neonatal BAV may be undertaken in a manner similar to that described above [5, 57–60]. However, injury to the femoral artery [8, 61] is of concern. Consequently, other routes of access, namely, subscapular [62], axillary [63], carotid [64], and umbilical [65] arterial, anterograde femoral venous [66, 67], and umbilical venous [9, 15] routes have been tried. Because of limitations of space, these will not be reviewed in this chapter. The interested reader may find the discussion of these procedures elsewhere [17, 18, 24, 29].

4. Immediate results

Immediate reduction in the peak-to-peak systolic pressure gradients across the aortic valve (**Figures 8–11**) along with a decrease in the LV peak systolic and end diastolic pressures with no substantial change in cardiac index occurred. There is

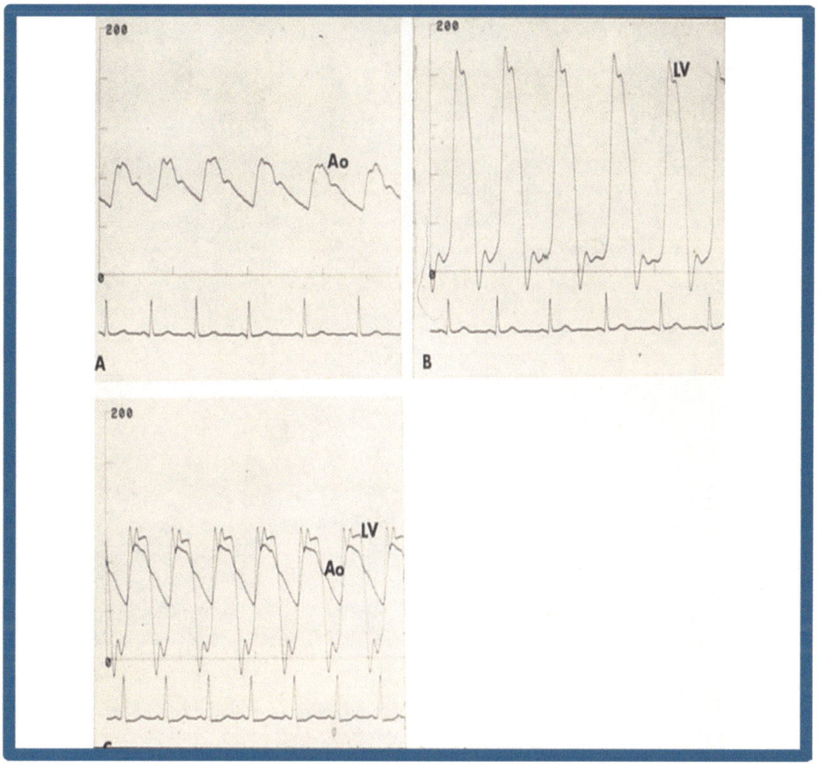

Figure 9.
Aortic (Ao) and left ventricular (LV) pressure tracings prior to (A and B) and 15 minutes following (C) balloon aortic valvuloplasty demonstrating almost complete abolition of the peak-to-peak pressure gradient across the aortic valve. (Reproduced from reference [5]).

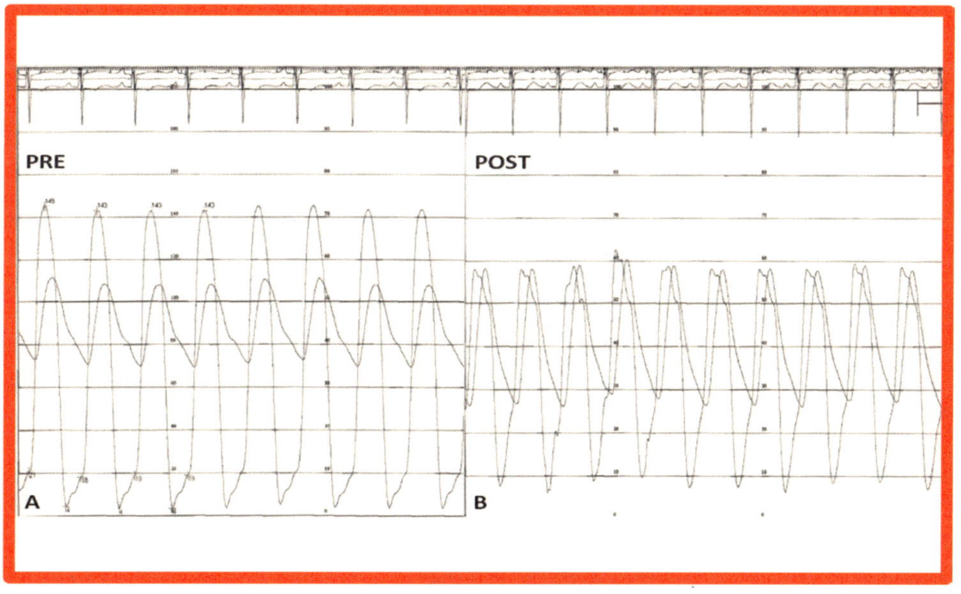

Figure 10.
Simultaneous pressure recordings from the left ventricle and aorta prior to (PRE—A) and 15 minutes following (POST—B) balloon aortic valvuloplasty demonstrating no residual gradient. There is a slight decrease in aortic diastolic pressure (B) suggesting aortic insufficiency. (Reproduced from reference [22]).

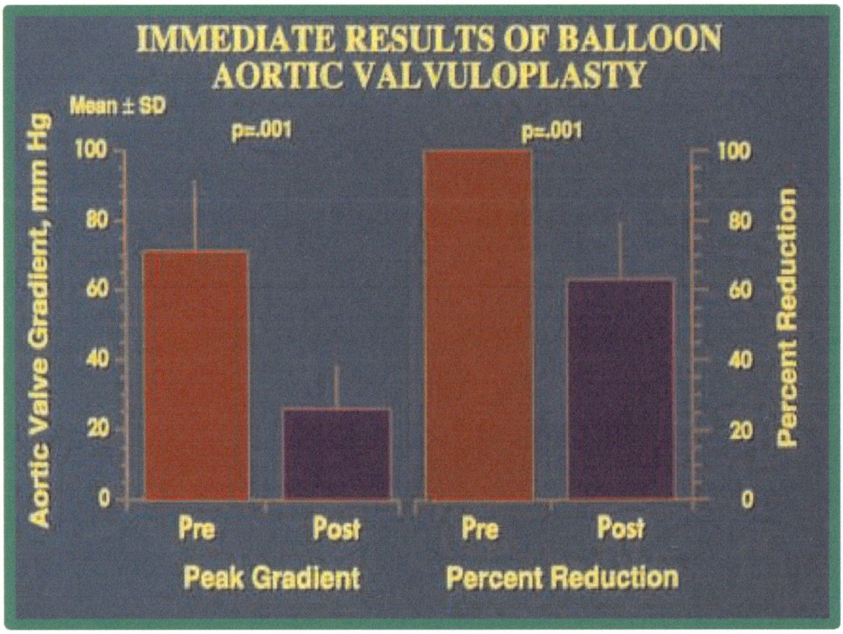

Figure 11.
Bar graph illustrating immediate results of balloon aortic valvuloplasty for aortic valve stenosis. Significant (p = 0.001) decrease in the peak-to-peak systolic pressure gradients (left panel) and percent reduction (right panel) were shown. Mean + standard deviation (SD) is marked. Pre, prior to; post, following balloon aortic valvuloplasty. (Reproduced from reference [22]).

nearly 60% decline in the systolic gradient when compared to the pre-valvuloplasty values (**Figure 11**).

The extent of AI did not worsen (**Figure 12**; pre vs. post) and there were no patients exhibiting grade 3+ AI. Actually, some improvement of aortic insufficiency was noticed in some patients which suggests restored coaptation of the aortic valve leaflets following BAV. Except for neonates, nearly all patients were sent home within 24 hours of BAV.

Lababidi et al. [47] were the first to document results of BAV in children; they reported the results of 23 consecutive patients with valvar AS. In this series, the peak-to-peak systolic pressure gradient through the aortic valve was reduced from 113 ± 48 to 32 ± 15 mmHg ($p < 0.001$) following BAV. Mild aortic regurgitation was seen in 10 (43%) patients. Two children needed surgical repair. The author of this chapter presented immediate results of BAV in 16 patients in the late-1980s [1, 3]; the results of larger number of patients (N = 26) became available [5, 7] subsequently. In the initial 16 children, decrease of peak-to-peak systolic pressure gradient through the aortic valve from 72 ± 21 to 28 ± 13 mmHg ($p < 0.001$) occurred (**Figures 8–11**). Similarly, LV peak systolic pressures decreased from 162 ± 21 to 124 ± 18 mmHg ($p < 0.001$) and LV end-diastolic pressures were reduced from 13 ± 5 to 9 ± 6 mmHg ($p < 0.01$). There was no significant change in cardiac index (3.4 ± 0.5 vs. 3.4 ± 0.4 liters/min/meter^2; $p > 0.1$) [1]. Generally, the gradients decreased by 60% of pre-valvuloplasty values (**Figure 11**). Similar reduction in peak-to-peak systolic pressure gradients across the aortic were observed in larger cohort (**Figure 13**) [7].

In the second cohort comprising of 26 children [7], the immediate outcome was like that observed by other workers, as tabulated elsewhere (Table I of reference [5]).

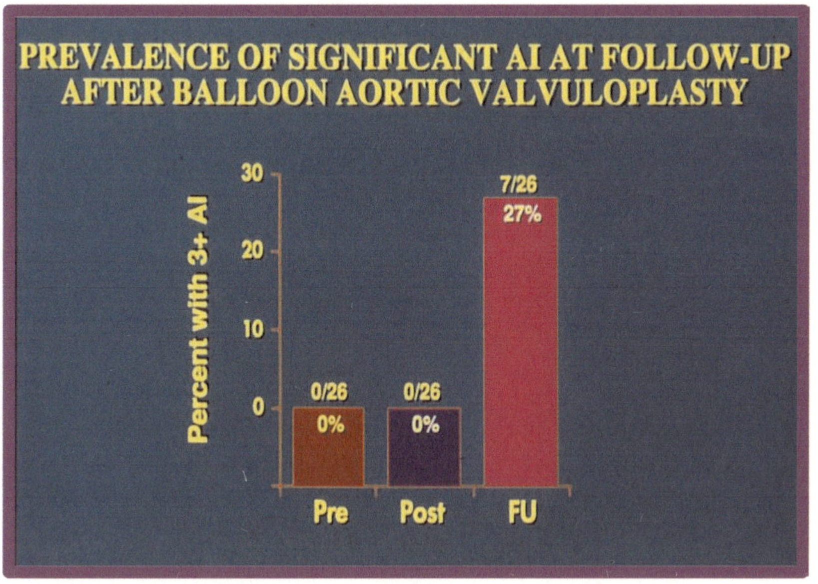

Figure 12.
Bar graph demonstrating the prevalence of grade III aortic insufficiency prior to (pre), immediately following (post) balloon aortic valvuloplasty and at late follow-up (FU). No change in aortic insufficiency is seen immediately after balloon valvuloplasty. However, significant increase occurred at late follow-up. (Modified from reference [10]).

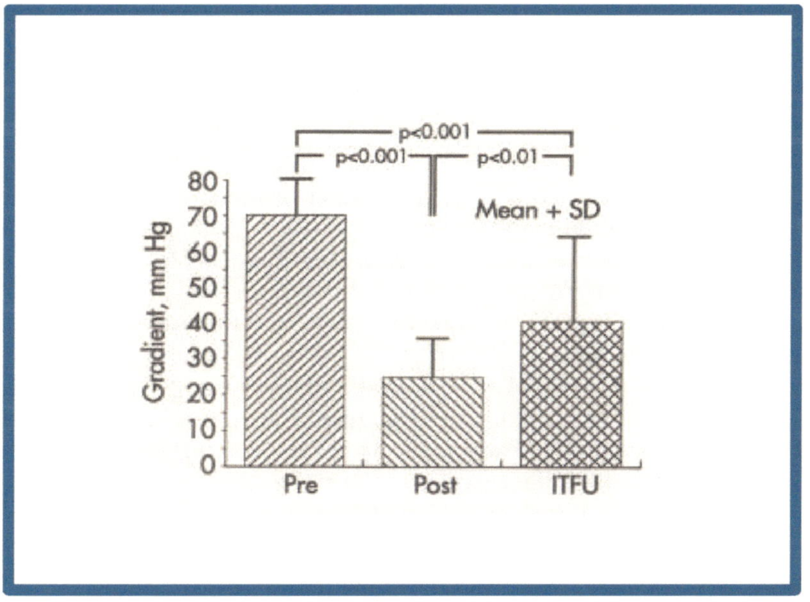

Figure 13.
Bar graph demonstrating immediate and follow-up results after balloon aortic valvuloplasty. Note significant ($p < 0.001$) decrease in peak-to-peak systolic pressure gradients across the aortic valve after balloon valvuloplasty (pre, before vs. post, immediately after). Gradient measured during repeat catheterization in 15 patients increased ($p < 0.01$) at intermediate-term follow-up (ITFU) of mean of 16 months. (Reproduced from reference [7]).

The occurrence of substantial (3+ or more) AI did not happen for the entire group (**Figure 12**). Echocardiographic studies revealed no change in the 1. LV end-diastolic dimension (36 ± 9 vs. 35 ± 10 mm; $p > 0.1$), 2. LV posterior wall thickness in diastole

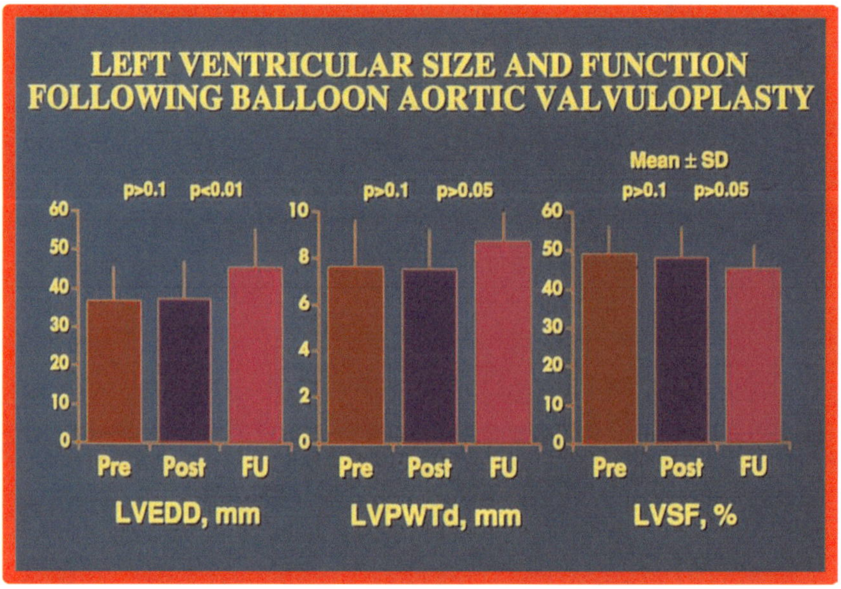

Figure 14.
Bar graph demonstrating left ventricular (LV) end-diastolic dimension (EDD) in mm (left panel), LV posterior wall thickness in diastole (PWTd) in mm (middle panel) and LV shortening fraction (SF) in % (right panel) prior to (pre), on the day after (post) balloon aortic valvuloplasty, and at late follow-up (FU). Mean + standard deviations (SD) are marked. Note that LVEDD, LVPWTd, and LVSF did not change ($p > 0.1$) immediately after balloon aortic valvuloplasty. At late follow-up the LVEDD increased ($p < 0.001$) while the LVPWTd and LVSF remain unchanged ($p > 0.05$). (Reproduced from reference [29]).

(7.2 ± 2.1 vs. 7.5 ± 1.9 mm; $p > 0.1$), and 3. LV fractional shortening (50 ± 8 vs. 47 ± 8%; $p > 0.1$) following BAV (**Figure 14**). But the Doppler flow velocity magnitudes across the aortic valve (4.0 ± 0.05 vs. 3.0 ± 0.8 m/s; $p < 0.001$) diminished as were the peak instantaneous Doppler gradients (**Figure 15**). No child from our study subjects required immediate surgical therapy. Immediate results after BAV documented during the decade of 1983–1992 were tabulated (Table I) in our book [5] for the interested reader. In the ensuing three decades, several interventionalists, too numerous to list, have reported their results of BAV and these are generally similar to those of the first three cohorts described above. However, more recent multi-institutional studies are worthy of review: In the first of these [68], results of BAV in 373 patients from 22 US institutions were examined. Success, defined as residual peak-to peak systolic pressure gradient across the aortic valve ≤35 mmHg and no greater than mild AI, was achieved in 71% patients. Adverse events were seen in 20% of patients. In the second study comprising of 1026 patients from the IMPACT (Improving Pediatric and Adult Congenital Treatments) Registry [69], procedural success was achieved in 71% of non-critical patients and 63% of critical AS patients.

5. Short-term follow-up results

At short-term follow up, defined as ≤2 years, peak-to-peak systolic pressure gradients across the aortic valve by cardiac catheterization (**Figure 13**) as well as by Doppler-calculated peak instantaneous gradients (**Figure 15**) either were unchanged or slightly increased when compared to acute results. These gradients continue to be pointedly

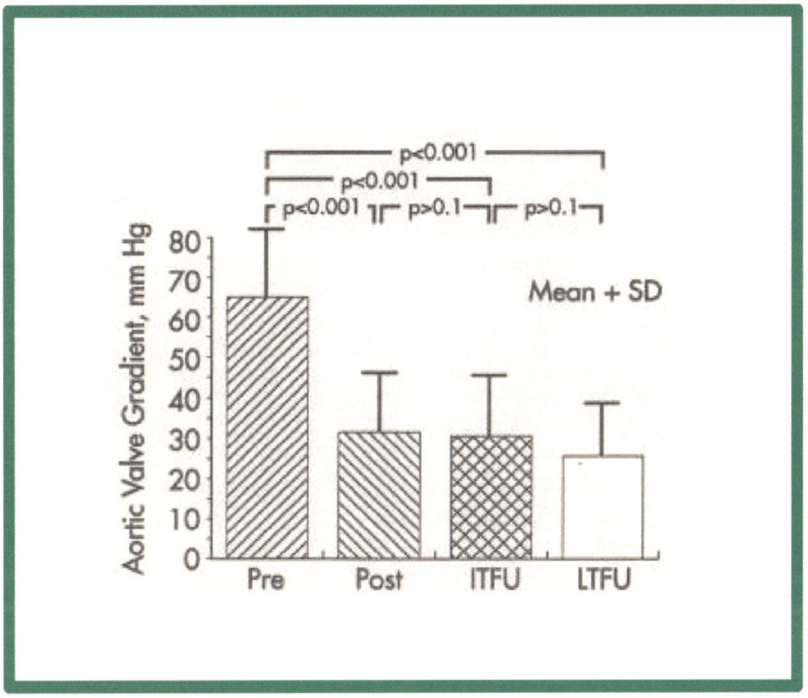

Figure 15.
Bar graph showing maximal peak instantaneous Doppler gradients before (pre) and 1 day after (post) balloon aortic valvuloplasty and at intermediate term (ITFU) and late (LTFU) follow-up. There was significant reduction ($p < 0.001$) in the gradient after balloon aortic valvuloplasty which remained essentially unchanged ($p > 0.1$) at ITFU (12 ± 5 months) and at LTFU (3–9 years [mean 6 years]). Doppler-derived maximal peak instantaneous gradients at follow-up continued to be lower ($p < 0.001$) than pre-valvuloplasty gradients. (Reproduced from reference [7]).

lower than pre-BAV values [7]. Aortic valve gradients measured by Doppler in 26 patients at a follow-up of 16 ± 11 months past BAV were 31 ± 15 mmHg. These data were similar ($p > 0.1$) to gradients recorded immediately following BAV and remain lower ($p < 0.001$) than pre-BAV gradients (**Figure 15**). Nevertheless, when the residual gradient of each patient was assessed, restenosis characterized as a peak gradient of more than 50 mmHg was noticed in 6 (23%) children (**Figure 16**). Early in our experience, four of these children had aortic valvotomy by surgery and two had repeat BAV at a median period of 9 months after the initial BAV. The extent of AI stayed steady at short-term follow-up [7]. Short-term follow up results described by other researchers were comparable to those of ours as tabulated (Table II) in our book [5].

5.1 Restenosis and predictors of restenosis

As pointed out in the previous segment, restenosis after BAV seems to occur (**Figure 16**). The reason why restenosis happens following BAV was examined by analyzing the follow-up outcomes of 16 children [1]. Based on the short-term follow-up results, the 16 patients were split into two groups: Group I who had good results (N = 12) with aortic valve peak gradients less than 50 mmHg at follow-up and Group II who had poor results (N = 4) with peak gradients more than 50 mmHg. In Group I patients, the peak pressure gradient across the aortic valve was reduced from 70 ± 21

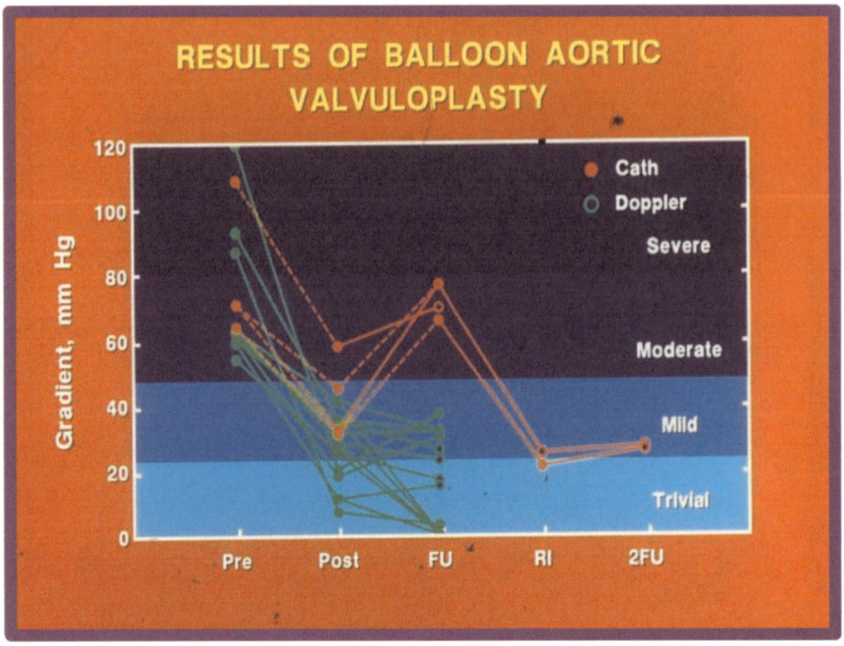

Figure 16.
Line graph showing aortic valve peak to peak systolic pressure gradients prior to (pre), immediately following (post) and at follow-up (FU) after balloon aortic valvuloplasty. Patients with good results are shown in green while those with poor results are shown in orange. Re-intervention (RI) (balloon valvuloplasty) was performed in some patients and the gradients fell. On further follow-up (2FU), the residual gradients remained low. When severity of the gradients was examined, the severity grade of the stenosis decreased in all patients going from severe to moderate, mild, or trivial and from moderate to mild or trivial. (Reproduced from reference [29]).

to 24 ± 11 mmHg ($p < 0.001$) at the time of BAV, which stayed unaltered (26 ± 10 mmHg; $p > 0.1$) at short-term follow-up (**Figure 17**, left panel). No child in this group needed re-intervention. In Group II patients, the aortic valve peak gradient was reduced (79 ± 20 mmHg vs. 42 ± 13 mmHg; $p < 0.001$) following BAV. Nevertheless, at short-term re-evaluation, the residual peak gradient increased substantially to 73 ± 5 mmHg ($p < 0.001$) (**Figure 17**, right panel). All four children underwent successful re-intervention, two by surgical valvotomy and two by repeat BAV [1].

Seventeen different variables (Tables I, II, and III of reference [1]) were scrutinized by multivariate stepwise logistic regression testing, as detailed earlier [1, 70, 71] to detect factors that can prognosticate recurrence in Group II subjects. This assessment detected age less than 3 years at the time of BAV and immediate post-BAV peak-to-peak gradient across the aortic valve ≥30 mmHg as prognosticators of recurrent obstruction [1]. In a later study [7, 10], while examining the long-term results of 26 children, the risk factors for recurrence at short-term re-evaluation were precisely identical to those observed in our first report [1]. Furthermore, this analysis [7, 10] indicated that the greater the number of risk factors, the higher the likelihood for restenosis (**Figure 18**).

Sholler et al. [72] studied the impact of different technological and morphologic issues on the acute outcomes of BAV. However, they were unable to demonstrate any statistically significant role of any factors examined. Other researchers, as reviewed previously [7, 10, 22], explored reasons of reappearance of aortic valve obstruction following BAV; however, they could not discern any factors causing recurrence. A

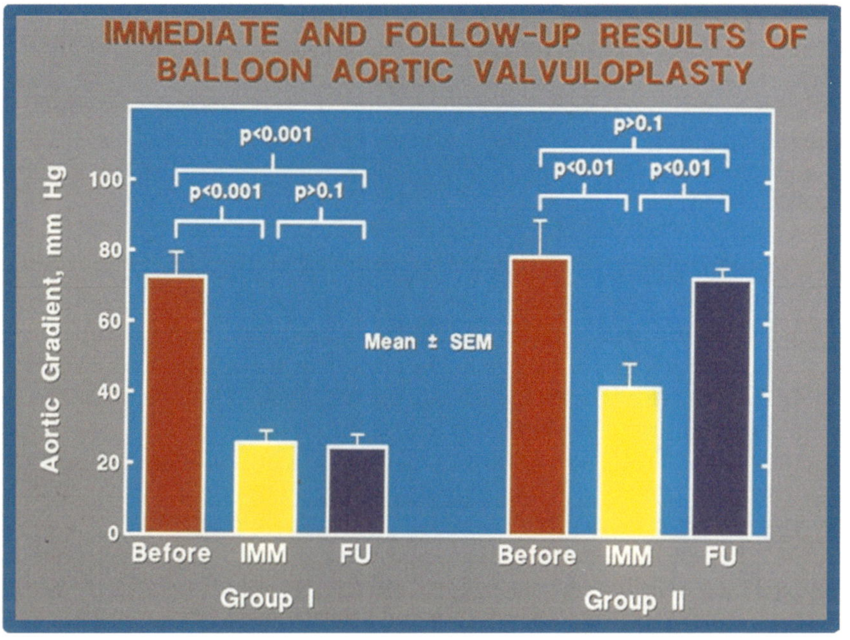

Figure 17.
Bar graph showing immediate (IMM) and follow-up (FU) results of balloon aortic valvuloplasty in group I with good results (left panel) and in group II with poor results (right panel). In group I with good results, the aortic valve gradient decreased significantly ($p < 0.001$) immediately after valvuloplasty and remained low ($p < 0.001$) at follow-up. In group II with poor results, the aortic valve gradient fell ($p < 0.01$) immediately after valvuloplasty and returned to pre-valvuloplasty values ($p > 0.1$) at follow-up. Mean + standard error of mean (SEM) is shown. (Reproduced from reference [29]).

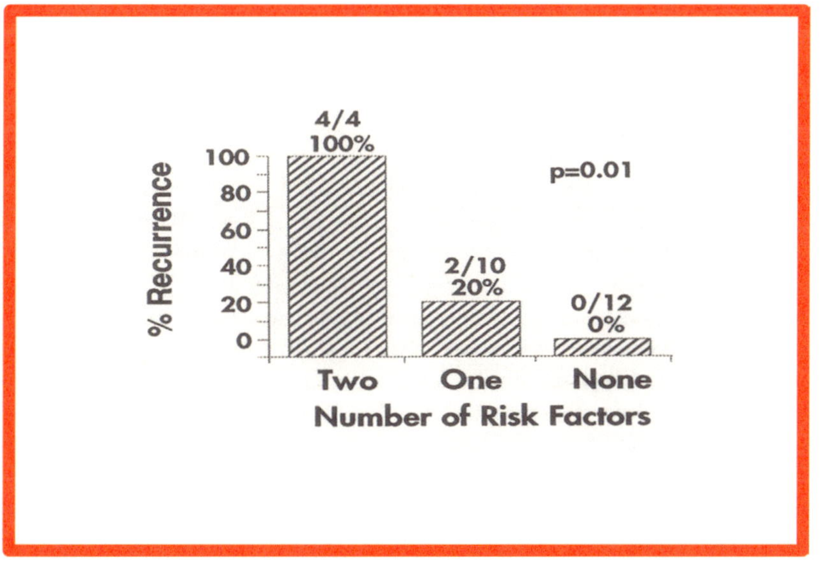

Figure 18.
Bar graph demonstrating influence of multiple risk factors on rates of recurrence of aortic stenosis after balloon aortic valvuloplasty. Note that the larger the number of risk factors, the greater is the probability for restenosis. Percentages and actual numbers are shown on the top of each bar. (Reproduced from reference [10]).

suggestion was made that double balloon BAV may be superior to BAV using one balloon [73]; but thorough assessment of these statistics [74] did not justify such a claim. Balloon/annulus ratios and morphology of the aortic valve may be central elements of restenosis phenomenon; though, the range of variability observed in our study and that of others was not able to establish noteworthy variances; it is likely that investigations involving larger number of patients may unearth other reasons for restenosis [7, 10, 22].

Based on the data presented [1, 5, 7], it was determined that age ≤ 3 years and immediate post-BAV peak-to-peak gradient across the aortic valve ≥30 mmHg may be predictive of aortic valve re-obstruction. It is further surmised that circumventing or reducing risk factors may prevent or lessen the rate of recurrence following BAV. Because the immediate post-BAV gradients across the aortic valve ≥30 mmHg is an alterable risk factor, we advocate use of balloons large enough to decrease the peak-to-peak systolic gradient to <30 mmHg [1, 5, 7].

5.2 Feasibility of repeat BAV for restenosis following prior BAV

As shown in a preceding section, reappearance of aortic obstruction following BAV was detected. We examined the feasibility and effectiveness of repeat BAV in patients who had recurrence after a prior BAV [75]. Twenty-six children with aortic stenosis had BAV between 1983 and 1993; peak gradients across the aortic valve decreased from 71 ± 20 to 26 ± 12 mmHg ($p < 0.001$). At short-term (10 ± 4 months) evaluation, residual gradients of 34 ± 20 mmHg stayed lesser ($p < 0.001$) than pre-BAV gradients but have risen ($p < 0.01$) when compared with acute post-BAV peak gradients. When each patient statistics were examined, six (23%) of the 26 developed re-obstruction, characterized as residual pressure gradients more than 50 mmHg. In our early experience, four patients had successful aortic valvotomy by surgery and two patients underwent a second BAV. Repeat BAV reduced peak gradients from 77 and 66 mmHg to 13 and 6 mmHg, respectively (**Figure 19**) [75]. Two additional children acquired re-obstruction during long-term follow-up and had repeat BAV successfully at 70 and 107 months after original BAV, respectively. The diameter of the balloons utilized in these 4 patients is a little bigger than that utilized at the time of first BAV.

Thus, our experience indicates that repeating BAV is both feasible and effective in managing recurring aortic valve obstruction after prior BAV. Based on these data we recommended that repeat BAV as the therapy of choice for such patients [7, 10, 22, 75]. It should be mentioned that our group of investigators [7, 75] were among the first to demonstrate that repeat BAV is possible and successful in alleviating residual/recurrent aortic stenosis following a previous BAV. In a single institutional study involving 509 patients [76], our findings of feasibility and effectiveness of repeat BAV were validated. These investigators undertook repeat BAV in 115 of 509 patients (23% of initial cohort) who had restenosis following first BAV. A subsequent recurrence occurred in 49 (10% of total). These patients were also effectively managed with a third BAV [76]. In another study of 43 patients [77], the study authors concluded that repeat BAV successfully addresses recurrence of aortic stenosis and delays the need for aortic valve surgery. Accordingly, it is now established that repeat BAV is feasible and effective in alleviating recurrent obstruction following original BAV and in the author's opinion, repeat BAV is the first choice in the treatment of patients with recurrent AS. The feasibility and effectiveness of repeat balloon dilatation was also

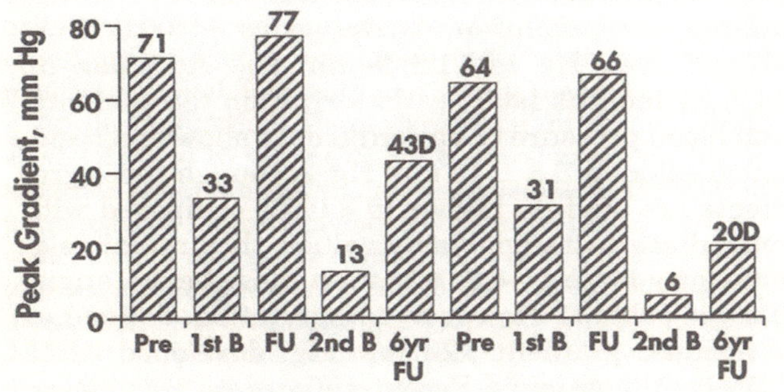

Figure 19.
Bar graph showing aortic valve peak to peak systolic pressure gradients before (pre), after initial balloon valvuloplasty (1st B), at follow-up (FU), after repeated balloon dilatation (2nd B), and at late follow-up at 6 and 7 years, respectively, in 2 patients with restenosis. Note significant decrease in gradient after each balloon valvuloplasty. Gradients remained low after second balloon valvuloplasty by Doppler (D) and at late follow-up 6 and 7 years later. (Reproduced from reference [75]).

demonstrated for other recurrent obstructive lesions such as pulmonary stenosis and coarctation of the aorta [11, 12, 75].

6. Long-term follow-up results

We evaluated long-term, defined as more than 5 years of mean follow-up, results of 26 patients who were restudied 3–10 years (6.7 ± 1.7 years) following BAV. Twenty-two of these patients were reinvestigated longer than 5 years after BAV [7]. In the following paragraphs, these data will be reviewed. Then a review of works of others reporting long-term results will be summarized.

6.1 Residual stenosis

The peak instantaneous Doppler gradients at long-term follow-up were low at 27 ± 17 mmHg (**Figure 15**). The aortic valve peak gradients were lower than pre-BAV gradients ($p < 0.001$) and are similar ($p > 0.1$) to both immediate post-valvuloplasty and short-term follow up values (**Figure 15**) [7].

6.2 Development of aortic insufficiency

The degree of AI was quantified by the ratio of the jet width on color Doppler of AI to dimension of the LV outflow tract, as described previously [7]. While there was minimal change in the degree of AI both immediately after BAV or at short-term follow-up (**Figure 12**), the number of patients with 3 + AI increased at long-term follow-up ($p < 0.01$) (**Figures 12** and **20**). In these seven (28%) patients with 3 + AI,

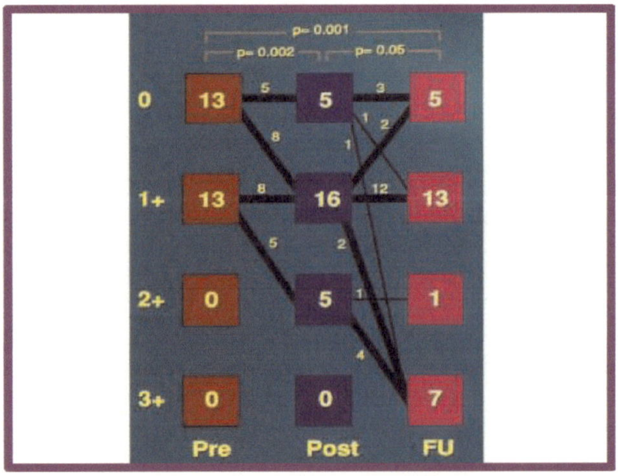

Figure 20.
Degree of aortic insufficiency by Doppler echocardiography before (pre), the day after (post), and at late follow-up (FU). There is a significant (p = 0.002) increase in aortic insufficiency from pre-valvuloplasty to post-valvuloplasty. Number of patients with grade 3+ aortic insufficiency (0 of 26 vs. 7 of 26) at follow-up (FU) increased (p < 0.02). (Modified from reference [7]).

the left ventricular end-diastolic dimension was at or larger than 90th percentile for the body surface area. Two (8%) of these children had successful Ross operation. The remaining 5 patients were being observed carefully [7]. It was concluded that AI is the most important long-term problem with BAV; this is not too dissimilar to the long-term follow-up outcomes of aortic valve surgery. Additional discussion of AI (probable causes) will be presented in a subsequent part of this chapter.

6.3 Ventricular dimensions and function

At long-term follow-up, the left ventricular end-diastolic diameter (45.4 ± 9.9 mm) was larger ($p < 0.01$) than both post-BAV (37.2 ± 0.5 mm) and pre-BAV (36.7 ± 8.5 mm) measurements (**Figure 14**, left panel). To avoid potential impact of growth, standardization of left ventricular measurements to square root of body surface area was made. The resultant values were: 38.5 ± 42 vs. 49.9 ± 5.7 mm/♪m^2 ($p < 0.001$); these data continue to show that the LV end-diastolic dimension is larger at late follow-up, presumably related to the adverse effect of AI. Nevertheless, the LV posterior wall thickness in diastole (8.3 ± 1.7 mm) (**Figure 14**, middle panel) and LV shortening fraction (45 ± 6%) (**Figure 14**, right panel) at long-term follow-up did not significantly ($p > 0.05$) change.

6.4 Re-interventions and actuarial event-free rates

Eight (31%) patients, six at the time of short-term follow-up and two during long-term follow-up developed restenosis; these patients were successfully managed with either surgical valvotomy (N = 4) or second BAV (N = 4). One patient had a left ventricular apex-to-descending aortic conduit to circumvent severe left ventricular mid-cavitary obstruction. Seven (27%) patients had severe AI during long-term follow-up (**Figures 14** and **20**). Two of these children had a successful Ross procedure. Based on these data, event-free rates were calculated (**Figure 21**).

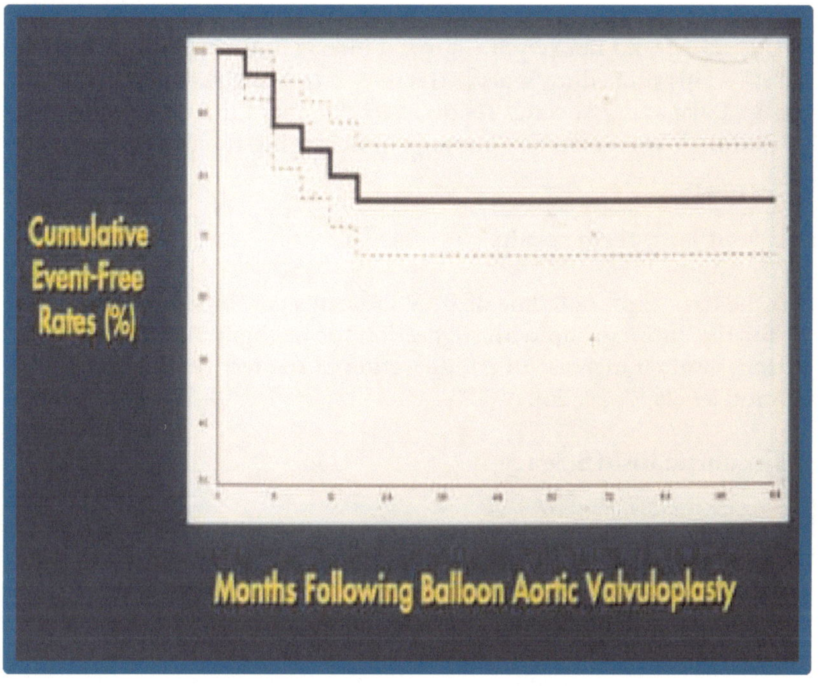

Figure 21.
Actuarial event-free rates after balloon aortic valvuloplasty. Seventy percent confidence limits are marked with dashed lines. Note intervention-free rates at 1, 2, 5, and 9 years are 80, 76, 76, and 76%, respectively. (Modified from reference [7]).

The probability of freedom from re-intervention at 1-, 2-, 5- and 10- year follow-up was 80, 76, 76 and 60%, respectively (**Figure 21**) [7].

6.5 Long-term results by other investigators

Awasthy et al. [78] compared the results of BAV of adolescents and adults with two other groups, namely, 1. Babies below 1 year of age and 2. Children between 1 and 11 years. The necessity for repeat BAV in 10.3–18.1% patients, occurrence of grade 3 or more of AI in 9–9.6% subjects and need for surgical intervention in 2.4–3.6% at follow-up were similar ($p > 0.1$) for all three age subsets. In an accompanying editorial published in Indian Heart Journal [25], long-term results of BAV described by several interventional cardiologists were tabulated and this table will not be reproduced here because of limitations of space, but can be found in our editorial [25].

Other studies reporting on long-term outcomes, not included in the table, will now be reviewed. In a single center study involving 78 patients by Sullivan and associates, the estimated freedom from re-intervention was 44% (95% CI: 20–65%) at 15 years and 62% (95% CI: 40–77%) patients remained free of aortic valve replacement. Post-BAV gradients greater than 30 mmHg and acute AI appear to predispose for aortic valve replacement [79]. In another single center study, Pillai et al. [80] followed 92 patients for 5.7 ± 1.3 years following BAV; 85% patients had successful outcome, 10% subjects developed re-stenosis requiring re-intervention, and 2.2% patients developed severe AI. Auld et al. [81] investigated long-term outcomes of sixty patients with a median follow-up of 6.8 years and found freedom from re-intervention in 75% of study subjects. Long-term results after BAV in 57 patients were examined by

Godlewski and Werner [82]; they found significant progression of AI and that 90, 77, and 59.5% of patients did not require surgical intervention at 5, 10, and 18 years following BAV. This procedure is also effective in treating rheumatic aortic valve stenosis; Pillai and associates followed 92 patients for a mean of 5.7 years and concluded that BAV is an effective strategy in managing rheumatic aortic valve stenosis [83].

6.6 Summary of long-term results

In brief, the long-term outcome of BAV indicates continued relief of narrowing for the entire group with suggestion for negligible additional re-obstruction, gradual increase of AI, dilatation of the left ventricle and high re-intervention levels [7, 22, 25].

6.7 Causes of aortic insufficiency

As shown in the preceding sections, significant AI was found at long-term evaluation following BAV (**Figures 12** and **20**). Many other investigations as well as that of ours demonstrate a tendency to increase in intensity of AI as time passes; the lengthier the follow up duration, the greater the degree of AI. Substantial AI was documented in 24–38% subjects with necessity for replacement of the aortic valve in 8–14% patients, as charted elsewhere (Table 4 of reference [10]).

Our study sought to examine the causes of AI [7]. The patients were split into two groups: Group I, 19 children with no significant AI (grade 2+ or less) and Group II, 7 children with 3+ AI. Fifteen biographic, anatomic, physiologic, and technical data (Table II of reference [7]) were assessed by multivariate logistic regression testing to detect factors causing AI [7]. This evaluation detected several factors that were statistically dissimilar between Groups I and II (Table IV of reference [7]). These are Doppler quantified AI both preceding and immediately after BAV and the procedure undertaken during the second half of our experience with BAV. These three items were entered into a multivariate logistic regression model with all feasible groupings. A model that comprises immediate post-BAV Doppler AI fits the information best. Adding pre-BAV Doppler AI and procedural experience to the model that includes post-BAV Doppler AI did not substantially increase its prognostic value [7]. Consequently, it was concluded that the degree of immediate post-BAV grade of AI is prognostic of late onset of substantial AI. The correlation among these two variables is demonstrated in **Figure 22**. Sullivan [79], Godlewski [82] and their associates also found that the degree of AI at the time of BAV is associated with late AI, confirming our observations.

Intra-operative balloon dilatation with large balloons (1.2–1.5 times the annulus of the aortic valve) both in experimental animal [84] and human [84, 85] models have been shown to result in injury and tears of the aortic valve leaflets producing AI. Hence, we plotted the level of AI at late follow-up along with the balloon/annulus ratio (**Figure 23**) and noticed no correlation between the size of the balloon and level of AI in our study subjects.

The causes for development of AI at late follow-up after BAV are not clearly known. The theories that have previously been advanced are: (1) Doppler-assessed degree of AI both before and immediately after BAV [7, 79, 82], (2) better relief of aortic valve gradient after BAV [84], (3) large balloon/annulus ratio [72, 86, 87], (4) poor morphology of the aortic valve [7] including uni-commissural aortic

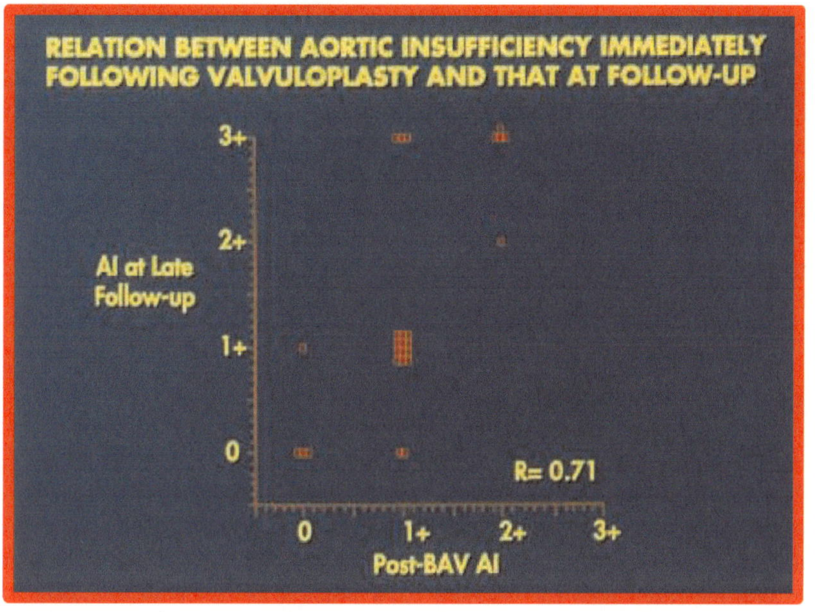

Figure 22.
Relationship of immediate post-valvuloplasty Doppler-estimated aortic insufficiency (AI) with AI at late follow-up after balloon aortic valvuloplasty (BAV). Note good correlation (R = 0.71) between the two. (Modified from reference [7]).

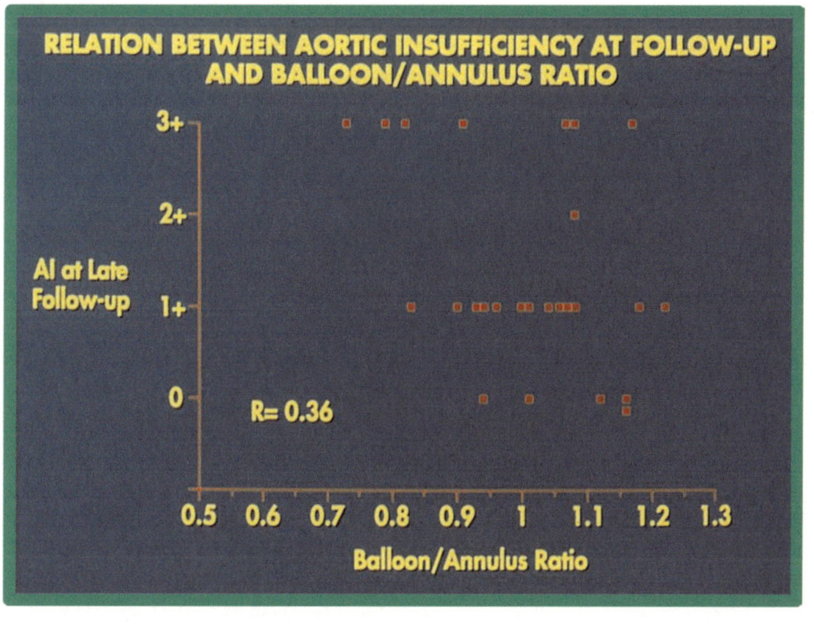

Figure 23.
Relationship of balloon/annulus ratio utilized during balloon aortic valvuloplasty (BAV) with the degree of Doppler-assessed aortic insufficiency (AI) at late follow-up. Note poor correlation (R = 0.36) between these two parameters. Also note grade 3+ AI occurred with wide range of balloon/annulus ratios. (Modified from reference [7]).

valve [72], and (5) prolapse of aortic valve leaflets [86]. However, none of these factors appear to have proof in support of their role in producing AI. Our data [7] and that of others [79, 82] suggested that the degree of AI immediately following BAV is prognostic for development of significant AI at long-term follow-up (**Figures 12**, **20** and **22**). We surmised that a mixture of poor aortic valve morphology and large sized balloons [7, 10, 22, 25] are likely to ultimately turn out to be causing AI at long-term follow-up. Further investigations of the above mentioned and additional causes for late AI and formulating techniques to avoid AI were suggested [7, 10, 22, 26].

7. Comparison with surgery

Evaluation of comparative results of BAV vs. surgery is fraught with challenges in that: (1) there are no randomized studies to deal with this issue, (2) difficulties exist for comparison of "older" historical surgical outcomes with "current" BAV results, (3) short duration of follow-up after BAV, and (4) a smaller quantity of BAV subjects accessible for follow up when compared with surgical patients. In the early-1990s, I analyzed the results of surgical therapy reported in 10 papers [5]. The authors of these 10 papers examined the outcomes of 41–179 patients who were followed for 0.3–26 years after surgical intervention. The surgical mortality for children ranged from 0 to 4% while late mortality was 4–22%. In the natural history survey [88], the surgical and late mortality rates were 1.2 and 1.9%, lower than that was reported in above papers. Sixteen to seventy-eight per cent (16–78%) of patients developed restenosis of the aortic valve and 6–65% of patients developed AI. Repeat surgery to alleviate restenosis or to repair/replace regurgitant aortic valve was required in 16–39% patients [5]. Thus, surgical outcomes were not as good as BAV results [5]. Gatzoulis et al. [89] observed no substantial variation in mortality, morbidity, or the need for re-intervention within 12 months of the surgery and BAV. Additional studies, as detailed elsewhere [10, 22] observed no important variation in mortality, morbidity or need for re-intervention among surgical and BAV groups. In addition, the two groups have comparable rates of freedom from re-intervention 5 years after both procedures. A meta-analysis of 2368 patients from 20 studies (1835 in the BAV group and 533 in the surgical group) found no differences in hospital mortality and prevalence of moderate AI between the groups [90]. In addition, they found no differences in long-term survival or freedom from replacement of the aortic valve. However, a greater number of patients required re-intervention in the BAV group. Given the less-invasive BAV, despite higher re-interventions rates, they concluded that a randomized controlled study is necessary. In another meta-analysis of 18 separate investigations consisting of a total of 4078 patients, survival rates, incidence of late AI, and need for aortic valve replacement were similar in both BAV and surgical groups; however, the need for reintervention was higher after BAV than after surgery [91]. These authors suggest comparison of in-hospital days and morbidity associated with both forms of therapy in future studies. However, single institutional studies differ in their conclusions with some suggesting comparable outcomes [92–94] and others favoring surgery [94–96]. Therefore, the author favors BAV because of considerable occurrence of mortality, both early and late, universal morbidity and the necessity for re-operation seen with surgical valvotomy. Therefore, BAV is a desirable alternative to surgery [5, 10, 22].

8. Complications seen with BAV

Complications may be observed at the time of BAV or may be detected during follow-up; these will be briefed here and for a more detailed description, the reader is referred to our prior publications [8, 29]. Complications at the time of BAV are transient bradycardia, premature beats, and a drop in arterial pressure during balloon inflation. These abnormalities are restored to normalcy after deflation of the balloon. A short period of balloon inflation (≤ 5 seconds), as suggested previously [5] is likely to lessen such complications. Additional complications are loss of blood necessitating blood transfusion; thrombotic occlusion of the femoral artery needing heparin, streptokinase or thrombectomy [97]; other rhythm abnormalities such as transient left bundle branch block [5], right bundle branch block, transient lengthening of QTc interval [98], short-lived atrioventricular block, supraventricular and ventricular tachycardias [5, 98, 99]; cardiac arrest [100]; perforation of cardiac structures [97, 101]; rupture of the balloon [47, 102]; dislodgement of the balloon [89]; tears of the aortic or mitral valve leaflets [89, 103]; right coronary artery occlusion; transitory ischemia of the myocardium [98]; cerebrovascular accidents [104]; and onset of subvalvar obstruction [105]; however, these complications are infrequent. Tears of the aortic valve were observed in animal models in whom large balloons (1.2–1.5 times the aortic valve annulus) were used [85]. Consequently, large balloons (larger than aortic valve annulus) should not be utilized during BAV. Deaths have been seen in association with BAV [72, 84, 103, 106, 107]; such events are caused by rupture of the aorta, temporary obstruction of severe/critical obstructions, aortic valve cusp perforation or avulsion, exsanguination from iliac/femoral vessel tears, and ventricular fibrillation. Sudden death which is unexplained has also been reported [107] but is very uncommon. Complications seen during follow up were occlusion of the femoral artery [3, 8], development of AI and reappearance of aortic valve obstruction; the latter two were examined in the preceding sections.

9. Miscellaneous issues

Additional issues associated with BAV, such as development of subvalvar obstruction [108, 109], mechanism of valvuloplasty [3, 5, 110–112], balloon characteristics utilized during BAV [1–3, 5] will not be reviewed because of limitations of space.

10. Balloon valvuloplasty in specific age groups

In the preceding review, discussion of BAV was primarily centered on infants, children, adolescents, and young adults with congenital AS. The indications, techniques, and outcomes of BAV in the fetuses, neonates, premature infants, and elderly adults with AS are somewhat different; however, will not be examined in this chapter because of limitations of space, but can be found elsewhere [29].

11. Transcatheter aortic valve replacement

Since the description of TAVR [48–50] in the early 2010s, TAVR has been used extensively to treat elderly patients with calcific AS. Given the enthusiasm with which the TAVR is being used at many institutions, it should be pointed out that the TAVR should only be used for calcific AS of the elderly subjects and the non-calcific AS in adolescents and adults should be addressed with the less invasive BAV [25]. The details of the procedure and results of TAVR are discussed in other chapters in this book and therefore, the discussion of TAVR will not be included in this chapter.

12. Summary and conclusions

After the report by Lababidi et al. of BAV in 1983, this procedure was applied by a number of other cardiologists for alleviation of aortic valve obstruction. This review focuses on congenital aortic valve stenosis. The indications for BAV are peak systolic aortic valve pressure gradients of more than 50 mmHg with symptoms or ECG changes or a peak gradient more than 70 mmHg regardless of the symptoms or ECG abnormalities. One or two balloon valvuloplasty catheters are positioned across the aortic valve, over extra-stiff guide wire(s) and the balloon(s) is/are inflated until the waist of the balloon(s) is eliminated. The recommended balloon/annulus ratio is 0.8–1.0. Femoral arterial access is the most utilized route for BAV; however, other routes of access such as trans-umbilical arterial or venous or trans-venous routes are favored in neonates and young infants to circumvent injury to the femoral artery.

Immediately following BAV, fall in peak systolic pressure gradient across the aortic valve in conjunction with decrease in LV peak systolic and end-diastolic pressures occurs in most patients. Development of AI is rare in children, although it may be seen in the newborn. At short-term follow-up, catheterization-measured and Doppler derived peak aortic valve gradients stay low for the entire cohort. However, when each patient's data is scrutinized, close to one-fourth of patients developed restenosis, defined as peak-to-peak gradient ≥50 mmHg. When the causes for re-stenosis were investigated, age ≤ 3 years and an immediate post-BAV gradient ≥30 mmHg were found to predict restenosis. Patients with restenosis may be treated with repeat BAV or surgery. Repeating BAV is effective in alleviating restenosis. Long-term follow-up information indicates minimal Doppler gradients, negligible further restenosis beyond what was seen at short-term follow-up and progression of AI in nearly 25% children. Kaplan-Myer event-free rates at 5- and 10-years following BAV are in mid 70s and low 60s respectively. These data indicate good outcomes and avoided or postponed surgical therapy. However, significant AI at long-term follow-up is of concern. Current recommendations favor BAV as first line therapy for alleviation of congenital aortic valve stenosis.

Conflict of interest

The author declares no conflict of interest.

Author details

P. Syamasundar Rao
Children's Heart Institute, Children's Memorial Hermann Hospital and McGovern Medical School, University of Texas Health Sciences Center at Houston, Houston, TX, USA

*Address all correspondence to: p.syamasundar.rao@uth.tmc.edu

IntechOpen

© 2023 The Author(s). Licensee IntechOpen. This chapter is distributed under the terms of the Creative Commons Attribution License (http://creativecommons.org/licenses/by/3.0), which permits unrestricted use, distribution, and reproduction in any medium, provided the original work is properly cited.

References

[1] Rao PS, Thapar MK, Wilson AD, Levy JM, Chopra PS. Intermediate-term follow-up results of balloon aortic valvuloplasty in infants and children with special reference to causes of restenosis. The American Journal of Cardiology. 1989;**64**:1356-1360

[2] Rao PS. Comparison of single and double balloon valvuloplasty in children with aortic stenosis (letter). Journal of the American College of Cardiology. 1989;**13**:1216-1217

[3] Rao PS. Balloon aortic valvuloplasty: A review. Clinical Cardiology. 1990;**13**: 458-466

[4] Rao PS. Percutaneous balloon valvuloplasty/angioplasty in congenital heart disease. In: Bashore TM, Davidson CT, editors. Percutaneous Valvuloplasty and Related Techniques. Baltimore, MD: Williams & Wilkins; 1990. pp. 251-277

[5] Rao PS. Balloon valvuloplasty for aortic stenosis. In: Rao PS, editor. Transcatheter Therapy in Pediatric Cardiology. New York: Wiley-Liss, Inc; 1993. pp. 105-127

[6] Singh GK, Marino CJ, Rao PS. Left heart outflow obstruction, aortic stenosis and coarctation of the aorta: An echocardiographic assessment. Pediat Ultrasound Today. 1996;**1**:61-76

[7] Galal O, Rao PS, Al-Fadley F, Wilson AD. Follow-up results of balloon aortic valvuloplasty in children with special reference to causes of late aortic insufficiency. American Heart Journal. 1997;**113**:418-427

[8] Lee HY, Reddy SCB, Rao PS. Evaluation of superficial femoral artery compromise and limb growth retardation following transfemoral artery balloon dilatations. Circulation. 1997;**95**:974-980

[9] Rao PS, Jureidini SB. Transumbilical venous anterograde, snare-assisted balloon aortic valvuloplasty in a neonate with critical aortic stenosis. Catheterization and Cardiovascular Diagnosis. 1998;**45**:144-148

[10] Rao PS. Balloon aortic valvuloplasty. Journal of Interventional Cardiology. 1998;**11**:319-329

[11] Chopra PS, Rao PS. Balloon aortic valvuloplasty in children (editorial). The Journal of Invasive Cardiology. 1999;**11**: 277-279

[12] Rao PS. Long-term follow-up results after balloon dilatation of pulmonic stenosis, aortic stenosis and coarctation of the aorta: A review. Progress in Cardiovascular Diseases. 1999;**42**:59-74

[13] Rao PS. Nonsurgical management of pulmonary and aortic stenosis in children with transluminal balloon dilatation techniques. Gulf Medical College Ajman Health Journal. 2000;**2**:18-24

[14] Singh GK, Rao PS. Left heart outflow obstructions. In: Crawford MH, JP DM, editors. Cardiology. London: Mosby International; 2001. pp. 7-11.1-7-11.9

[15] Rao PS. Anterograde transumbilical venous balloon aortic valvuloplasty (letter). Catheterization and Cardiovascular Interventions: Official Journal of the Society for Cardiac Angiography & Interventions. 2002;**56**: 439

[16] Singh GK, Rao PS. Left heart outflow obstructions. In: Crawford MH, JP DM,

Paulus WJ, editors. Cardiology. Second ed. Edinburgh: Mosby International; 2004. pp. 1317-1326

[17] Rao PS. Role of interventional cardiology in neonates: Part II—Balloon angioplasty/ valvuloplasty. Neonatology Today. 2007;**2**(10):1-12

[18] Rao PS. Role of interventional cardiology in neonates: Part II—Balloon angioplasty/valvuloplasty. Congenital Cardiol Today. 2008;**6**(1):1-14

[19] Singh GK, Rao PS. Left heart outflow obstructions. In: Crawford MH, JP DM, Paulus WJ, editors. Cardiology. Third ed. Edinburgh, UK: Mosby Elsevier, ISBN 978-0-7234-3485-6; 2010. pp. 1507-1518

[20] Samraj R, Rao PS. Concurrent transcatheter therapy of valvar aortic stenosis and patent ductus arteriosus: Case report and review. The Journal of Invasive Cardiology. 2011;**23**(4):E72-E75

[21] Rao PS. Consensus on timing of intervention for common congenital heart diseases: Part I—Acyanotic heart defects. Indian Journal of Pediatrics. 2013;**80**:72-78

[22] Agu NC, Rao PS. Balloon aortic valvuloplasty. Pediatrics and Therapeutics. 2012;**S5**:004. DOI: 10.4172/2161-0665.S5-004

[23] Rao PS. Catheter interventions in the neonate: Part II – Balloon angioplasty/ valvuloplasty. In: Rao PS, Vidyasagar D, editors. Perinatal Cardiology: A Multidisciplinary Approach. Minneapolis, MN: Cardiotext Publishing; 2015. Chapter 20

[24] Rao PS. Neonatal catheter interventions. In: Vijayalakshmi IB, editor. Cardiac Catheterization and Imaging (from Pediatrics to Geriatrics). New Delhi, India: Jaypee Publications; 2015. pp. 388-432

[25] Rao PS. Balloon aortic valvuloplasty (editorial). Indian Heart Journal. 2016; **68**:592-595. DOI: 10.1016/j.ihj.2016.03.018

[26] Rao PS. Management of congenital heart disease: State of the art—Part I—Acyanotic heart defects. Children (Basel). 2019;**6**:42. DOI: 10.3390/children6030042

[27] Singh GK, Mowers KL, Marino C, Balzer D, Rao PS. Effect of pressure recovery on pressure gradients in congenital stenotic outflow lesions in pediatric patients-clinical implications of lesion severity and geometry: A simultaneous Doppler echocardiography and cardiac catheter correlative study. Journal of the American Society of Echocardiography. 2020;**33**:207-217. DOI: 10.1016/j.echo.2019.09.001

[28] Rao PS. Aortic stenosis. In: Pediatric Cardiology: How it Has Evolved over the Last 50 Years. New Castle upon Tyne: Cambridge Scholars Publishing; 2020. pp. 231-256. ISBN-13: 9781527548886

[29] Rao PS. Role of balloon aortic valvuloplasty in the management of aortic stenosis. Journal of Clinical Cardiology and Cardiovascular Interventions. 2021;**4**(12):1-28. DOI: 10.31579/2641-0419/171

[30] Rao PS. Diagnosis and management of acyanotic heart disease: Part I—Obstructive lesions. Indian Journal of Pediatrics. 2005;**72**:496-502

[31] Rao PS. Congenital heart defects – A review. In: Rao PS, editor. Congenital Heart Disease—Selected Aspects, ISBN 978-953-307-472-6. London, UK, Rijeka, Croatia: InTech; 2012

[32] Alexiou C, Langley SM, Dalrymple-Hay MJ, Salmon AP, Keeton BR, Haw MP, et al. Open commissurotomy for critical isolated aortic stenosis in neonates. The Annals of Thoracic Surgery. 2001;**71**:489-493. DOI: 10.1016/S0003-4975(00)02232-3

[33] El Khoury G, de Kerchove L. Principles of aortic valve repair. Elsevier. 2013;**145**:S26-S29. DOI: 10.1016/j.jtcvs.2012.11.071

[34] Poncelet AJ, El Khoury G, De Kerchove L, Sluysmans T, Moniotte S, Momeni M, et al. Aortic valve repair in the paediatric population: Insights from a 38-year single-Centre experience. European Journal of Cardio-Thoracic Surgery. 2017;**51**:43-49. DOI: 10.1093/ejcts/ezw259

[35] Wiggins LM, Mimic B, Issitt R, Ilic S, Bonello B, Marek J, et al. The utility of aortic valve leaflet reconstruction techniques in children and young adults. The Journal of Thoracic and Cardiovascular Surgery. 2020;**159**:2369-2378. DOI: 10.1016/j.jtcvs.2019.09.176

[36] Wang S, Nento D, Singh H, Agarwal A. Advances in the management of congenital aortic valve disease. In: Rao PS, editor. Congenital Heart Defects—Recent Advances. London, UK, Rijeka, Croatia: InTechOpen; 2022

[37] Solymar L, Rao PS, Mardini MK, Fawzy ME, Guinn G. Prosthetic valves in children and adolescents. American Heart Journal. 1991;**121**:557-568

[38] Popov AF, Coskun KO, Tirilomis T, Schmitto JD, Hinz J, Kriebel T, et al. Mechanical aortic valve replacement in children and adolescents after previous repair of congenital heart disease. Artificial Organs. 2009;**33**:915-921. DOI: 10.1111/j.1525-1594.2009.00886.x

[39] Ross DN. Homograft replacement of the aortic valve. Lancet. 1962;**2**(7254):487. DOI: 10.1016/s0140-6736(62)90345-8

[40] Barratt-Boyes BG, Lowe JB, Cole DS, Kelly DT. Homograft replacement for aortic valve disease. Thorax. 1965;**20**:489-504

[41] Ross DN. Aortic root replacement with a pulmonary autograft—Current trends. The Journal of Heart Valve Disease. 1994;**3**:358-360

[42] Sharabiani MT, Dorobantu DM, Mahani AS, Turner M, Peter Tometzki AJ, Angelini GD, et al. Aortic valve replacement and the Ross operation in children and young adults. Journal of the American College of Cardiology. 2016;**67**:2858-2870. DOI: 10.1016/j.jacc.2016.04.021

[43] Dotter CT, Judkins MP. Transluminal treatment of arteriosclerotic obstruction: Description of a new technique and a preliminary report of its application. Circulation. 1964;**30**:654-670

[44] Gruntzig AR, Senning A, Siegothaler WE. Non-operative dilatation of coronary artery stenosis: Percutaneous transluminal coronary angioplasty. The New England Journal of Medicine. 1979;**301**:61-68

[45] Kan JS, White RI, Mitchell SE, et al. Percutaneous balloon valvuloplasty: A new method for treating congenital pulmonary stenosis. New England Journal of Medicine. 1982;**307**:540-542

[46] Lababidi Z. Aortic balloon valvuloplasty. American Heart Journal. 1983;**106**:751-752

[47] Lababidi Z, Wu J, Walls JT. Percutaneous balloon aortic valvuloplasty: Results in 23 patients. The American Journal of Cardiology. 1984; **54**:194-197

[48] Leon MB, Smith CR, Mack M, Miller DC, Moses JW, Svensson LG, et al. Transcatheter aortic-valve implantation for aortic stenosis in patients who cannot undergo surgery. The New England Journal of Medicine. 2010;**363**:1597-1607

[49] Mack MJ, Leon MB, Thourani VH, Makkar R, Kodali SK, Russo M, et al. Transcatheter aortic-valve replacement with a balloon-expandable valve in low-risk patients. The New England Journal of Medicine. 2019;**380**:1695-1705

[50] Nishimura RA, Otto CM, Bonow RO, Carabello BA, Erwin JP 3rd, Fleisher LA, et al. 2017 AHA/ACC focused update of the 2014 AHA/ACC guideline for the management of patients with valvular heart disease: A report of the American college of cardiology/american heart association task force on clinical practice guidelines. Circulation. 2017;**135**:e1159-e1195

[51] Rao PS. Influence of balloon size on the short-term and long-term results of balloon pulmonary valvuloplasty. Texas Heart Institute Journal. 1987;**14**:57-61

[52] Narang R, Das G, Dev V, Goswami K, Saxena A, et al. Effect of the balloon-anulus ratio on the intermediate and follow-up results of pulmonary balloon valvuloplasty. Cardiology. 1997; **88**:271-276

[53] De Giovanni JV, Edgar RA, Cranston A. Adenosine induced transient cardiac standstill in catheter interventional procedures for congenital heart disease. Heart. 1998;**80**: 330-333

[54] Daehnert I, Rotzsch C, Wiener M, Schneider P. Rapid right ventricular pacing is an alternative to adenosine in catheter interventional procedures for congenital heart disease. Heart. 2004;**90**: 1047-1050

[55] Sanborn TA. Vascular closure devices for transarterial interventions. In: Rao PS, Kern MJ, editors. Catheter Based Devices for Treatment of Noncoronary Cardiovascular Disease in Adults and Children. Philadelphia, PA: Lippincott, Williams & Wilkins; 2003. pp. 493-494

[56] Kiramijyan S, Magalhaes MA, Ben-Dor I, et al. The adjunctive use of Angio-seal in femoral vascular closure following percutaneous transcatheter aortic valve replacement. EuroIntervention. 2016;**12**: 88-93. DOI: 10.4244/EIJV12I1A16

[57] Lababidi Z, Weinhaus L. Successful balloon valvuloplasty for neonatal critical aortic stenosis. American Heart Journal. 1986;**112**:913-916

[58] Wren C, Sullivan I, Bull C, Deanfield J. Percutaneous balloon dilatation of aortic valve stenosis in neonates and infants. British Heart Journal. 1987;**58**:608-612

[59] Kasten-Sportes CH, Piechaud J, Sidi D, Kachaner J. Percutaneous balloon valvuloplasty in neonates with critical aortic stenosis. Journal of the American College of Cardiology. 1989;**13**:1101-1105

[60] Zeevi B, Keane JF, Castaneda AR, Perry SB, Lock JE, et al. Neonatal critical valvar aortic stenosis: A comparison of surgical and balloon dilatation therapy. Circulation. 1989;**80**:831-839

[61] Vermillion RP, Snider AR, Bengur AR, et al. Doppler evaluation of femoral arteries in children after aortic balloon valvuloplasty or coarctation

balloon angioplasty. Pediat Cardiology. 1993;**14**:13-18

[62] Alekyan BG, Petrosyan YS, Coulson JD, Danilov YY, Vinokurov AV. Right subscapular artery catheterization for balloon valvuloplasty of critical aortic stenosis in infants. The American Journal of Cardiology. 1995;**76**:1049-1052

[63] Austoni P, Figini A, Vigrati G, Donatelli F. Emergency aortic balloon valvotomy in critical aortic stenosis of the neonates (letter). Pediat Cardiology. 1990;**11**:59-60

[64] Fischer DR, Ettedgui JA, Park SC, et al. Carotid artery approach for balloon dilatation of aortic valve stenosis in the neonate: A preliminary report. Journal of the American College of Cardiology. 1990;**15**:1633-1636

[65] Beekman RH, Rocchini AP, Andes A. Balloon valvuloplasty for critical aortic stenosis in the newborn, influence of new catheter technology. Journal of the American College of Cardiology. 1991;**17**: 1172-1176

[66] Hausdorf G, Schneider M, Schrimer KR, Schulze-Neick I, Lange PE. Anterograde balloon valvuloplasty of aortic stenosis in children. The American Journal of Cardiology. 1993;**71**: 560-562

[67] O'Laughlin MP, Slack MC, Grifka R, Mullins CE. Pro-grade double balloon dilatation of congenital aortic valve stenosis: A case report. Catheterization and Cardiovascular Diagnosis. 1993;**28**: 134-136

[68] Torres A, Vincent JA, Everett A, Lim S, Foerster SR, Marshall AC, et al. Balloon valvuloplasty for congenital aortic stenosis: Multi-center safety and efficacy outcome assessment. Catheterization and Cardiovascular Interventions. 2015;**86**:808-820. DOI: 10.1002/ccd.25969

[69] Boe BA, Zampi JD, Kennedy KF, Jayaram N, Porras D, Foerster SR, et al. Acute success of balloon aortic valvuloplasty in the current era: A national cardiovascular data registry study. JACC. Cardiovascular Interventions. 2017;**10**:1717-1726. DOI: 10.1016/j.jcin.2017.08.001

[70] Rao PS, Thapar MK, Kutayli F. Causes of restenosis following balloon pulmonary valvuloplasty for valvar pulmonary stenosis. The American Journal of Cardiology. 1988;**62**:979-982

[71] Rao PS, Thapar MK, Kutayli F, et al. Causes of recoarctation following balloon angioplasty of unoperated aortic coarctation. Journal of the American College of Cardiology. 1989;**13**:109-115

[72] Sholler GF, Keane JF, Perry SB, Sanders SP, Lock JE. Balloon dilatation of congenital aortic valve stenosis: Results and influence of technical and morphological features on outcome. Circulation. 1988;**78**:351-360

[73] Beekman RH, Rocchini AP, Crowley DC, et al. Comparison of single and double balloon valvuloplasty in children with aortic stenosis. Journal of the American College of Cardiology. 1988;**12**:480-485

[74] Rao PS. Double balloon aortic valvuloplasty in children (letter). Journal of the American College of Cardiology. 1989;**13**:1216-1217

[75] Rao PS, Galal O, Wilson AD. Feasibility and effectiveness of repeat balloon dilatation of restenosed obstructions following previous balloon valvuloplasty/angioplasty. American Heart Journal. 1996;**132**:403-407

[76] Brown DW, Dipilato AE, Chong EC, et al. Aortic valve reinterventions after balloon aortic valvuloplasty for congenital aortic stenosis at intermediate and late follow-up. Journal of the American College of Cardiology. 2010; **56**:1740-1749

[77] Petit CJ, Maskatia SA, Justino H, Mattamal RJ, Crystal MA, Ing FF. Repeat balloon aortic valvuloplasty effectively delays surgical intervention in children with recurrent aortic stenosis. Catheterization and Cardiovascular Interventions. 2013;**82**:549-555. DOI: 10.1002/ccd.24562

[78] Awasthy N, Garg R, Radhakrishnan S, Shrivastava S. Long-term results of percutaneous balloon valvuloplasty of congenital aortic stenosis in adolescents and young adults. Indian Heart Journal. 2016; **68**:604-611. DOI: 10.1016/j.ihj.2016.03.001

[79] Sullivan PM, Rubio AE, Johnston TA, Jones TK. Long-term outcomes and re-interventions following balloon aortic valvuloplasty in pediatric patients with congenital aortic stenosis: A single-center study. Catheterization and Cardiovascular Interventions. 2017;**89**:288-296. DOI: 10.1002/ccd.26722

[80] Pillai AA, Balasubramanian VR, Sharma DK. Immediate and long-term follow up results of balloon aortic valvuloplasty in congenital bicuspid aortic valve stenosis among young patients. The Journal of Heart Valve Disease. 2018;**27**:17-23

[81] Auld B, Carrigan L, Ward C, Justo R, Alphonso N, Anderson B. Balloon aortic valvuloplasty for congenital aortic stenosis: A 14-year single Centre review. Heart, Lung & Circulation. 2019;**28**: 632-636. DOI: 10.1016/j.hlc.2018.02.014

[82] Godlewski K, Werner B. Long-term results of percutaneous balloon aortic valvuloplasty in children with aortic stenosis: A single-center experience. Kardiologia Polska. 2020;**78**:559-566. DOI: 10.33963/KP.15245

[83] Pillai AA, Ramasamy C, Saktheeshwaran M, Selvaraj R, Satheesh S, Jayaraman B. Balloon valvuloplasty in rheumatic aortic valve stenosis: Immediate and long-term results. Cardiovascular Intervention and Therapeutics. 2015;**30**:45-50. DOI: 10.1007/s12928-014-0286-0

[84] Helgason H, Keane JF, Fellows KE, Kulik TJ, Lock JE. Balloon dilation of the aortic valve: Studies in normal lambs and in children with aortic stenosis. Journal of the American College of Cardiology. 1987;**9**:816-822. DOI: 10.1016/s0735-1097(87)80237-1

[85] Phillips RR, Gerlis LM, Wilson N, Walker DR. Aortic valve damage caused by operative balloon dilatation of critical aortic valve stenosis. British Heart Journal. 1987;**57**:168-170. DOI: 10.1136/hrt.57.2.168

[86] Shaddy RE, Boucek MM, Sturtevant JE, Ruttenberg HD, Orsmond GS. Gradient reduction, aortic valve regurgitation and prolapse after balloon aortic valvuloplasty in 32 consecutive patients with congenital aortic stenosis. Journal of the American College of Cardiology. 1990;**16**:451-456

[87] Rochini AP, Beekman RH, Shachar GB, Benson L, Schwartz D, et al. Balloon aortic valvuloplasty: Results of the Valvuloplasty and angioplasty of congenital anomalies registry. The American Journal of Cardiology. 1990; **65**:784-789

[88] Wagner HR, Ellison RC, Keane JF, et al. Clinical course in aortic stenosis. Circulation. 1987;**56**:I47-I56

[89] Gatzoulis MA, Rigby ML, Shinebourne EA, Redington AN. Contemporary results of balloon valvuloplasty and surgical valvotomy for congenital aortic stenosis. Archives of Disease in Childhood. 1995;**73**:66-69

[90] Hill GD, Ginde S, Rios R, Frommelt PC, Hill KD. Surgical valvotomy versus balloon valvuloplasty for congenital aortic valve stenosis: A systematic review and meta-analysis. Journal of the American Heart Association. 2016;**5**(8):e003931. DOI: 10.1161/JAHA.116.003931

[91] Saung MT, McCracken C, Sachdeva R, Petit CJ. Outcomes following balloon aortic Valvuloplasty versus surgical Valvotomy in congenital aortic valve stenosis: A meta-analysis. The Journal of Invasive Cardiology. 2019;**31**:E133-E142

[92] Prijic SM, Vukomanovic VA, Stajevic MS, Bjelakovic BB, Zdravkovic MD, Sehic IN, et al. Balloon dilation and surgical valvotomy comparison in non-critical congenital aortic valve stenosis. Pediatric Cardiology. 2015;**36**:616-624. DOI: 10.1007/s00246-014-1056-6

[93] Justo RN, McCrindle BW, Benson LN, Williams WG, Freedom RM, Smallhorn JF. Aortic valve regurgitation after surgical versus percutaneous balloon valvotomy for congenital aortic valve stenosis. The American Journal of Cardiology. 1996;**77**:1332-1338. DOI: 10.1016/s0002-9149(96)00201-9

[94] Atik SU, Eroğlu AG, Çinar B, Bakar MT, Saltik İL. Comparison of balloon dilatation and surgical valvuloplasty in non-critical congenital aortic valvular stenosis at long-term follow-up. Pediatric Cardiology. 2018;**39**: 1554-1560. DOI: 10.1007/s00246-018-1929-1

[95] Brown JW, Rodefeld MD, Ruzmetov M, Eltayeb O, Yurdakok O, Turrentine MW. Surgical valvuloplasty versus balloon aortic dilation for congenital aortic stenosis: Are evidence-based outcomes relevant? The Annals of Thoracic Surgery. 2012;**94**:146-153; discussion 153-155. DOI: 10.1016/j.athoracsur.2012.02.054

[96] Herrmann JL, Clark AJ, Colgate C, Rodefeld MD, Hoyer MH, Turrentine MW, et al. Surgical valvuloplasty versus balloon dilation for congenital aortic stenosis in pediatric patients. World Journal for Pediatric and Congenital Heart Surgery. 2020;**11**: 444-451. DOI: 10.1177/2150135120918774

[97] Wessel DL, Keane JF, Fellows KE, Robichaud H, Lock JE. Fibrinolytic therapy for femoral arterial thrombosis after cardiac catheterization in infants and children. The American Journal of Cardiology. 1986;**58**:347-351

[98] Ewert P, Bertram H, Breuer J, Dähnert I, Dittrich S, et al. Balloon valvuloplasty in the treatment of congenital aortic valve stenosis — A retrospective multicenter survey of more than 1000 patients. International Journal of Cardiology. 2011;**149**:182-185

[99] Weesner KM. Ventricular arrhythmias after balloon aortic valvuloplasty. The American Journal of Cardiology. 1990;**66**:1534-1535

[100] Shrivastava S, Das GS, Dev V, Sharma S, Rajani M. Follow-up after percutaneous balloon valvoplasty for noncalcific aortic stenosis. The American Journal of Cardiology. 1990;**65**:250-252

[101] Waller BF, Girod DA, Dillon JC. Transverse aortic wall tears in infants after balloon angioplasty for aortic valve stenosis: Relation of aortic wall damage

to diameter of inflated angioplasty balloon and aortic lumen in seven necropsy cases. Journal of the American College of Cardiology. 1984;**4**:1235-1241

[102] Loya Y, Sharma S. Balloon tear during valvuloplasty. American Heart Journal. 1991;**121**:1841-1842

[103] Fellows KE, Radtke W, Keane JF, Lock JE. Acute complications of catheter therapy for congenital heart disease. The American Journal of Cardiology. 1987; **60**:679-683

[104] Ed T, Duncan WJ, Tyrell MJ, Lowry NJ. Neurological complications of balloon angioplasty in children. Pediatric Cardiology. 1991;**12**:98-101

[105] Luomirssky A, O'Laughlin MP, Nihill MS, Mullins CE. Left ventricular mid-cavity obstruction after balloon dilatation in isolated aortic valve stenosis in children. Catheterization and Cardiovascular Diagnosis. 1991;**22**:89-92

[106] Booth P, Redington AN, Shinebourne EA, Rigby MW. Early complications of interventional balloon catheterization in infants and children. British Heart Journal. 1991;**65**: 109-112

[107] Brown DW, Dipilato AE, Chong EC, Gauvreau K, McElhinney DB. Sudden unexpected death after balloon valvuloplasty for congenital aortic stenosis. Journal of the American College of Cardiology. 2010;**56**:1939-1946

[108] Fontes VF, Esteves CA, Eduardo J, et al. Regression of infundibular hypertrophy after pulmonary valvotomy for pulmonic stenosis. The American Journal of Cardiology. 1988;**62**:977-979

[109] Thapar MK, Rao PS. Significance of infundibular obstruction following balloon valvuloplasty for valvar pulmonic stenosis. American Heart Journal. 1989;**118**:99-103

[110] Rao PS, Linde LM. Pressure and energy in the cardiovascular chambers. Chest. 1974;**66**:176-178

[111] Rao PS. Balloon angioplasty and valvuloplasty in infants, children and adolescents. Current Problems in Cardiology. YearBook Medical Publishers, Inc. Chicago, 1989; 14(8): 417-500

[112] Thapar MK, Rao PS. Mechanism of valvuloplasty/angioplasty. In: Rao PS, editor. Transcatheter Therapy in Pediatric Cardiology. New York: Wiley-Liss; 1993. pp. 45-58

Chapter 6

Catheter-Based Therapies: Current Practices and Considerations

Sidra R. Shah, Hafez Golzarian and Sandeep M. Patel

Abstract

In just over a decade, there have been paradigm shifts globally in the catheter-based therapies available for the management of patients with severe aortic stenosis. The use of transcatheter aortic valve replacement (TAVR) has been a crucial turning point in the field of cardiology as it granted an option for a minimally invasive method to replace a valve for patients who may or may not be suitable for cardiac surgery. In this chapter, we discuss the current practices and considerations as well as the ongoing evolution of catheter-based approaches for TAVR. The predominant focus of the chapter will be on aortic valve device modifications, prototypes of valves, device delivery systems, and the various techniques. However, discussions on indications/contraindications, proper work-up, preparation, equipment and personnel, complications, and post-procedural management & surveillance will also be reviewed.

Keywords: aortic stenosis (AS), transcatheter aortic valve implantation (TAVI), transcatheter aortic valve replacement (TAVR), surgical aortic valve replacement (SAVR), percutaneous, transcatheter

1. Introduction

Aortic valve stenosis is a common valvular disease that occurs due to narrowing and stiffening of the valve which restricts blood flow in the body. It is a systolic murmur heard loudest at the 2nd intercostal space in the right upper sternal border. The murmur radiates to the carotids and is described as crescendo-decrescendo. Some causes of the narrowing include calcification of the valve due to aging, congenital valve abnormalities, and rheumatic heart disease. Most people with aortic stenosis can be asymptomatic for years before developing worsening symptoms such as shortness of breath, syncope, fatigue, palpitations, and/or angina. The valve can be repaired or replaced with different procedures depending on the patient's condition. Valve replacement is done by aortic valve replacement surgery or transcatheter aortic valve replacement (TAVR). TAVR is a minimally invasive procedure that replaces the aortic valve in patients who are not candidates for surgery. This procedure has significantly evolved over the years and has become part of the standard of care to improve patient outcomes in aortic stenosis.

2. History

For decades since the inception of the first surgical aortic valve repair in 1962, the only treatment option available for surgically high-risk patients suffering from severe aortic stenosis (AS) was medical management. In 1985, Alain Cribier performed the first catheter-based balloon aortic valvuloplasty in a 77-year-old inoperable female [1]. Unfortunately, this still provided little to no long-term improvements in outcomes for patients. On May 1, 1989, Henning R. Andersen successfully developed and implanted the first percutaneous synthetic aortic valve in an 80-kg closed chest pig in Aarhus University Hospital of Denmark (**Figure 1**) [2, 3].

His inspiration stemmed from the works of Andreas Grüntzig and Charles Dotter who pioneered and performed the first-in-man percutaneous transluminal coronary angioplasty in 1977 in Zurich, Switzerland. Their works led to their nomination for the Nobel Prize in Medicine the following year. Augmenting what these two pioneers established, it was their student Julio Palmaz who then went on to invent and successfully implant the first balloon-expandable coronary stents. According to Andersen, it was in February 1989 during a conference lecture about balloon-expandable stents led by Palmaz in Scottsdale, Arizona when he suddenly thought of the idea of attempting such balloon-expandable stents but with larger diameters with collapsible valve tissue on the inside to mimic the structure and function of heart valves [2]. Andersen believed that if he utilized a very similar technique as Grüntzig and Palmaz, then he would be able to also perform percutaneous artificial heart valve implantations without the need for surgery. Upon returning to Denmark from the conference, Andersen spent several months creating his own valve prototypes utilizing iron and steel wires of various thickness and stiffness which he would buy from local hardware stores. These early valves were roughly ~25 mm in diameter and consisted of 15–16 loops closed by soldering [2]. Over the next 3 years, Andersen continued to optimize durability and functionality of his device on pigs. Eventually he went on to add high loops for the commissure posts to be able to mount biological leaflets which he would harvest from pig hearts purchased from a local slaughterhouse (**Figure 2**).

Andersen credited J. Michael Hasenkam, a young cardiovascular surgeon in-training at the time, for this idea of mounting on biological leaflets to his new device.

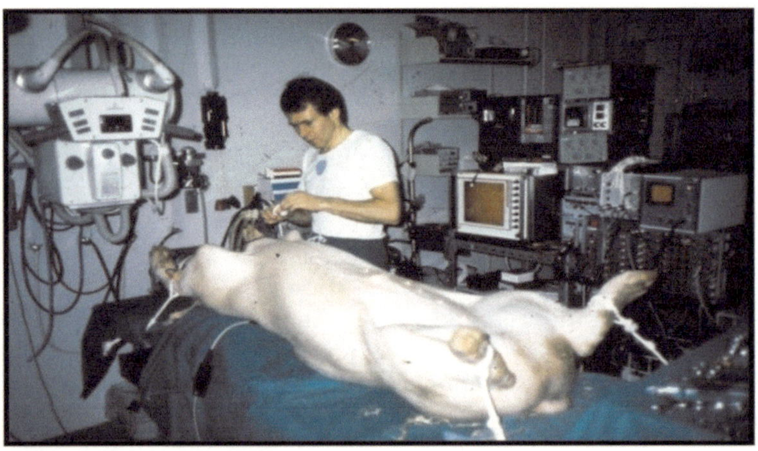

Figure 1.
Henning Rud Andersen preparing an 80 kg pig in 1989 in the animal lab of Aarhus University Hospital (image obtained from Ref. [2]).

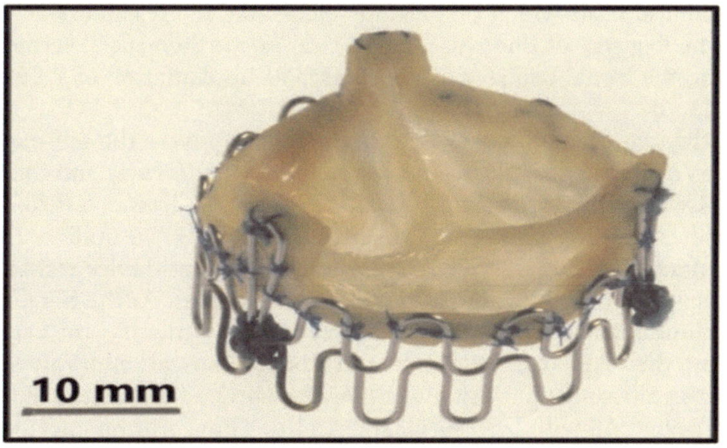

Figure 2.
Early handmade prototype of an aortic valve with three high loops for mounting leaflets harvested from pig valves (image obtained from Ref. [2]).

He also credited his medical student, Lars Lyhne Knudsen, for assisting him in developing various stents and mounting the leaflets and valves within. Andersen et al. went on to implant 35 more devices in-vitro in pigs. Their work was initially widely rejected and even ridiculed by journals, as well as many cardiothoracic surgeons around the world. In May 1992, their work was finally accepted and published by European Heart Journal [3]. In 1995, Andersen, Hasenkam, and Knudsen obtained a patent for their new invention. Over the next few years, their work rapidly began to gain recognition and other groups replicated their techniques utilizing both self-expandable and balloon-expandable valves on dogs, sheep, and pigs, all with positive outcomes.

On April 16, 2002, at the Charles Nicolle University Hospital in Rouen, France, Alain Cribier became the first to successfully perform aortic valve placement in an adult human patient [4]. Cribier went on to repeat his success utilizing both the traditional retrograde approach as well as the antegrade atrial trans-septal approach [5, 6]. All his implantations were performed under conscious sedation without the need for extracorporeal circulation and on high-risk inoperable patients, some of which were already in a state of cardiogenic shock. His trans-septal approach proved to be time-consuming, complex, and associated with more complications. Furthermore, interventionalists were becoming more comfortable with percutaneous techniques via various arterial access sites (more recently including the carotid artery). Thus, the anterograde methodology was abandoned. In 2003, Cribier's startup company, Percutaneous Valve Technologies, was acquired by Edwards Lifesciences for $125 million. Thus, the Cribier-Edwards bioprosthetic valve became the first-generation of in-human transcatheter aortic valve replacement (TAVR) valves. In 2004, the first TAVR procedure was performed in the United States by Dr. William O'Neill at Henry Ford Hospital.

In the subsequent years, many clinical scientists, biotechnological companies, investors, and physicians joined this attractive and fiercely growing industry. Many augmented the devices and delivery systems while others continued to work on improving the technique itself. In 2007, the Edwards SAPIEN valve, made of bovine pericardium, was introduced as a life-saving option for prohibitive high surgical risk patients [7, 8]. Meanwhile that same year, Webb et al. demonstrated the feasibility and efficacy of the retrograde approach for TAVR [9].

The first clinical trials which successfully elucidated the feasibility and safety of TAVR were the Registry of Endovascular Critical Aortic Stenosis Treatment (RECAST) and the Initial Registry of EndoVascular Implantation of Valves in Europe (I-REVIVE) [5, 6].

By 2009, the two predominant valves in the industry were the self-expandable CoreValve ReValving system (CoreValve Inc., Irvine, California) and the balloon-expandable Edwards SAPIEN valve (Edwards Lifescience, Irvine, California). In 2009, CoreValve Inc. was acquired by Medtronic for over $700 million, thus allowing rapid global marketing, larger clinical trials, and continuous device refinement to minimize procedural complications and optimize outcomes. At the time, two momentous clinical trials which enrolled nearly 10,000 patients—the CoreValve/Evolut trial and the PARTNER (Placement of Aortic Transcatheter Valves) trial—demonstrated significant superiority with TAVR compared to medical management in patients with severe AS with high surgical risk [10]. Thus, prompt approval for TAVR by the U.S. Food and Drug Administration followed in 2011. By 2014, TAVR was being performed in over 50 countries, in over 720 centers around the world [11].

In 2016, positive results from the PARTNER II and the Surgical Replacement and Transcatheter Aortic Valve Implantation (SURTAVI) trials proved the balloon expandable Edwards SAPIEN XT and Medtronic's CoreValve self-expanding valve to be non-inferior to surgery with respect to stroke and mortality even in patients who were intermediate surgical risk [12]. In 2019, published results from the PARTNER 3 trial revealed that the newer-generation SAPIEN 3 Ultra TAVR valve demonstrated superiority to surgery in both primary and numerous secondary endpoints in even low surgical patients [13]. As of 2023, the three-year follow-up outcomes from the ongoing Evolut Low Risk trial paired with the PARTNER 3 outcomes, continue to demonstrate overall non-inferiority of TAVR to SAVR in low-risk patients [14]. These promising results continue to be sustained. By 2025, over a quarter million TAVRs are projected to be performed annually around the world [11]. As more other ongoing global clinical trials continue to suggest both feasibility and safety of TAVR regardless of surgical risk, the paradigm global shifts towards perfecting the solution to severe aortic stenosis are expected to continue.

3. Indications

Today, TAVR is an FDA-approved treatment option for patients with severe native calcific AS of all risk profiles and for patients with failed surgical bioprosthetic valves. Preliminary results from clinical trials investigating outcomes in patients with low surgical risks are ongoing. We determine this risk using the Society of Thoracic Surgeon (STS) scoring system. A score greater than or equal to 4% (predicted risk of surgical mortality at 30 days) is the cutoff in today's practice in determining eligibility for TAVR. The EuroSCORE II is an alternative scoring system that can be used for risk stratification. An STS score of ≥8% or a EuroSCORE II >15–20% indicates high risk.

According to the American Heart Association (AHA) guidelines and the European Society of Cardiology (ESC) guidelines, patients with severe low-flow low-gradient AS who have a left ventricular ejection fraction of less than 50% should also undergo TAVR regardless of the presence or absence of symptomatology [15]. If ejection fraction is preserved in these patients, the AHA issues a class 1 recommendation for intervention whereas Europe issues a class IIa recommendation. Asymptomatic patients with severe AS who have a preserved ejection fraction, should only undergo intervention on a case-by-case basis such as in patients with rapid rates of stenosis, severely elevated serum levels of B-type natriuretic peptide (Pro-BNP), or exercise intolerance [15–19].

Both North American and European guidelines mutually share the same criteria to classify severity and type of AS. We define severe high gradient AS a maximum velocity greater than or equal to 4.0 m/s with a mean transaortic gradient greater than or equal to 40 mmHg typically associated with an aortic valve area of <1.0 cm^2. We define low-flow low gradient severe AS having a valve area of less than 1.0 cm^2 with a concomitant maximum velocity less than 4.0 m/s and a mean transaortic gradient less than 40 mmHg. Although both North American and European societies agree on the indication of TAVR for older and high-risk patients. The European guidelines currently remain more conservative in their approach in younger patients requiring bioprosthetic valves. TAVR is generally considered in these patients only after the age of 75. The AHA however, recommends considerations of TAVR in patients above the age of 65 [15]. A schematic for diagnosis and treatment of AS adopted from the 2020 AHA guidelines is shown in **Figure 3** [16].

Factors that favor TAVR over SAVR include age, frailty, higher surgical risk, redo surgery, patients with prior radiation therapy to the chest, presence of a porcelain aorta, and the availability of a healthy percutaneous access sites. Factors that favor SAVR include younger age, bicuspid aortic valve, multivessel CAD, aortopathy requiring intervention, and concomitant significant valvulopathy necessitating cardiac surgery. As of now, there are no recommendations for early transcatheter intervention in patients with moderate AS. Clinical trials such as the TAVR UNLOAD trial in which we are assessing the safety and efficacy of TAVR in patients with moderate AS have been initiated and are currently ongoing. The indications for TAVR are anticipated to continuously evolve in years to come.

4. Contraindications

It is imperative for clinicians to be aware of both absolute and relative contraindications for TAVR. Absolute clinical contraindications include patient life expectancy of less than 12 months, myocardial infarction within the last 30 days, stroke within the last 6 months, patient intolerance to an anticoagulation/antiplatelet regimen, the absence of a Heart Team and cardiothoracic surgical team, and active bacteremia or endocarditis. Absolute anatomical contraindications include heavy aortic or left ventricular outflow tract disease and calcification, a short distance between the coronary ostia and the native aortic annulus, annulus size that is too small (less than 18 mm) or too large (greater than 29 mm), and the presence of mobile plaques and thrombi in the aorta and unsuitable access options [20].

Relative contraindications for TAVR include severe left ventricular dysfunction (EF <20%), inadequate heavily calcified femoral arteries, hemodynamic instability, severe pulmonary hypertension resulting in right ventricular dysfunction, hypertrophic cardiomyopathy, and severe mitral regurgitation.

5. Pre-procedural work-up

Appropriate patient selection via individual risk stratification, optimal valve sizing, and determining feasibility of different access routes are all factors that are

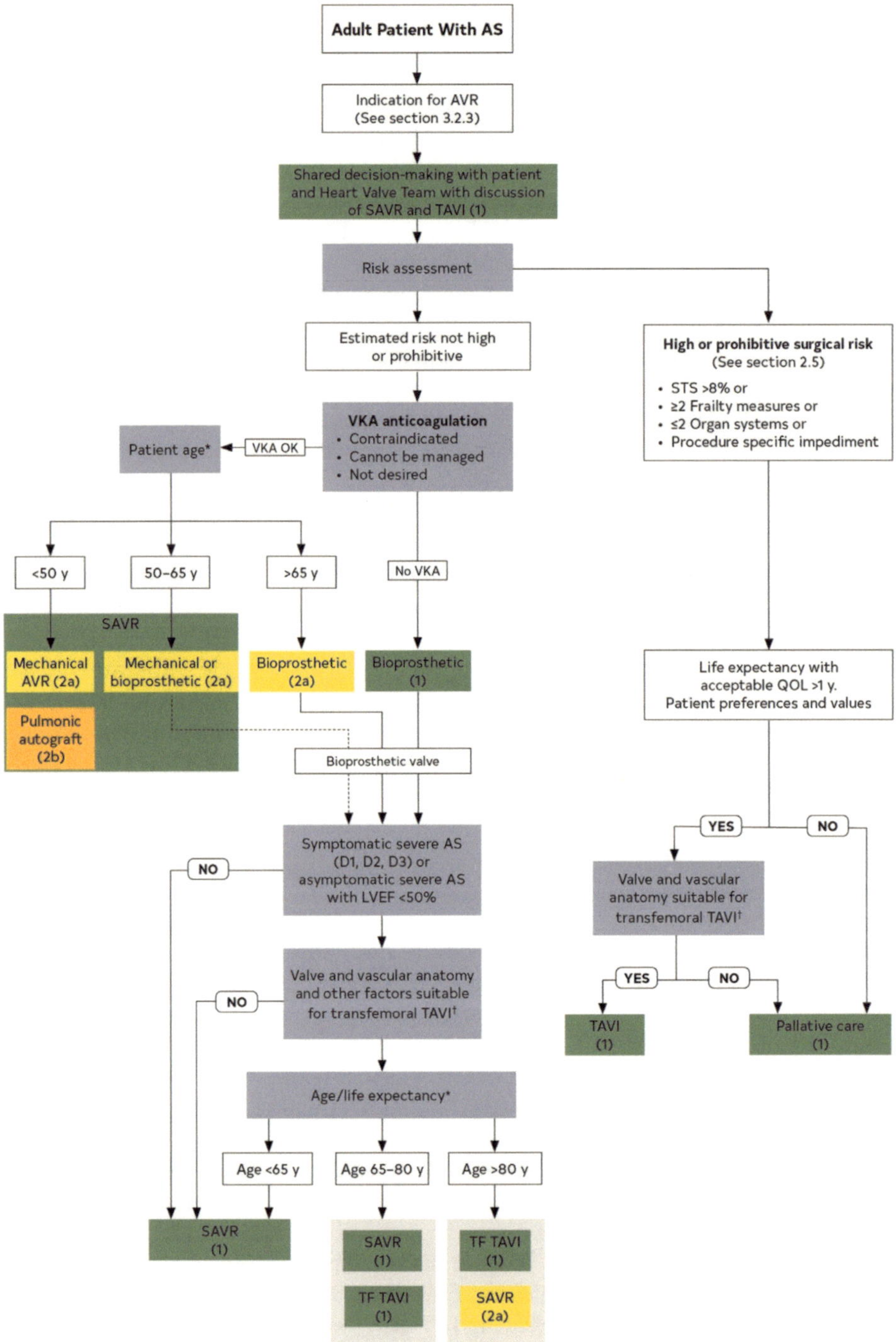

Figure 3.
A schematic for management of AS adopted from the 2020 AHA guidelines (image obtained from Ref. [16]).

carefully and meticulously worked up prior to TAVR. This pre-screening is an ever-changing multifaceted selection process that utilizes a multidisciplinary approach. A Heart Team consisting of an interventional cardiologist, cardiac surgeon, clinical cardiologist, and anesthetist are responsible for actively performing the pre-procedural screening and work-up. However, because these patients are generally elder with many comorbidities, physicians from even other specialties often participate in pre-procedural optimization.

The confirmation of severe AS is done with echocardiography demonstrating a valve area of <1.0 cm^2 mean pressure gradient of 40 mmHg or greater or a maximum aortic velocity of 4.0 m/s or greater. This step is heavily operator dependent as any misalignment of the probe can result in underestimation of the pressure gradient and jet velocity. The measured valve area should be indexed to the patient's body surface area ≤ 0.6 cm^2/m^2 in patients with normal left ventricular ejection fraction. Note that patients with low-flow, low gradient severe AS may have aortic velocities and valve gradients that are falsely lower. If these patients demonstrate a reduced ejection fraction, then we use low-dose dobutamine echocardiography (maximum dose 20 μg/kg/min) to mimic normal physiological flow and obtain accurate values. If valve area remains $\leq$1.0 cm^2 and peak velocity exceeds 4.0 m/s, then a diagnosis of true severe AS is made regardless of the flow rate. If the aortic valve area increases to greater than 1.0 cm^2 during dobutamine echocardiography, then a diagnosis of pseudo-severe AS or moderate AS can be assumed, and the patient should undergo heart failure therapy and close clinical follow-up.

Transesophageal echocardiography tends to underestimate the severity of AS when compared to transthoracic echocardiography [21]. In the majority of patients, transthoracic echocardiography is adequate enough to confidently establish a diagnosis of severe AS. However, when there are discordant findings, we look for other tests to help guide our decision-making. Thus, in addition to echocardiography, we utilize computed tomography to confirm the severity of AS. Similar to that of coronary calcium scoring, computed tomography allows us to use the Agatston algorithm to quantitate the severity of aortic valve calcifications. We utilize calcium score cutoffs of 2065 in males and 1275 in females for severe AS [22]. Recent studies have revealed that an elevated pre-TAVR calcium score from computed tomography is an independent risk factor for acute stroke, thus providing prognostication capabilities as well [23]. Computed tomography also provides the added benefit of a three-dimensional visualization of the valve and left ventricular outflow tract as two-dimensional imaging often results in underestimation of the severity of stenosis. This is largely due to the fact that the continuity equation which we use to calculate valve area from stroke volume states that flow passing through the outflow tract equals the flow through the aortic valve and assumes a circular outflow tract though in reality, the tract is frequently oval. Computed tomography angiography of the chest, abdomen, and pelvis is generally also done to help confirm valve size but more importantly, to visualize the patient's vasculature and determine the optimal entry point for access, if any.

Because the association of coronary artery disease and AS is strong, conventional guidelines recommended left heart catheterization prior to TAVR in order to assess presence of unstable coronary disease and determine if revascularization or bypass grafting should be performed prior to AVR. Depending on heart catheterization findings, the Heart Team may elect to proceed with SAVR versus TAVR. However, recent studies published by AHA revealed that revascularization TAVR did not result in improved clinical outcomes and in fact, was associated with an increased risk of major vascular complications and 30-day mortality [24].

Other conventional preprocedural testing includes carotid duplex ultrasonography, pulmonary function testing, and assessing baseline ambulatory function status, complete blood counts, and renal function. Carotid ultrasonography allows clinicians to screen for internal carotid artery stenosis which is believed by many to correlate with risk of periprocedural stroke. However, some studies have since emerged showing no statistically significant benefit in performing carotid ultrasonography [25, 26]. For now however, it remains a part of preprocedural workup at many centers. Pulmonary function testing remains a routine part of the risk stratification and STS scoring of patients undergoing valve replacement as the severity of the patient's lung disease continue to show direct correlation to peri-procedural mortality [27].

We universally assess for baseline functional status with a simple outpatient six-minute walk test during which we assess both speed, gait, and ability to complete the test. It is a simple and cheap test that helps us further risk stratify patients and to monitor functional status pre and post procedurally. Among high-risk adults undergoing TAVR, the six-minute walk test does not predict post-procedural outcomes but does however predict long-term mortality [28].

Renal function is also important to assess as both acute and chronic kidney disease are associated with adverse events in patients undergoing valve replacement [29]. In patients who develop acute kidney injuries, studies have shown a four-fold increase in postoperative mortality [30, 31]. A baseline complete blood count allows to assess platelet counts and for any anemia. Finally, a preprocedural international normalized ratio and type and screen are also obtained as part of preprocedural blood work.

6. Contemporary devices

Contemporary TAVR devices consist of balloon-expandable valves, self-expanding valves, mechanically expanding valves, and delivery systems/sheaths. In the last two decades, technological advancements have significantly improved devices by incorporating and enhancing features that allow for recapture, easier deployment, repositioning, all while reducing associated complications such as perivalvular leaks and stroke [32]. As TAVR continues to undergo procedural modifications and indications, these devices are expected to continue to evolve. As of 2023, there are three newer-generation valves that are FDA-approved for commercial TAVR in the US: the SAPIEN 3 Ultra (Edwards Lifesciences), Evolut PRO+ (Medtronic), and Portico (Abbott Laboratories). Other valves such as the ACURATE Neo/Neo2 (Boston Scientific), JenaValve (JenaValve Technology), Myval THV (Meril Life Sciences), Allegra (New Valve Technologies) have Conformite Europeenne (CE) markings by the European Union and actively undergoing review for potential US FDA-approval in the near future.

Balloon-expandable valves are intra-annular valves that include the Sapien system and the Myval system. They require transient rapid ventricular pacing with concomitant valve-balloon inflation. Close monitoring of the pacer lead is imperative in order to avoid risk of pacing lead perforation. The cons of these valves are that they are not able to be repositioned. Additionally, sicker patients may not be able to tolerate rapid ventricular pacing, thus hemodynamics must be very closely monitored. One major advantage of these valves is that they have a lower frame height thus allowing for easier coronary access [33, 34]. They have delivery sheaths that typically allow for better controllable flexibility and steerability, and thus are preferred in patients with difficult vascular anatomy.

Self-expanding valves are typically supra-annular but newer prototypes that are intra-annular are now being manufactured. These valves do not require rapid ventricular pacing. They offer the advantage of being able to be repositioned and

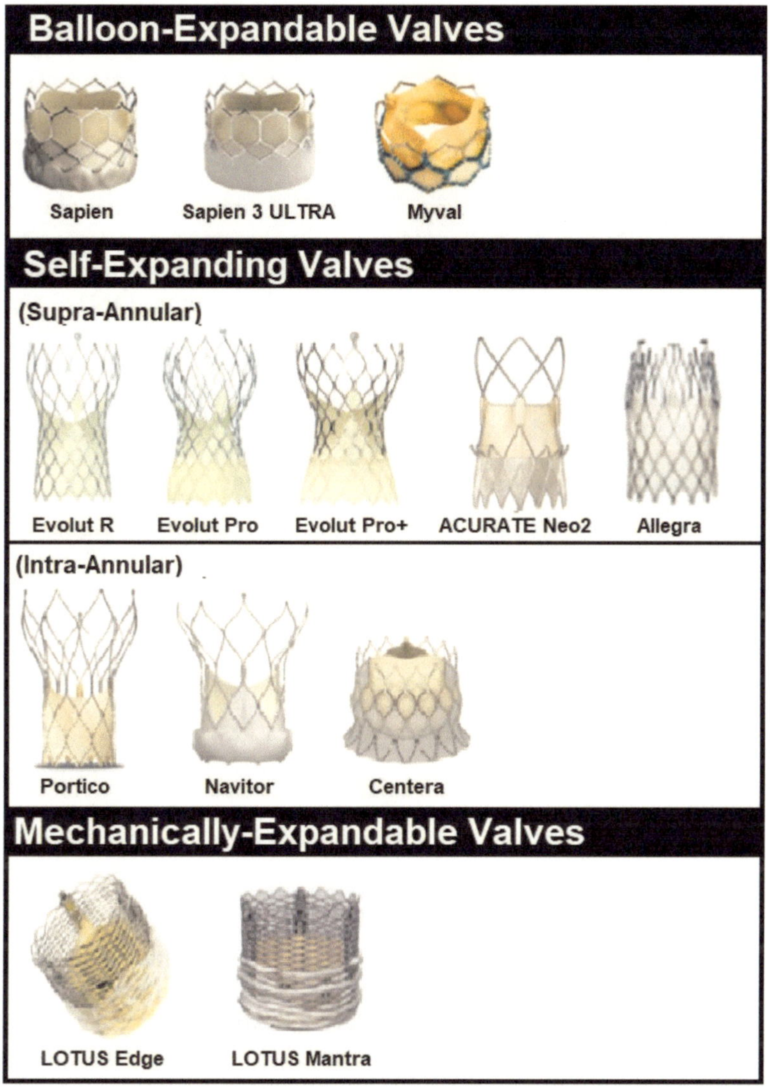

Figure 4.
Various types of contemporary transcatheter aortic valves.

retrievable. The cons of these valves include limited maneuverability. They also tend to create a greater challenge for coronary access due to their larger frame sizes. Self-expanding valves tend to have higher rates of pacemaker implantations and paravalvular leaks (**Figure 4**) [35].

6.1 SAPIEN 3 Ultra (Edwards Lifesciences)

The balloon-expandable SAPIEN 3 Ultra transcatheter aortic valve is the fifth-generation valve in the Sapien series and is available in four sizes (20, 23, 26, and 29 mm). Its design consists of three bovine pericardial tissue leaflets with a cobalt-chromium frame. The novel modifications of this device include the polyethylene terephthalate cuff that has significantly minimized the rate and degree of paravalvular leaks. The Ultra has a greater frame height than the previous generation, allowing an even greater reduction of paravalvular leaks [36]. It is neither retrievable nor repositionable. The Commander Delivery System (Edwards Lifesciences) consists of an inner balloon on which the valve is crimped prior to advancement. A transfemoral approach is preferred using a 14 or 16 French (F) Edwards eSheath and crimper. In cases in which femoral access is not feasible or appropriate, a transaortic or transapical approach may also be utilized. In such cases, a Certitude delivery system is needed. This system is compatible with 18 and 21-F sheaths. The 21-F sheath is reserved for the larger 29 mm valve. The PARTNER trials are the largest clinical trials that have reported outcomes of the SAPIEN 3 which led to FDA approvals in all four risk profiles. When compared to the SAVR cohort from PARTNER II, TAVR with the SAPIEN 3 valve demonstrated lower rates of mortality (7% vs. 12.4%) and stroke (4.5% vs. 7.9%) at 1-year follow up in low-risk patients [13].

6.2 Myval (Meril Life Sciences)

The balloon expandable Myval heart valve obtained its CE mark in 2019. It consists of a tri-leaflet made of bovine pericardium on a cobalt alloy frame as well as a polyethylene terephthalate cuff similar to the SAPIEN 3 that is in place both internally and externally to reduce paravalvular leaks. It comes in nine sizes (20, 21.5, 23, 24.5, 26, 27.5, 29, 30.5, and 32 mm). The valves should be crimped over Navigator THV Balloon Delivery System (Meril Life Sciences) prior to advancement through the introducer.

6.3 Evolut PRO+/FX (Medtronic)

The self-expanding supra-annular Evolut Pro+ is a new generation FDA-approved valve in the Evolut series and offers the lowest delivery profile for 23–29 mm valves, capable of treating vessels down to 5.0 mm. Valves from this series have been the most extensively studied and most commonly implanted. It is available in four sizes (23, 26, 29, and 34 mm). Its design consists of three porcine pericardial tissue leaflets mounted on a frame made of nitinol. The novel modification of this device is the newly added porcine external skirt which minimizes paravalvular leaks [37]. Valves of the Evolut series have been shown to cause greater rates of conduction disturbances and pacemaker dependency compared to some of the other valves [38]. However, the data available on the Pro+ thus far has shown lower rates of pacemaker implantation. The delivery system allows the valve to be recaptured up to three times. In the US Evolut PRO Study, zero patients experienced moderate paravalvular leak during the same follow-up period used in the PARTNER II SAPIEN 3 trial, in which moderate paravalvular leak was seen in 3.4% of patients. In 2022, Medtronic announced their next generation of Evolut valve—the Evolut FX. They have significantly improved commissural alignment which we anticipate will allow better coronary flow and access when needed. The FX also allows for easier tracking as it now has gold markers built into the frame. These prototype modifications should overall help improve alignment

DOI: http://dx.doi.org/10.5772/intechopen.113334

and allow for symmetric implantations. Multicenter studies are ongoing but preliminary data has thus far shown favorable outcomes.

6.4 ACURATE Neo/Neo2 (Boston Scientific)

The ACURATE Neo2 is a self-expanding supra-annular nitinol alloy stent available in three sizes: small (21–23 mm), medium (23–25 mm), and large (25–27 mm). Its design consists of porcine leaflets mounted on a large-cell nitinol frame that allows for easy coronary access. An 18-F sheath is required for transfemoral approach. A simple two-step deployment provides the operator with greater ease of deployment. The global SAVI registry revealed very positive outcomes in terms of pacemaker implantation rates and stroke (8.2% and 1.9% respectively) [39].

6.5 Portico (Abbott Laboratories)

The self-expanding intra-annular Portico TAVI system was approved by the FDA in 2021. It is available in four sizes (23, 25, 27, and 29 mm). Its design consists of bovine leaflets mounted on a large-cell nitinol frame. The annular and large-cell design allows for easy coronary access. It is fully re-sheathable. An 18-F sheath is required and used with its FlexNav delivery system which Abbott claims to need 76% less insertion force than the Evolut PRO.

6.6 LOTUS Edge (Boston Scientific)

The LOTUS Edge is the second of the LOTUS mechanically expandable valve series that allows for hemodynamic evaluation and repositioning as needed prior to deployment. The expansion is mediated by a mechanical controlled system. Mortality rates in patients who have undergone TAVR with LOTUS were very comparable to the rates from SAPIEN 3 [40]. The LOTUS edge was FDA-approved in 2019. Since then, the newest generation (Mantra) has been created as well. At this time however, these valves have been recalled due to issues with its delivery system, but due to a substantial number of patients in whom the valve was implanted, operators need to be familiar with the valve and its design.

7. Equipment and personnel

The care of a patient with severe aortic stenosis should be collaboratively under a Heart Team that consists of a primary cardiologist, an interventional cardiologist, cardiothoracic surgeon, radiologist, and anesthetist. We discussed the meticulous workup and pre-screening measures necessary prior to fully committing to a transcatheter approach. Depending on the comorbidities of the patient, additional specialists may be invited to help fine-tune and optimize patients prior to undergoing TAVR. This multidisciplinary team is needed even post-procedurally to ensure proper follow-up and care should any complications arise.

Centers who wish to pursue TAVR are recommended to have an active valvular heart disease program with at least two surgeons experienced in valvular surgery.

A heart catheterization laboratory, high quality radiology and imaging department should also available. Access to multiple echocardiographic modalities is also necessary. A hybrid operating room is preferred but not mandatory.

The American College of Cardiology, along with partnering societies (AATS, SCAI, STS, ACCF) clearly delineate the components needed for centers to establish and maintain a TAVR program. Quality is the primary endpoint. These are assessed with several various metrics. Due to the learning curves associated with the procedure, having adequate volume of patients is necessary. It has been shown that roughly 30–45 cases are needed for operators to plateau in their procedure times and success rates [41, 42]. The slope for major post-procedural outcomes however remains steep for roughly the first 100 cases [43]. Thus, proceduralists are expected to have documented involvement with 100 cases with half (50) requiring them to be the primary operator. **Table 1** summarizes current requirements to establish TAVR programs.

ACC requirements for new TAVR programs [45]
There should be documentation of a multidisciplinary approach and of patient access to all forms of therapy for aortic valve disease (TAVR, SAVR, and palliative and medical care) using an SDM process. • For all patients with aortic stenosis meeting criteria for valve replacement, there should be documentation of the following: ◦ Completion of an evaluation by both a cardiac surgeon and a cardiologist with knowledge and experience in both TAVR and SAVR ◦ Education of patients regarding the treatment recommendations and options by the multidisciplinary team ◦ Use of an SDM process incorporating patient preference • For patients undergoing TAVR, there should be documentation of evaluation by 1 surgeon involved in the TAVR program ◦ For this requirement to fulfill CMS coverage criteria, the NCD should be updated as it currently recommends evaluation by surgeons for all patients having TAVR
The proposed TAVR proceduralist for a new TAVR program should document the following: • Prior TAVR experience with participation in 100 transfemoral TAVRs lifetime, including 50 TAVRs as primary operator • Being board eligible or certified in either interventional cardiology or cardiothoracic surgery • Certification of device-specific training on device(s) to be used.
The TAVR sites must have: • The site must have documented expertise, state of the art technology and dedicated board-certified imager. • Echocardiography: TTE, TEE and 3D • CT Scan and MR imaging
The proposed TAVR surgeon for a new TAVR program should document the following: • 100 lifetime SAVRs or 25 per prior year or 50 over 2 years and ≥20 SAVRs in the year prior to TAVR program initiation Board eligible or certified by the American Board of Thoracic Surgery or equivalent
The institution should document the following prior to expanding into alternative-access TAVR (e.g., transapical, direct aortic, brachiocephalic arteries, transcaval): • Completion of 80 TAVRs using transfemoral access with an STS/ACC TVT Registry 30-day risk-adjusted TAVR all-cause mortality “as expected” or “better than expected”
The institution should document the following concerning its SAVR program: • ≥2 hospital-based cardiac surgeons who both spend ≥50% time at the hospital with the proposed TAVR program • Minimum hospital SAVR volume†: 40 per prior year or 80 over 2 years • Quality assessment/quality improvement program:

ACC requirements for new TAVR programs [45]
◦ Active participation in the STS National Database or a validated state/multi-institutional consortium that gathers and reports risk adjusted and benchmarked outcomes ◦ Quality metric: STS 2- or 3-star rating for isolated AVR and AVR plus CABG in both reporting periods during the most recent reporting year
The institution should document the following resources and experience: • PCI ◦ Minimum volume: 300 PCI/year ◦ Active participation in the NCDR/Cath PCI Registry or a validated state/multi-institutional consortium that gathers and reports risk-adjusted and benchmarked outcomes ◦ Quality metric: PCI in-hospital risk-adjusted mortality (NQF endorsed) above the bottom 25th percentile for the most recent 4 consecutive quarters. • Vascular interventions ◦ Physicians experienced and competent in vascular arterial interventions • Pacemaker capabilities ◦ Experienced and competent physicians for temporary and permanent pacemaker placement and management ◦ On-site services should be available 24 hours/day and 7 days/week to handle conduction disturbances as a result of TAVR
Quality assessment/quality improvement program requirements: • Active participation of institution in STS/ACC TVT Registry and STS National Database or a validated state/multi-institutional consortium registry ◦ Registry submission of all cases using FDA-approved TAVR/SAVR technology, including off-label uses ◦ Registry documentation that data submissions meet performance metrics for completeness and accuracy as defined by each registry • Multidisciplinary team quarterly meetings with documentation of the following: ◦ Review of institutional reports for TAVR (quarterly) and SAVR (semi-annually) from the STS/ACC TVT Registry and STS National Database or an alternative approved registry ◦ Assessment and proposed actions if site performance for TAVR and SAVR is suboptimal relative to volume and quality requirements, including national benchmarking of performance metrics ◦ Presentation of selected TAVR/SAVR cases at quarterly mortality/morbidity conferences

Table 1.
TAVR program recommendations and requirements in the United States as of 2018 per official statement by ACC and its partnering societies. Obtained from Bavaria et al. (obtained from Ref. [44]).

8. Techniques

The TAVR procedure is commonly performed in a hybrid room that has both Cath lab and operating room abilities, although some are performing the procedure in a standard cardiac catheterization laboratory. Primarily driven by visualization on fluoroscopy correlating to previously performed CT scan. At times, various Heart Teams will use transesophageal echocardiographic coregistration with fluoroscopy. There are various accesses used, with transfemoral arterial approach being the most common one. Approximately more than 95% of cases are completed this way. The femoral route has also shown lower rates of complications. However, when this method cannot be used due to severe tortuosity or diseased iliofemoral arterial vessels, an alternative route can be chosen based on the particular valve being used, patient's risk factors, or if a patient has unfavorable iliofemoral artery characteristics [44].

The alternative common access options include transubclavian access, transthoracic approach (transapical antegrade and transaortic retrograde), and transcarotid approach.

- *Transsubclavian/transaxillary approach* is done by a surgical cut-down to the subclavian artery or percutaneous axillary artery access for insertion of the valve. The axillary artery's proximal third (between the medial border of pectoralis minor and lateral border of the first rib) demonstrates an ideal area for both surgical and percutaneous methods.

- *Transaortic approach* is performed by a direct insertion of the valve delivery system into the ascending aorta via a sheath in the aorta from a lateral thoracotomy or median sternotomy.

- *Transapical approach* is best for patients who have severe peripheral artery disease or heavily calcified aorta/ascending arch. These patients typically are at a higher risk for stroke or other embolic events.

- *Transcarotid approach* is done with a surgical-cut of the common carotid artery. It is important to use neurologic monitoring with this approach.

- *Transcaval approach* involves the femoral vein and percutaneous electrosurgical techniques to puncture from the inferior vena cava into the aorta (**Table 2**) [44].

Access	Procedural success (%)	30 D mortality	Major and life-threatening bleeding	Neurological events (TIA/ stroke)	New pacemaker implantation (%)
Trans-femoral (3–14)	95–100	2.1–5%‡ 5.2–9.7%†	9.3–28.1%‡ 3.5–11.4%†	1.4–6.7% (30 days stroke) 2.3–4.1% (1 year stroke)	3.4–34.1 5.9–20.1
Trans-axyllarian (16)	97.9	5.7%	7.8% life threatening 36.2% major bleeding	2.1%	24.7
Trans-aortic (17–24)	87–100	6.1–13%	0.3–12%	0–3.2%	0–14
Trans-apical (13, 25–28)	90–96	4.6–14%	3.6–6.1%	1.3–4.1%	5.4–11.0
Trans-carotid (29)	100	6.3%	4.2%	3.1% (all TIAs, stroke not reported)	26.5
Trans-caval (30, 31)	100	8%	12% (6% transcaval related)	5%	16

†Data derived from TVT. Gary. UK TAVI. Observant and France2 registries.‡Data derived from Partner A, Partner B, Partner II, Notion and SURTAVI trials.

Table 2.
Procedural outcomes per access site [46].

DOI: http://dx.doi.org/10.5772/intechopen.113334

9. Procedure

9.1 Edwards SAPIEN 3 transcatheter heart valve (THV)

Sterile technique is to be followed during the device preparation and implantation (**Figure 5**) [47].

Rinsing procedure:

1. The THV comes in a jar. Examine the valve before opening the device for any signs of damage. If there are signs of leaking, missing seals, etc. the valve should not be used for implantation.

2. Place two sterile bowls with approximately 500 mL of sterile saline to fully rinse out the glutaraldehyde sterilant from the heart valve.

3. Next, carefully remove the THV from the jar without touching the tissue. Compare the THV serial identification number with the one on the jar lid. Check again for any damage to the THV.

4. Rinse the THV in first bowl of sterile saline. Make sure the saline completely covers the THV and the holder. Submerge both and slowly swirl the saline for approximately 1 minute. Transfer the THV and holder to second bowl. Again, slowly swirl the saline for another minute. Leave the THV in the second bowl until needed. This is to keep the THV hydrated and prevent the tissue from drying. CAUTION: The THV should be the only thing placed in the rinse bowl. Direct contact should also be avoided during the rinse process [47].

Preparing the device components:

1. Inspect all the components for any signs of damage. Check to see if the Edwards Commander delivery system is unflexed and make sure the balloon catheter is advanced in the flex catheter.

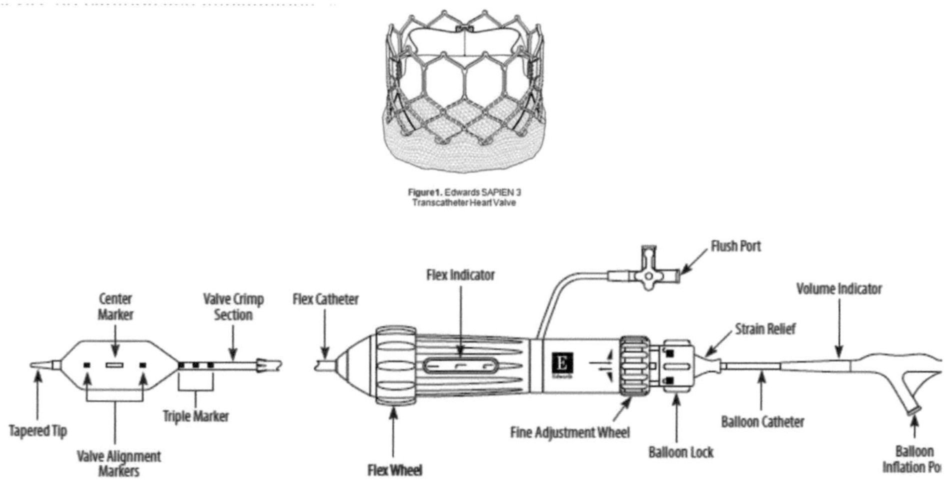

Figure 5.
Edwards commander delivery system [47].

2. Flush out the flex catheter.

3. Remove the distal balloon cover carefully from the delivery system.

4. From the distal end of the guidewire, remove the stylet and put aside. Flush the guidewire with heparinized saline and insert the stylet back through the distal portion of guidewire lumen.

5. Cover the flex catheter tip with proximal balloon cover and put the delivery system in default position. Unscrew the loader cap located in loader tube and flush it. Place this loader cap on the proximal balloon cover and on the flex catheter.

6. Advance the balloon catheter into the flex catheter. Remove the proximal balloon over the balloon shaft in the blue section.

7. Put a 3-way stopcock to the balloon inflation port. Fill a syringe with about 20 mL diluted contrast medium and attach that to the 3-way stopcock as well.

8. Fill the inflation device and then lock it and attach to stopcock.

9. Close the 3-way stopcock to inflation device and then de-air the system using a 500 cc syringe. Release the plunger slowly and have zero-pressure in the system.

10. Close the 3-way stopcock towards the delivery system. Transfer contrast medium to the syringe based on the delivery system and THV size.

11. Close stopcock to the syringe and remove the syringe. Lock the Inflation device until THV deployment (**Table 3**) [47].

Mount the THV onto the delivery system:

1. Place two sterile bowls with approximately 100 mL of sterile saline to rinse the Qualcrimp crimping accessory.

2. Submerge this accessory in the first bowl and slowly swirl it for about 1 minute. Repeat this in the second bowl.

THV size (mm)	Inflation volume (mL)
20	11
23	17
26	23
29	33

Table 3.
Inflation volume with corresponding THV size.

3. Remove ID tag from the THV. Attach the crimp stopper to the base and click into place.

4. Have the crimper in the open position and place the THV in the crimper aperture.

5. Make sure the THV is parallel to the Qualcrimp edge. Place both the Qualcrimp accessory and the THV in the crimper aperture. The delivery system should be inserted within the THV in the Valve Crimp section by having the inflow of the THV on the distal end of the delivery system.

6. The THV should be crimped until it is at the Qualcrimp Stop which is on the 2 piece Crimp stopper.

7. Carefully remove the Qualcrimp crimping accessory from the THV and remove the Qualcrimp Stop therefore leaving the Final Stop in place.

8. Crimp the THV fully until it also reaches the Final Stop. Repeat the crimp of the THV two more times.

9. Next, pull at the balloon shaft and lock it in the default position.

10. With heparinized saline, flush the loader and advance the THV into the loader until the tip is exposed.

11. Place the loader cap to the loader, re-flush the delivery system, and close the stopcock to the delivery system. Remove stylet and flush the guidewire of the system [47].

THV delivery:

1. Prepare the Edwards eSheath introducer and insert the loader into the sheath.

2. Advance the delivery system through the sheath until the THV is out of the sheath. Then retract the loader to be at the proximal end of the delivery system.

3. Begin valve alignment in a straight section of the aorta by unlocking the balloon lock and pulling the balloon catheter back. Engage the balloon lock and position the THV in between the valve alignment markers.

4. Advance the catheter with using the flex wheel. Confirm the position of the THV with the aortic annulus. Adjust position as necessary.

5. Begin the THV deployment by unlocking the inflation device. Start rapid pacing; balloon inflation can begin once the systolic blood pressure is down to 50 mmHg or lower. Inflate the balloon and deploy the THV. Hold for 3 seconds and make sure the inflation device barrel is empty. Deflate the balloon and turn off the pacemaker [47].

System removal:

1. Retract the device while unflexing the delivery system. Remove the devices when the ACT level is appropriate. Close the access site [47].

9.2 Medtronic Evolut FX transcatheter aortic valve

See **Figures 6–8**.

9.2.1 Anatomical criteria

See **Table 4**.
Inspection and rinsing:

1. Carefully inspect the device packaging for any signs of damage. Remove the product from the package.

2. Inspect the product for any signs of defects.

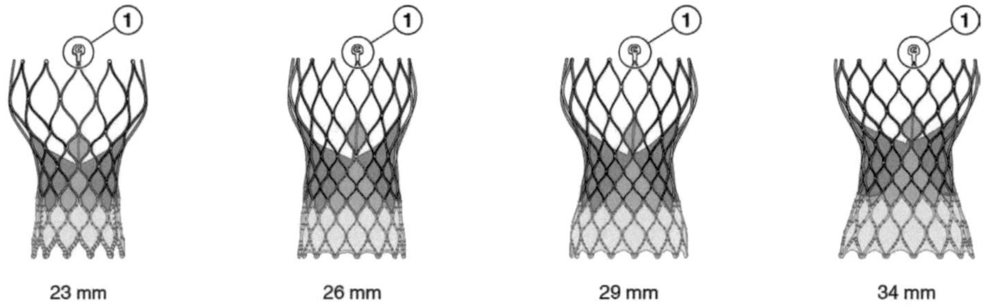

1- C paddle

Figure 6.
Available valve sizes.

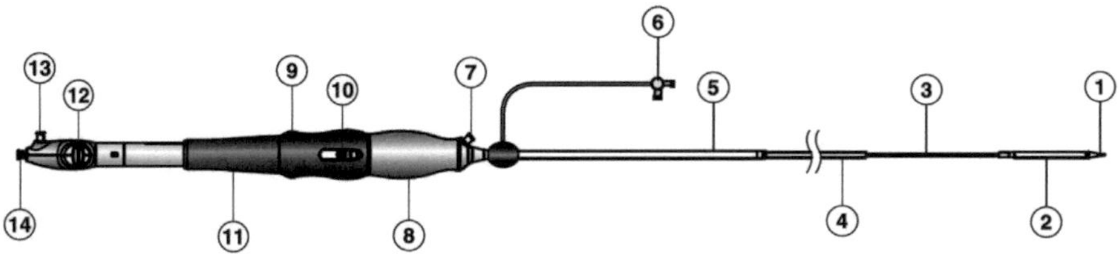

1 Catheter tip
2 Capsule (Model D-EVOLUTFX-2329: 18 Fr [6.0 mm] outer diameter [OD]; Model D-EVOLUTFX-34: 22 Fr [7.33 mm] OD)
3 Catheter shaft
4 Stability layer
5 Model D-EVOLUTFX-2329: 14 Fr equivalent Evolut FX inline sheath (18 Fr [6.0 mm] OD); Model D-EVOLUTFX-34: 18 Fr equivalent Evolut FX inline sheath (22 Fr [7.33 mm] OD)
6 Evolut FX inline sheath flush port
7 Stability layer flush port
8 Gray front grip
9 Deployment knob
10 Trigger
11 Dark blue hand rest
12 Tip-retrieval mechanism
13 Capsule flush port
14 Wire lumen flush port

Figure 7.
Delivery catheter system (catheter) [48].

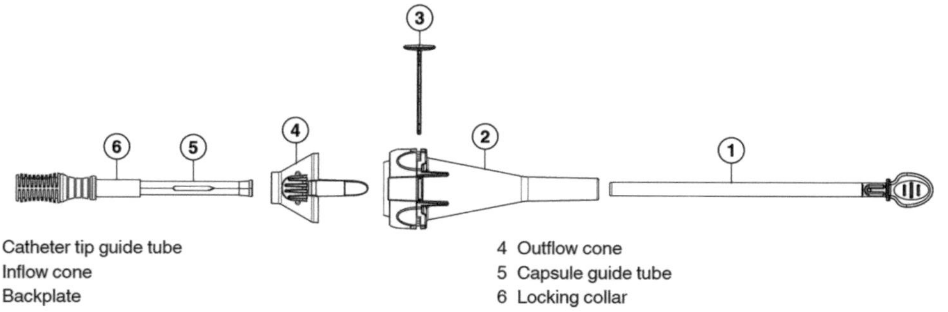

Figure 8.
Evolut FX loading system [48].

Size	Aortic annulus diameter	Aortic annulus perimeter ($\pi \times$ aortic annulus diameter)
23 mm	17[a]/18 mm to 20 mm	53.4[a]/56.5 mm to 62.8 mm
26 mm	20 mm to 23 mm	62.8 mm to 72.3 mm
29 mm	23 mm to 26 mm	72.3 mm to 81.7 mm
34 mm	26 mm to 30 mm	81.7 mm to 94.2 mm

Table 4.
Anatomical aortic annulus diameter and perimeters with corresponding valve sizes.

3. Remove the locking clips on the rinsing bowls and remove the bowls from the integrated loading bath.

4. Detach the locking clips from the distal and proximal trays.

5. From the distal tray, raise the tray tab to the tray tab holder on the proximal tray.

6. Add cold, sterile saline to the integrated loading bath [48].

Catheter and loading system preparation:

1. Attach a 10 mL syringe with sterile saline on the proximal end of the handle to the capsule flush port. Keep the syringe attached until the loading is complete.

2. Lift the distal end of catheter to a vertical direction. Open the capsule to reveal the paddle attachment.

3. Next flush the capsule flush port. Make sure there is no leakage noted during flushing. If any leakage is noted, use a new system.

4. While flushing the capsule flush port, immerse the capsule in the cold saline bath.

5. Use a locking clip to position the catheter tip into the loading bath.

6. Put the loading system in the integrated loading bath [48].

Rinsing of the bioprosthesis:

1. Place 500 mL of sterile saline into three rinsing bowls.

2. Carefully remove the bioprosthesis from the packaging by using blunt foreceps.

3. Check the serial number attached on the tag of the bioprosthesis with the serial number on the container.

4. Remove the serial number tag from the bioprosthesis cautiously.

5. Place the bioprosthesis in one of the sterile rinsing bowls.

6. Carefully mix the bioprosthesis by hand in order to remove the glutaraldehyde.

7. Rinse the bioprosthesis in the second and third rinsing bowls. Leave it in the third bowl until ready to be used [48].

Loading procedure of bioprosthesis:

1. Immerse the bioprosthesis in the integrated loading bath.

2. Make sure the capsule guide tube is open (unlocked) with the locking collar at proximal end of capsule guide tube.

3. Advance the capsule guide tube over the catheter shaft and across the catheter tip.

4. Once across, advance the locking collar to the distal end of the capsule guide tube until it is locked (closed). Continue advancing until it reaches the distal end of the capsule.

5. Make sure the backplate is placed in the inflow cone and the uncovered part is facing up.

6. Place the inflow portion into the inflow cone. Check to make sure the bioprosthesis frame paddle has a "C" facing up and it is aligned with the paddle attachment pockets.

7. Place the outflow cone into the inflow cone until it is locked.

8. In the distal end of the inflow cone place the catheter tip guide tube. Place the distal catheter tip in the catheter tip guide tube.

9. Withdraw the catheter tip guide tube to place the bioprosthesis frame paddles in the attachment pockets.

10. Advance the capsule guide tube so the distal part covers the paddle attachment pockets as well as the top part of the outflow struts.

11. Continue advancing until the capsule catches the bioprosthesis outflow struts and until the distal end of the capsule guide tube covers the commissure pad.

12. From the outflow cone, remove the backplate and the catheter tip guide tube.

13. Advance the inflow cone to crimp the inflow portion of bioprosthesis frame. Move the locking collar to the proximal end of the guide tube.

14. Continue progressing until the capsule comes out 5 mm of the catheter tip.

15. Disconnect the capsule guide tube with the outflow and inflow cone.

16. Next, advance the capsule until the gap closes between the capsule and catheter tip.

17. Rotate the deployment knob towards the arrows to relive stress.

18. Inspect the capsule to make sure it is not misloaded and dree of bends.

19. Place a 10 mL syringe of sterile saline to the stability layer flush port.

20. Remove the loading stylet from guidewire lumen.

21. Place a 10 mL syringe of sterile saline on the proximal end of the handle to the wire lumen flush port.

22. Place a 10 mL syringe of sterile saline to the Evolut FX inline sheath flush port and flush it.

23. Check the loaded bioprosthesis under fluoroscopy before placing in the patient. After checking, leave the bioprosthesis immersed in sterile saline [48].

Implantation of bioprosthesis:

1. Achieve vascular access with a primary and secondary access artery. The primary access will place the Evolut FX device and the secondary access will place the reference pigtail.

2. Place a central line and insert a temporary pacemaker.

3. Place an introducer sheath into both accesses. Give anticoagulant, maintain ACT greater than 250 seconds.

4. Advance a pigtail catheter to the ascending aorta and fix the distal tip in the noncoronary cusp of the aortic valve.

5. Place an angiographic catheter over a J-tip guidewire in the primary access and progress to the ascending aorta.

6. Next, exchange the J-tip guidewire for a straight-tip guidewire and advance it across the aortic valve into the left ventricle. Then advance the angiographic catheter into the left ventricle.

7. Replace the straight-tip guidewire with an exchange length J-tip guidewire. Replace the angiographic catheter for a 6 french pigtail.

8. Take out the guidewire and connect the catheter to the transducer. Advance the pigtail catheter and place into the apex of the left ventricle. Remove the pigtail catheter with the guidewire in the left ventricle.

9. Advance the device over the guidewire with the delivery catheter flush ports towards the left side of the patient for better commissure alignment. Place the catheter tip and capsule through the access site and insert the Evolut FX inline sheath. Use fluoroscopy to watch the guidewire in the left ventricle.

10. With fluoroscopic assistance, advance the guidewire to the aortic annulus and advance the device through the valve. With angiogram make sure the pigtail catheter is in the correct position in the noncoronary cusp of the aortic root. The bioprosthesis should be at a target dept. of 3 mm in comparison to the valve annulus.

11. Rotate the deployment knob towards the arrows to deploy the bioprosthesis. Adjust valve position as needed and position the bioprosthesis in order for the radiopaque markers to be at the level of the native valve annulus.

12. Confirm the deployment with fluoroscopy or a second radiographic view [48].

9.3 Commissural alignment

ALIGN TAVR was a study done in 2020 which was the first complete evaluation of the importance of commissural alignment in TAVR. The study compared the effect of the initial deployment orientation of the 483 SAPIEN 3, 100 ACURATE-neo, and 245 Evolut transcatheter heart valves on the final orientation of commissural alignment. 828 patients from 5 centers were studied who had undergone the TAVR procedure from March 2016 to September 2019. The patient's pre-TAVR computed tomography (CT) imaging and procedure fluoroscopy were studied. The pre-TAVR CT had coplanar fluoroscopic views added to it to help determine the commissural alignment. The severe overlap in between the coronary arteries and neocommisural posts were defined as 0° to 20° apart. The different types of valves were classified differently. The Evolut and ACURATE-neo deployment commissural post were defined as center back (CB), center front (CF), inner curve (IC), and outer curve (OC). The Sapien 2 valve had commissural post at clock position 3, 6, 9, and 12. This study showed that valve alignment can be optimized. The SAPIEN 3's orientation did not have an impact on alignment. While ACURATE-neo commissural post showed less coronary artery overlap at the CB or IC in deployment versus in CF or OC. The Evoult "Hat" had less overlap at OC or CF at initial deployment versus IC or CB. This study showed the significance of optimizing valve alignments in order to avoid coronary artery overlap [49].

9.4 To TEE or not to TEE

Commonly the TAVR procedure is performed with a transesophageal echocardiography (TEE) probe in place. However there has been recent studies that suggest a different approach with similar results. This "Minimalist TAVR approach" is completed with no continuous TEE and the valve is placed with just angiography. A post-TAVR transthoracic echo (TTE) is done to allow for signs of early complications and view any para-valvular leaks. This is then followed by long term echocardiography completed within 1 month and 1 year to view the function of the prosthetic valve and see if there were any other changes due to the procedure such as pulmonary hypertension, mitral regurgitation, or tricuspid regurgitation [50].

10. Complications

As in any procedure, complications with TAVR can occur intra- and post-procedure. Some common complications include: (1) valve function (Paravalvular leakage (PVL)), (2) vascular access/bleeding complications (injury at arterial access site and/or vascular closure problems), (3) valve deployment (including malpositioning, annular rupture), (4) organ injuries (such as stroke, myocardial ischemia/injury, and acute kidney injury), (5) arrhythmic abnormalities like high-degree atrioventricular block and atrial fibrillation, and (6) in some cases death.

10.1 Paravalvular aortic regurgitation

Longer-Term complications include PVR. Patients with moderate and severe PVR had a three-time increase in 30-day mortality. Diagnosis of PVR includes multiple modalities such as doppler echocardiography, cardiac magnetic resonance, and angiography.

10.2 Vascular access bleeding

Access complications 30 days post procedure have ranged from 11% for high-risk cohorts [51]. Risk factors include severe tortuosity, percutaneous preclosure device failure, sheath-to-artery ratio, and presence of circumferential calcification. A mechanical factor that may increase bleeding risk is use of large delivery catheters. Of the various techniques, the transapical approach has been associated with related risk of myocardial tears [52]. Due to new technological advances, newer TAVR devices now have a 14F inner diameter instead of a 24–26F inner diameter sheaths required in the first TAVR systems. This has correlated with a decrease in vascular complications by 11–14%.

10.3 Valve deployment

Transcatheter heart valve malpositioning can occur due to lack of proper visualization or in inadequate ventricular pacing. Valve migration can also occur. Annular rupture is a very rare, unpredictable, and life-threatening complication typically related to balloon aortic valvuloplasty or balloon-expandable valves.

10.4 Aortic dissection

Aortic dissection is a rare and possibly fatal complication of the procedure. Approximately 0.6–1.9% incidence rate has been shown after a TAVR procedure. Any part of the ascending or descending aorta can be involved in the dissection depending on which access approach was used. If post procedure an aortic dissection is suspected, aortic angiography can be used. The patient can have various symptoms and signs including chest pain, abdominal pain, and hypotension. It is important to note that the treatment of aortic dissection will vary based on the site and type of dissection. Type A dissections need to be treated with surgery while Type B can be medically managed [53].

10.5 Organ injuries

Stroke and brain injury: Stroke is a feared neurological complication to suffer from after a TAVR. Incidence of stroke is approximately 1.6% and can be a source of morbidity [54].

Myocardial ischemia/injury: Coronary obstruction may occur after a TAVR and can be treated with percutaneous coronary intervention (PCI), coronary artery bypass graft (CABG), or valve repositioning/retrieval.

- With native aortic valve procedures—Coronary obstruction can happen rarely after a TAVR in approximately 0.7% of cases [51].

- With valve-in-valve procedures—Coronary obstruction is more commonly seen up to 3.5 [55].

Acute kidney injury (AKI): A significant amount of TAVR patients do suffer from renal insufficiency. AKI have been associated with a worse outcome and approximately 2.24% of patients required dialysis. A study titled the PROTECT-TAVI (PROphylactic effecT of furosEmide-induCed diuresis with matched isotonic intravenous hydraTion in Transcatheter Aortic Valve Implantation) had 112 patients undergoing TAVR who were randomly assigned to intravenous hydration with normal saline matched with urine output with diuresis (RenalGuard group) versus a control group of just normal saline. The study showed the rate of AKI was lower in the RenalGuard group than the control group [51, 55].

10.6 Arrhythmic complications

High grade heart block: Having a history of baseline conduction abnormalities (such as bundle branch blocks) have been a known risk factor for having a post-procedural pace maker (PPM) placed. It may also depend on the type of valve placed, Sapien vs. CoreValve. One study noted, that post TAVR, PPM was placed in 1.8–8.5% of patients who received the Sapien versus 19.1–42.5% of patients who received CoreValve [56].

New onset atrial fibrillation (NOAF): This is also commonly seen after a TAVR. In one study it was identified that 31.9% of patients had NOAF in a 46-hour time period postoperatively [57].

10.7 Valve-in-valve implantation complications

For patients with a failed bioprosthetic valve, the types of complications are similar to those patients with native aortic valve stenosis. However, coronary artery obstruction is more common and paravalvular regurgitation and PPM placement are less frequent [58].

Due to new transcatheter heart valves that now have external covering sealing skirts, these new devices have led to a lower rate of PVL from 8.3% of the first-generation device to 5.4% with the second-generation device and down to 3.4% with the third-generation device.

11. Adjunctive devices: cerebral embolic protection devices

Cerebral embolic protection devices (CEPD) are used in order to prevent cerebral embolization during the procedure and thus may help lower the stroke risk with the TAVR procedure. There are many types of CEPD that have their own set of pros and cons. Overall the filtration needs to protect the major cerebral arteries throughout the entire procedure [59].

11.1 Sentinel CEPD

This device is the most studied CEPD and only FDA-approved device for commercial use. It can be implanted through a 6-French sheath through a radial or brachial access. There are two filters in the delivery system. One filter is to be placed in the brachiocephalic trunk and the other is placed in the left common carotid artery. With this the left subclavian artery is not covered. Therefore, there is not a complete cerebral protection with this device. There have been a few clinical trials comparing the Sentinel to unprotected groups. The CLEANTAVI and MISTRAL-C randomized controlled trials showed a reduction in the amount of new ischemic brain lesions in the protected areas in the Sentinel versus the unprotected groups. The PROTECTED TAVR trial studied whether TAVR reduces the risk of periprocedural stroke with CEP use. This was a large, randomized, prospective trial in which CEP was successfully deployed in 94.4% of patients. The results showed that the incidence of procedural complications did not differ significantly between patients who underwent TAVR with CEP versus without CEP. However, there was a 95% confidence interval with the outcome therefore it did not rule out the overall benefit of use of CEP in TAVR procedure [60].

11.2 TriGUARD embolic deflector device

This system contains a single-use, biocompatible filter mesh. It can be implanted through a 9-French transfemoral sheath using fluoroscopy to be deployed in the aortic arch. This device covers the right brachiocephalic, left common carotid, and subclavian artery. Therefore, it prevents cerebral embolization by redirecting the debris to the descending aorta. The device is stabilized in a stable position by being anchored in the right brachiocephalic artery ostium. The TriGUARD's safety was initially confirmed in the DEFLECT 1 trial as it also showed 80% of patients had successful coverage of all three branches. The second-generation of this device, TriGUARD HDH was invented and then also evaluated in other studies. The DEFLECT III trial showed less neurological deficits as defined by the National Institutes of Health Stroke Scale (NIHSS) and cognitive function improvement [59]. *TriGUARD 3* is an update of the current TriGUARD HDH that provides easier usage, extensive coverage of all three major branches, and less interference with the TAVR. This device contains a biocompatible nitinol filter mesh which has a smaller pore size compared to the previous TriGUARD HDH which helps prevent smaller particles from getting into the cerebral circulation. It can be delivered through an 8-French transfemoral sheath. This device does not need a stabilizer as there is enough stability offered through the nitinol shaft and from the circumferential device pressure from the aortic arch. The REFLECT II trial proved that the TriGUARD group had higher safety when compared to the unprotected group (15.9% vs. 7%). This study had successful device positioning in 59.3% of the patients [59].

11.3 Point-guard system™ dynamic cerebral embolic protection (Transverse Medical, Inc, Denver, CO, USA)

This device has a filter mesh in a flexible nitinol frame that can cover all the major branches of the aortic arch. This is stabilized during positioning through its isolation zone. Currently this system is not widely available for use as there is not enough clinical data. The CENTER trial will be initiated to evaluate this system [59].

11.4 Emblok embolic protection system (Innovatice Cardiovascular Solutions, Grand Rapids, MI, USA)

This system not only offers cerebral protection during TAVR but also protects the abdominal and peripheral vasculature. The device can be implanted through an 11-French transfemoral sheath with a pigtail catheter and is then advanced into the aorta. This device was studied and proven to have successful deployment. The study noted that no cerebrovascular or cardiovascular events were seen at 30 days follow-up. However further studies need to be done to see improvement in clinical outcomes using this device [59].

Overall, the introduction of CEPD was done in order to help lower the risk of stroke after the TAVR procedure and to help prevent cerebral embolization. However, in studies involving CEPD, there has not been a significant reduction noticed in stroke rate. This could be seen due to limiting number of studies and sample size used. The PROTECTED TAVR trial had a 95% confidence interval therefore it did not rule out the overall benefit of the use of CEP in TAVR procedure [60]. Nevertheless, CEPD may be an asset in the future for cerebral embolic protection with technical improvements.

12. Post-procedure management

Post TAVR care includes routine follow-up clinically. This includes getting an echocardiogram prior to discharge, at 1 month follow-up, then at 6–12 months, and followed by annually. Echocardiogram is used to watch for long term complications as well as assess the transvalvular gradient over time.

12.1 Antithrombotic treatment

Antithrombotic therapy post TAVR depends on a few factors such as the simultaneous indication of antiplatelet therapy (history of recent coronary artery stent placement) and/or the simultaneous indication of anticoagulation (history of atrial fibrillation). Regardless it is important for patients to be on antithrombotic therapy at least for the first 3–6 months following the procedure.

For patients without a simultaneous indication of antiplatelet therapy or dual antiplatelet therapy (DAPT), it is recommended to treat with a single antiplatelet therapy (SAPT) for life. Typically, this includes Aspirin 75–100 mg daily. If aspirin is contraindicated for the patient, the alternative is clopidogrel (Plavix) 75 mg daily.

For patients with no indication of anticoagulation, it is recommended to be on DAPT with Aspirin and Plavix during the first 3–6 months (depending on valve type). Then followed by lifelong SAPT.

For patients with a simultaneous indication of dual antiplatelet therapy such that they had a recent coronary artery stenting, the duration of DAPT and the specific agents depends on the concurrent indication. After that period, it is recommended to continue with daily SAPT for life rather than anticoagulation.

Generally triple antithrombotic therapy (anticoagulation and DAPT) is typically avoided due to increase bleeding risks [61].

12.2 Endocarditis prophylaxis

Patients with prosthetic valves are at high risk for endocarditis. Rates are the highest during the first year of placement and then decrease over time. Therefore, it is vital to properly educate patients about infective endocarditis. This includes discussing the importance of regular dental care and antimicrobial prophylaxis before procedures that may lead to bacteremia. Recommended prophylaxis for penicillin tolerant and penicillin allergic patients included Amoxicillin and Clindamycin, respectively [62].

12.3 Durability of valves at 5–10 years

There are not many studies completed so far that show data regarding the long-term durability of the valve. In a study completed in the UK, using the UK TAVR registry, looked into patients who underwent TAVR over a span of 5 years. The study had 241 patients with 149 patients having the self-expandable valve and 80 patients with a balloon-expandable valve. The patients were evaluated post-procedure and echocardiographic follow-up ranging from 5 to 10 years. Most of the patients had none to trivial aortic regurgitation at follow-up. This study concluded that 91% of the patients did not have structural valve degeneration at 5 and 10 years post- TAVR follow up [63]. The NOTION trial spans over 10 years and is the longest clinical trial comparing randomized patients undergoing a TAVR versus SAVR. It was completed in Denmark and Sweden and enrolled patients between 2009 and 2013. The study shows patients who had a TAVR procedure had comparable risk for all-cause mortality, myocardial infarction, and stroke as patients who had a SAVR completed.

12.4 Redo TAVR (ViV TAVR)

Failed TAVRs can be challenging to approach and involve many factors to consider such as patient's advancing age, co-morbidities, transcatheter heart valve (THV) design, and tissue ingrowth. Late degeneration of THVs in patients will likely increase in the future therefore it is vital to know how to fix this issue. Redo TAVR has shown to be an effective and safe treatment in these situations [64].

12.5 Cardiac rehabilitation

Inpatient cardiac rehabilitation (CR) after TAVR has been shown to be strongly associated with improved clinical performance. One prospective cohort multicenter study looked at the multicomponent cardiac rehab effects on 136 patients. They took into consideration of the Frailty-Index, Short Form-12, six-minute walk distance, and work load on a bicycle. This study showed an improvement on physical activity and functional capacity after TAVR [65].

13. Future directions

TAVR is an innovative procedure that will always play a significant role in revolutionizing the management of aortic stenosis. This procedure has become more common and usually the first choice for many patients. There have been many successes in clinical outcome and cost effectiveness. Although the indication, procedure, and devices have evolved, we forsee that TAVR will continue to iterate in order to strive for perfection.

Author details

Sidra R. Shah[1], Hafez Golzarian[1] and Sandeep M. Patel[2]*

1 Internal Medicine Residency Program, Mercy Health—St. Rita's Medical Center, Lima, OH, USA

2 Structural Heart and Intervention Center, Mercy Health—St. Rita's Medical Center, Lima, OH, USA

*Address all correspondence to: smpatel@mercy.com

IntechOpen

© 2023 The Author(s). Licensee IntechOpen. This chapter is distributed under the terms of the Creative Commons Attribution License (http://creativecommons.org/licenses/by/3.0), which permits unrestricted use, distribution, and reproduction in any medium, provided the original work is properly cited.

References

[1] Harken DE, Taylor WJ, Lefemine AA, et al. Aortic valve replacement with a caged ball valve. The American Journal of Cardiology. 1962;**9**:292-299

[2] Andersen HR. How transcatheter aortic valve implantation (TAVI) was born: The struggle for a new invention. Frontiers in Cardiovascular Medicine. 2021;**8**:722693

[3] Andersen HR, Knudsen LL, Hasenkam JM. Transluminal implantation of artificial heart valves. Description of a new expandable aortic valve and initial results with implantation by catheter technique in closed chest pigs. European Heart Journal. 1992;**13**:704-708. DOI: 10.1093/oxfordjournals.eurheartj.a060238

[4] Cribier A, Eltchaninoff H, Bash A, Borenstein N, Tron C, Bauer F, et al. Percutaneous transcatheter implantation of an aortic valve prosthesis for calcific aortic stenosis: First human case description. Circulation. 2002;**106**:3006-3008. DOI: 10.1161/01.CIR.0000047200.36165.B8

[5] Cribier A, Eltchaninoff H, Tron C, Bauer F, Agatiello C, Sebagh L, et al. Early experience with percutaneous transcatheter implantation of heart valve prosthesis for the treatment of end-stage inoperable patients with calcific aortic stenosis. Journal of the American College of Cardiology. 2004;**43**:698-703. DOI: 10.1016/j.jacc.2003.11.026

[6] Cribier A, Eltchaninoff H, Tron C, Bauer F, Agatiello C, Nercolini D, et al. Treatment of calcified aortic stenosis with the percutaneous heart valve. Mid-term follow-up from the initial feasibility studies: The French experience. Journal of the American College of Cardiology. 2006;**47**:1214-1223. DOI: 10.1016/j.jacc.2006.01.049

[7] Leon MB, Smith CR, Mack M, et al. Transcatheter aortic-valve implantation for aortic stenosis in patients who cannot undergo surgery. The New England Journal of Medicine. 2010;**363**(17):1597-1607

[8] Smith CR, Leon MB, Mack MJ, et al. Transcatheter versus surgical aortic-valve replacement in high-risk patients. The New England Journal of Medicine. 2011;**364**:2187-2198

[9] Webb JG, Chandavimol M, Thompson CR, et al. Percutaneous aortic valve implantation retrograde from the femoral artery. Circulation. 2006;**113**(6):842-850

[10] Barbash I, Waksman R. Overview of the 2011 Food and Drug Administration circulatory system devices panel of the medical devices advisory committee meeting on the Edwards SAPIEN transcatheter heart valve. Circulation. 2012;**125**:550-555

[11] Bana A. TAVR-present, future, and challenges in developing countries. Indian Journal of Thoracic and Cardiovascular Surgery. 2019;**35**(3):473-484. DOI: 10.1007/s12055-018-00786-8. Epub 2019 Feb 13

[12] Leon MB, Smith CR, Mack MJ, et al. Transcatheter or surgical aortic-valve replacement in intermediate-risk patients. The New England Journal of Medicine. 2016;**374**:1609-1620

[13] Mack MJ, Leon MB, Thourani VH, et al. Transcatheter aortic-valve replacement with a balloon-expandable valve in low-risk patients. The New England Journal of Medicine. 2019;**380**(18):1695-1705

[14] Forrest JK, Deeb GM, Yakubov SJ, et al. On behalf of the low-risk trial

investigators, three-year outcomes after transcatheter or surgical aortic valve replacement in low-risk patients with aortic stenosis. Journal of the American College of Cardiology. 2023;**81**: 1663-1674

[15] Mesnier J, Panagides V, Nuche J, Rodés-Cabau J. Evolving indications of transcatheter aortic valve replacement-where are we now, and where are we going. Journal of Clinical Medicine. 2022; **11**(11):3090

[16] Otto C, Nishimura R, et al. 2020 ACC/AHA guideline for the management of patients with valvular heart disease. Journal of the American College of Cardiology. 2021;**77**(4): e25-e197

[17] Garry JD, Goldman M, Kohlwes J, Sidebotham D, Morrow CD, Drake DH, et al. Early surgery or conservative care for asymptomatic aortic stenosis. The New England Journal of Medicine. 2020; **383**:91-93

[18] Nakatsuma K, Taniguchi T, Morimoto T, Shiomi H, Ando K, Kanamori N, et al. B-type natriuretic peptide in patients with asymptomatic severe aortic stenosis. Heart. 2018;**105**: 384-390

[19] Taniguchi T, Morimoto T, Shiomi H, Ando K, Kanamori N, Murata K, et al. Initial surgical versus conservative strategies in patients with asymptomatic severe aortic stenosis. Journal of the American College of Cardiology. 2015; **66**:2827-2838

[20] Vahanian A, Alfieri O, Andreotti F, et al. Guidelines on the management of valvular heart disease (version 2012): the Joint Task Force on the Management of Valvular Heart Disease of the European Society of Cardiology (ESC) and the European Association for Cardio-Thoracic Surgery (EACTS). European Journal of Cardio-Thoracic Surgery. 2012;**42**(4):S1-S44. DOI: 10.1093/ejcts/ezs455

[21] Nanditha S, Malik V, Hasija S, Malhotra P, Sreenivas V, Chauhan S. Comparison of grading of aortic stenosis between transthoracic and transesophageal echocardiography in adult patients undergoing elective aortic valve replacement surgeries: A prospective observational study. Annals of Cardiac Anaesthesia. 2019;**22**(2):194-198

[22] Clavel M-A, Messika-Zeitoun D, Pibarot P, Aggarwal SR, Malouf J, Araoz PA, et al. The complex nature of discordant severe calcified aortic valve disease grading: New insights from combined doppler echocardiographic and computed tomographic study. Journal of the American College of Cardiology. 2013;**62**(24):2329-2338

[23] Foley M, Hall K, Howard JP, et al. Aortic valve calcium score is associated with acute stroke in transcatheter aortic valve Replacement patients. Society for Cardiovascular Angiography & Intervention. 2022;**1**(4):100349

[24] Kotronias RA, Kwok CS, George S, Capodanno D, Ludman PF, Townend JN, et al. Transcatheter aortic valve implantation with or without percutaneous coronary artery revascularization strategy: A systematic review and meta-analysis. Journal of the American Heart Association. 2017;**6**(6):13

[25] St Hilaire C, DeRieux J, Shenoda M, Casey K. Carotid duplex poorly predicts stroke risk during transcatheter aortic valve replacement. Annals of Vascular Surgery. 2022;**84**:107-113

[26] Condado JF, Jensen HA, Maini A, et al. Should we perform carotid doppler screening before surgical or

transcatheter aortic valve replacement? The Annals of Thoracic Surgery. 2017; **103**(3):787-794

[27] Henn MC, Zajarias A, Lindman BR, et al. Preoperative pulmonary function tests predict mortality after surgical or transcatheter aortic valve replacement. The Journal of Thoracic and Cardiovascular Surgery. 2016;**151**(2): 578-586.e5862

[28] Green P, Cohen DJ, Généreux P, et al. Relation between six-minute walk test performance and outcomes after transcatheter aortic valve implantation (from the PARTNER trial). The American Journal of Cardiology. 2013; **112**(5):700-706

[29] Makki N, Lilly SM. Advanced chronic kidney disease: Relationship to outcomes post-TAVR, a meta-analysis. Clinical Cardiology. 2018;**41**(8): 1091-1096

[30] Bagur R, Webb JG, Nietlispach F, et al. Acute kidney injury following transcatheter aortic valve implantation: Predictive factors, prognostic value, and comparison with surgical aortic valve replacement. European Heart Journal. 2010;**31**(7):865-874

[31] Sinning JM, Ghanem A, Steinhäuser H, et al. Renal function as predictor of mortality in patients after percutaneous transcatheter aortic valve implantation. JACC. Cardiovascular Interventions. 2010;**3**(11):1141-1149

[32] Rotman OM, Bianchi M, Ghosh RP, Kovarovic B, Bluestein D. Principles of TAVR valve design, modelling, and testing. Expert Review of Medical Devices. 2018;**15**:771-791

[33] Cahill TJ, Chen M, Hayashida K, Latib A, Modine T, Piazza N, et al. Transcatheter aortic valve implantation: Current status and future perspectives. European Heart Journal. 2018;**39**:2625-2634

[34] Claessen BE, Tang GHL, Kini AS, Sharma SK. Considerations for optimal device selection in transcatheter aortic valve replacement: A review. JAMA Cardiology. 2021;**6**:102-112

[35] Abdelghani M, Mankerious N, Allali A, Landt M, Kaur J, Sulimov DS, et al. Bioprosthetic valve performance after transcatheter aortic valve replacement with self-expanding versus balloon-expandable valves in large versus small aortic valve annuli: Insights from the CHOICE trial and the CHOICE-extend registry. JACC. Cardiovascular Interventions. 2018;**11**(24):2507-2518

[36] Binder RK, Rodés-Cabau J, Wood DA, Webb JG. Edwards SAPIEN 3 valve. EuroIntervention. 2012;**8**:Q83-Q87

[37] Forrest JK, Mangi AA, Popma JJ, Khabbaz K, Reardon MJ, Kleiman NS, et al. Early outcomes with the Evolut PRO repositionable self-expanding transcatheter aortic valve with pericardial wrap. JACC. Cardiovascular Interventions. 2018;**11**(2):160-168

[38] Perrin N, Perrin T, Hachulla AL, et al. Conduction disorders using the Evolut R prosthesis compared with the CoreValve: Has anything changed? Open Heart. 2018;**5**(1):e000770

[39] Möllmann H, Hengstenberg C, Hilker M, Kerber S, Schäfer U, Rudolph T, et al. Real-world experience using the ACURATE neo prosthesis: 30-day outcomes of 1,000 patients enrolled in the SAVI TF registry. EuroIntervention. 2 Feb 2018;**13**(15):e1764-e1770. DOI: 10.4244/EIJ-D-17-00628. PMID: 29131801

[40] Seeger J, Gonska B, Rottbauer W, Wohrle J. Outcome with the repositionable and retrievable Boston

Scientific Lotus valve compared with the balloon-expandable Edwards SAPIEN 3 valve in patients undergoing transfemoral aortic valve replacement. Circulation. Cardiovascular Interventions. 2017;**10**(6):e004670

[41] Suri RM, Minha S, Alli O, et al. Learning curves for transapical transcatheter aortic valve replacement in the PARTNER-I trial: Technical performance, success, and safety. Journal of Thoracic and Cardiovascular Surgery. 2016;**152**:773-80 e14

[42] Alkhouli MA, Raybuck BD, Badhwar V. Navigating the s-curve of transapical therapy. The Journal of Thoracic and Cardiovascular Surgery. 2016;**152**:781-782

[43] Carroll J, Vemulapalli S, Dai D, et al. The association between procedural experience for transcatheter aortic valve replacement and outcomes: Insights from the STS/ACC TVT registry. Journal of the American College of Cardiology. 2017

[44] Mahmaljy H, Tawney A, Young M. Transcatheter aortic valve replacement. In: StatPearls [Internet]. Treasure Island (FL): StatPearls Publishing. p. 2023

[45] Tommaso CL, Bolman RM 3rd, Feldman T, Bavaria J, Acker MA, Aldea G, et al. Multisociety (AATS, ACCF, SCAI, and STS) expert consensus statement: Operator and institutional requirements for transcatheter valve repair and replacement, part 1: Transcatheter aortic valve replacement. Journal of the American College of Cardiology. 2012;**59**(22):2028-2042

[46] Biasco L, Ferrari E, Pedrazzini G, Faletra F, Moccetti T, Petracca F, et al. Access sites for TAVI: Patient selection criteria, technical aspects, and outcomes. Frontiers in Cardiovascular Medicine. 2018;**5**:88. DOI: 10.3389/fcvm.2018.00088

[47] Transcatheter SAPIEN 3. Transcatheter SAPIEN 3 | Edwards Lifesciences. n.d. Available from: https://www.edwards.com/healthcare-professionals/products-services/transcatheterheart/transcatheter-sapien-3

[48] Medtronic. Transcatheter Aortic Heart Valves. Medtronic. n.d. Available from: https://www.medtronic.com/us-en/healthcare-professionals/products/cardiovascular/transcatheter-aortic-heart-valves.html

[49] Tang GHL, Zaid S, Fuchs A, Yamabe T, Yazdchi F, Gupta E, et al. Alignment of transcatheter aortic-valve neo-commissures (ALIGN TAVR): Impact on final valve orientation and coronary artery overlap. JACC. Cardiovascular Interventions. 2020;**13**(9):1030-1042. DOI: 10.1016/j.jcin.2020.02.005. Epub 2020 Mar 16

[50] Caldararu C, Balanescu S. Modern use of echocardiography in transcatheter aortic valve replacement: An up-date. Maedica (Bucur). 2016;**11**(4):299-307

[51] Généreux P, Head SJ, Van Mieghem NM, Kodali S, Kirtane AJ, Xu K, et al. Clinical outcomes after transcatheter aortic valve replacement using valve academic research consortium definitions: A weighted meta-analysis of 3,519 patients from 16 studies. Journal of the American College of Cardiology. 2012;**59**(25):2317-2326. DOI: 10.1016/j.jacc.2012.02.022. Epub 2012 Apr 11

[52] Rodés-Cabau J, Dauerman HL, Cohen MG, Mehran R, Small EM, Smyth SS, et al. Antithrombotic treatment in transcatheter aortic valve implantation: Insights for cerebrovascular and bleeding events. Journal of the American College of Cardiology. 2013;**62**(25):2349-2359. DOI: 10.1016/j.jacc.2013.03.029. Epub 2013 Apr 10

[53] Chaudhry MA, Sardar MR. Vascular complications of transcatheter aortic valve replacement: A concise literature review. World Journal of Cardiology. 2017;**9**(7): 574-582. DOI: 10.4330/wjc.v9.i7.574

[54] O'Brien SM, Shahian DM, Filardo G, et al. The Society of Thoracic Surgeons 2008 cardiac surgery risk models: Part 2-isolated valve surgery. The Annals of Thoracic Surgery. 2009;**88**(1 Suppl): S23-S42. DOI: 10.1016/j.athoracsur.2009.05.056

[55] Webb JG, Dvir D. Transcatheter aortic valve replacement for bioprosthetic aortic valve failure: The valve-in-valve procedure. Circulation. 2013;**127**(25):2542-2550

[56] Holmes DR Jr, Mack MJ, Kaul S, et al. 2012 ACCF/AATS/SCAI/STS expert consensus document on transcatheter aortic valve replacement. Journal of the American College of Cardiology. 2012;**59**(13):1200-1254. DOI: 10.1016/j.jacc.2012.01.001

[57] Amat Santos IJ, Rodés Cabau J, Urena M, et al. Incidence, predictive factors, and prognostic value of new-onset atrial fibrillation following transcatheter aortic valve implantation. Journal of the American College of Cardiology. 2012;**59**(2):178-188. DOI: 10.1016/j.jacc.2011.09.061

[58] Webb JG, Blanke P, Meier D, Sathananthan J, Lauck S, Chatfield AG, et al. TAVI in 2022: Remaining issues and future direction. Archives of Cardiovascular Diseases. 2022;**115**(4): 235-242

[59] Halim J, Cheng JM, den Heijer P, Schölzel BE, Vos J, Meuwissen M, et al. The role of cerebral embolic protection in transcatheter aortic valve replacement. Journal of Clinical Cardiology. 2021;**2**(4):88-95

[60] Kapadia SR, Makkar R, Leon M, Abdel-Wahab M, Waggoner T, Massberg S, et al. Cerebral embolic protection during transcatheter aortic-valve replacement. The New England Journal of Medicine. 2022;**387**(14):1253-1263. DOI: 10.1056/NEJMoa2204961. Epub 2022 Sep 17

[61] Kuno T, Takagi H, Sugiyama T, Ando T, Miyashita S, Valentin N, et al. Antithrombotic strategies after transcatheter aortic valve implantation: Insights from a network meta-analysis. Catheterization and Cardiovascular Interventions. 2020;**96**(2):E177-E186

[62] Zakhour J, Allaw F, Kalash S, Wehbe S, Kanj SS. Infective endocarditis after transcatheter aortic valve Replacement: Challenges in the diagnosis and management. Pathogens. 2023;**12**(2):255. DOI: 10.3390/pathogens12020255

[63] Blackman DJ, Saraf S, MacCarthy PA, Myat A, Anderson SG, Malkin CJ, et al. Long-term durability of transcatheter aortic valve prostheses. Journal of the American College of Cardiology. 2019;**73**(5):537-545

[64] Grube E, Sinning J, et al. The "big five" complications after transcatheter aortic valve replacement. JACC: Cardiovascular Interventions. 2019;**12**(4):370-372

[65] Eichler S, Salzwedel A, Reibis R, Nothroff J, Harnath A, Schikora M, et al. Multicomponent cardiac rehabilitation in patients after transcatheter aortic valve implantation: Predictors of functional and psychocognitive recovery. European Journal of Preventive Cardiology. 2017;**24**(3):257-264. DOI: 10.1177/2047487316679527. Epub 2016 Nov 16

Chapter 7

Valve-in-Valve Transcatheter Aortic Valve Replacement: Challenges for Now and the Future

Manoraj Navaratnarajah, Amit Modi and Sunil Ohri

Abstract

The recent years have seen a huge expansion in the number of bioprostheses implanted, and this number is likely to increase further in the future. This is likely to lead to a pandemic of patients requiring reoperation/re-intervention for structural deterioration of the valve. Valve-in-valve transcatheter aortic valve replacement (ViV-TAVR) has become a safe and effective alternative to redo aortic valve surgery and has gained approval for use in high-risk patients with prohibitive operative risk. ViV-TAVR is a complex procedure requiring rigorous planning, technical expertise and patient anatomical appreciation. In this chapter, we examine the evidence supporting the use of ViV-TAVR along with the primary technical issues surrounding this procedure such as: elevated postprocedural gradients, coronary obstruction and valve-related thrombosis. TAVR use is also expanding towards an increasingly young patient profile with extended life expectancy, likely to outlive the implanted bioprosthesis. We therefore also examine the huge current challenge of establishing what is the best lifetime strategy for the management of aortic valve disease in younger patients.

Keywords: transcatheter aortic valve replacement, valve-in-valve, structural valve deterioration, bioprosthetic valve failure, redo surgical aortic valve replacement

1. Introduction

The global burden of aortic valvular disease continues to rise due to an increasingly aged population [1]. The traditional treatment of aortic valve disease involved surgical aortic valve replacement (SAVR). However, with the arrival of transcatheter aortic valve replacement (TAVR), the therapeutic landscape has dramatically changed. SAVR is often precluded in patients at a very high risk for surgery, for example, frailty, extreme obesity, porcelain aorta, severe pulmonary hypertension, severe right ventricular dysfunction, severe liver disease, severe lung disease, poorly controlled diabetes and impaired renal function [2]. TAVR's indication has now been expanded to intermediate and low-risk patients [3]. This is based on a series of clinical trials comparing TAVR with SAVR [4–9]. Thus, TAVR is now approved for all patient risk profiles, representing a therapeutic option for all patients regardless of age [3].

IntechOpen

However, in young, low-risk patients with severe aortic stenosis, current guidelines recommend shared decision making, centred around patient preferences and beliefs [10, 11].

Of note, recent years, have seen an ever-increasing number of bioprostheses being implanted [12, 13]. More than 85% of implanted SAVRs are bioprosthetic [14]. This will inevitably lead to an enlarging population and potential future pandemic of patients requiring reoperation/reintervention for structural valve deterioration. Valve-in-valve transcatheter aortic valve replacement (ViV-TAVR) is a safe and effective alternative to redo SAVR and is currently approved for higher-risk patients deemed inoperable.

In this chapter, we examine the literature in detail and study the major reported technical issues with ViV-TAVR, the evidence supporting its use and the critical issue of what is the current optimum lifetime treatment strategy for aortic valve disease, particularly in younger patients. The advent of wider TAVR implantation in increasingly younger patients, having a longer life expectancy than the expected longevity of the bioprosthesis, has mandated a focused discussion of this issue. This is because the primary aortic valve intervention significantly influences subsequent valve therapies and what is best strategy, if indeed there is a single best strategy, is not yet established.

1.1 Structural valve degeneration

Bioprosthetic valve dysfunction is simply categorised as either (A) non-structural valve deterioration: valve thrombosis or endocarditis, paravalvular regurgitation, patient-prosthesis mismatch, *or* (B) structural valve deterioration: irreversible permanent degenerative intrinsic valve alterations [15, 16].

Of note, there is a wide variation in structural valve deterioration definition in the literature, leading to similar variations in reported valve failure incidences. The majority of SAVR studies define valve failure based on the need for reintervention. This likely underestimates the true incidence of structural valve deterioration, which is heavily dependent on manufacturer and prosthesis type.

2021 Valve Academic Research Consortium 3 (VARC-3) guidelines use 3 stages to define bioprosthetic valve failure: (1) any bioprosthetic valve dysfunction with clinically expressed criteria dysfunction, (2) valve intervention and (3) valve-related death [16, 17].

The optimum treatment of structural valve deterioration is yet to be defined and is likely to be bespoke and personalised according to anatomical, original valve- and patient-risk-related criteria. Approaches broadly compete between (A) traditional or (B) minimally invasive redo-SAVR and (C) ViV-TAVR valve.

1.2 Valve in valve TAVR versus redo SAVR: the evidence

There are no randomised controlled trials studying the best treatment of structural valve deterioration. There is also an obvious scarcity of long-term data on ViV-TAVR. Most studies are less than 5 years' duration, and there are no head-to-head comparison studies with redo-SAVR.

At present, ViV-TAVR is the treatment of choice for patients with structural valve deterioration considered high risk for redo-SAVR. However, redo-SAVR remains the first choice among patients at low-intermediate surgical risk unless unfavourable anatomies are present, for example, calcified aortic root or hostile chest.

Several meta-analyses demonstrate lower incidence of post-operative complications and 30-day mortality and similar 1-year and mid-term mortality rates for ViV-TAVR versus redo SAVR [18–20].

Pompeu et al. analysed 12 studies with 16,207 patients, comparing ViV-TAVR with redo-SAVR, published between 2015 and 2020. In their pooled analysis, ViV-TAVR was associated with significantly lower rates of 30-day mortality, major bleeding and shorter hospital stay. However, patients receiving ViV-TAVR were 4 times more likely to have severe patient prosthesis mismatch [18]. No difference in mortality was seen at 1 year. Thandra et al. analysed 9 observational studies with 2891 patients and a mean follow-up of 26 months. They too demonstrated significantly lower 30-day mortality, bleeding and length of stay but higher post-operative gradients with ViV-TAVR compared with redo-SAVR [19]. Saleem et al. analysed 11 studies including 8326 patients and showed similar findings. At 30-days, the risk of all-cause mortality, cardiovascular mortality and major bleeding were significantly lower with ViV-TAVR. At up to a 5-year follow-up, no significant difference in all-cause mortality, cardiovascular mortality and stroke was seen. However, again, ViV-TAVR showed a higher risk of patient prosthesis mismatch and greater transvalvular pressure gradients [20]. Hirji et al. looked at more than 3000 US patients, comparing ViV-TAVR versus redo-SAVR using the National Readmissions Database. Using propensity score matching, VIV-TAVR showed superiority over redo-SAVR in terms of 30-day mortality, 30-day morbidity, bleeding and hospital length of stay [21].

In the absence of good randomised control trials, later published meta-analyses draw similar conclusions [22–24]. Raschpichler et al. analysed 15 studies and 8881 patients; 50.2% underwent ViV TAVR and 49.8% redo-SAVR. Short-term mortality was 2.8% with ViV-TAVR compared with 5.0% with redo-SAVR, and again, mid-term mortality did not significantly differ (maximum follow-up 5 years). Again, significant, prosthetic valve regurgitation was 4 times more likely with ViV-TAVR, and severe patient prosthesis mismatch was 3 times more likely [22].

Formica analysed 12 studies with 3457 patients. The redo-SAVR group included 1783 patients and ViV-TAVR 1764. Redo-SAVR showed a higher incidence of all-cause mortality within 30 days with no difference observed between 30 days and 1 year and at a 5-year follow-up [23].

Bruno et al. analysed 11 studies with 8570 patients, 4224 undergoing ViV-TAVR and 4346 redo-SAVR. The studies focussed on intermediate-high-risk patients. 30-day all-cause and cardiovascular mortality were significantly lower with ViV-TAVR. At a mean follow-up of 717 days, there was no mortality difference between techniques. Major bleeding and new-onset atrial fibrillation were significantly lower with ViV-TAVR [24].

1.2.1 Limitations

These meta-analyses include non-randomised retrospective studies and are vulnerable to the inherent weaknesses of observational data. Therefore, results are to be interpreted with caution. In addition, clinically relevant and important valve-associated factors such as size, design and the precise manner of deterioration were rarely analysed and are of vital importance.

Other limitations include limited follow-up (<1 year in many studies), small sample sizes, a lack of randomisation and the inclusion of many retrospective observational studies. The lack of clear reported selection criteria in many included studies as well as a wide variation of inclusion criteria among studies are other limitations.

This gives rise to the obvious negatives of selection and allocation bias. As mentioned earlier, lack of data relating to degenerated prosthesis type; implanted bioprosthesis type, for example, stented, stentless and rapid deployment; the type of implanted TAVR (self-expanded versus balloon-expandable) and TAVR approach route renders meaningful scientific hard conclusions difficult to make. Randomised control trials with longer follow-ups and large multi-centre registries are essential to better analyse and define the differences in survival between these two procedures.

The overall broad conclusion of these large meta-analyses is that ViV-TAVR demonstrates better short-term mortality compared with redo-SAVR, but mid-term mortality is similar. Higher rates of severe patient prosthesis mismatch, high transvalvular gradients and post-procedural aortic regurgitation are associated with ViV-TAVR. Given the likely selection/allocation bias in the included studies and limitations mentioned earlier, authors universally advocate an adequately powered multi-centre randomised control trial with sufficiently long follow-up.

In a recent retrospective, propensity score-matched, multi-centre UK study, 911 patients were studied between 2005 and 2021. 125 pairs for analysis were created with a mean age of 75 years. In-hospital mortality was 7.2% for redo-AVR versus 0% for ViV-TAVR ($p = 0.002$). Intensive care unit and hospital length of stay and post-operative complications were significantly reduced with ViV- TAVR, but rates of moderate aortic regurgitation at discharge and elevated post-procedural gradients were increased [25]. Median follow-up was 4.2 years for redo-AVR and 3.1 years for ViV-TAVR, and no difference in mid-term survival was found in discharged patients. **Table 1** summarising the publications comparing ViV-TAVR with redo-SAVR.

1.3 Bioprosthetic valve failure

1.3.1 Pre-disposing factors

Minimising the chances of bioprosthetic valve failure is critical, and modifiable factors should be addressed to the maximum if possible, to avoid/retard structural valve degeneration. Patient characteristics, comorbidities, the type and size of implanted valve contribute to valve failure. Ochi et al. identified multiple risk factors for structural valve degeneration. Presence of patient prosthesis mismatch, sub-coronary implantation technique, absence of anti-calcification preparation, concomitant coronary artery bypass graft surgery, small valve sizes, high post-implantation gradients and renal disease were all implicated.

Meta-analysis identified younger age, increased body surface area, smoking and patient prosthesis mismatch as significant drivers of structural valve degeneration [26].

1.3.2 Patient-prosthesis mismatch

Discussion relating to patient prosthesis mismatch is complex and extensive and is not the focus of this chapter. However, review of the literature suggests that patient prosthesis mismatch is likely a critical factor contributing to structural valve degeneration [27]. Patient prosthesis mismatch can be and must be mitigated at the time of initial SAVR by implanting an appropriately sized valve, selecting the optimum valve design profile and/or surgical intervention to facilitate the implantation of an appropriately sized valve. Patients at high risk of significant patient prosthesis mismatch ideally should be identified pre-operatively, with the application of a targeted

DOI: http://dx.doi.org/10.5772/intechopen.112764

Study	(n)	Outcomes	Conclusions
Pompeu et al. [18] 2021 Meta-analysis 12 studies	16,207	ViV-TAVR was associated with lower rates of 30-day mortality, permanent pacemaker implantation, major bleeding and shorter hospital stay. ViV-TAVR was associated with higher rates of myocardial infarction, and severe patient prosthesis mismatch. No difference in mortality was seen at 1 year.	ViV-TAVR is a valuable option in the treatment of degenerated aortic bioprosthesis, especially in patients with high operative risk due to a lower incidence of peri-operative complications and better early survival compared with redo-SAVR ViV-TAVR is associated with higher rates of myocardial infarction and severe patient-prosthesis mismatch.
Thandra et al. [19] 2021 Meta-analysis 9 studies	2891	30-day mortality rate was significantly lower in ViV-TAVR group. No significant difference in mid-term and 1-year mortality between ViV-TAVR and redo- SAVR ViV-TAVR group had lower 30-day bleeding rate and length of stay. ViV-TAVR had higher post-operative gradients.	ViV-TAVR should be preferred over redo- SAVR particularly in those at intermediate-high surgical risk.
Saleem et al. [20] 2021 Meta-analysis 11 studies	8326	30-day all-cause mortality cardiovascular mortality and major bleeding rate were significantly lower in ViV-TAVR group. No difference in stroke rate, myocardial infarction and permanent pacemaker rate. No differences for all-cause mortality, cardiovascular mortality and stroke rate at 6 month-5 year follow up. ViV-TAVR had higher risk of patient-prosthesis mismatch and greater transvalvular pressure gradients post-implantation.	ViV-TAVR compared to redo-SAVR is associated with significant improvement in short-term mortality and major bleeding. For mid to long-term follow up, the outcomes were similar for both groups.
Hirji et al. [21] Multicentre US National database propensity-score matched analysis	6815	ViV-TAVR showed lower 30-day morbidity, and major bleeding. ViV-TAVR displayed shorter length of stay.	ViV-TAVR appears to confer an advantage over redo-SAVR in terms of 30-day mortality, morbidity, and bleeding complications in high-risk patients. Further studies are warranted to benchmark in low- and intermediate-risk patients and to adequately assess longer-term efficacy.
Raschpichler et al. [22]	8881	Short-term mortality was 2.8% in ViV-TAVR group compared to 5.0% redo-SAVR group (P = 0.02).	Better short-term mortality after ViV-TAVR compared with redo-SAVR. Mid-term mortality was similar between groups.

Study	(n)	Outcomes	Conclusions
2022 Meta-analysis 15 studies		Midterm mortality did not differ between groups. Rate of acute kidney injury was lower following ViV-TAVR. Prosthetic aortic valve regurgitation and severe patient-prothesis mismatch occurred more frequently after ViV-TAVR. No significant differences between groups with respect to stroke, myocardial infarction and pacemaker implantation	An adequately powered multi-center randomized clinical trial with sufficiently long follow-up in patients with low-to-intermediate surgical risk is warranted.
Formica et al. [23] 2023 Meta-analysis 12 studies	3547	Redo-SAVR group showed higher 30-day all-cause mortality. No mortality difference was observed between 30 days and 1 year. From 1 to 5 years redo-SAVR showed a survival benefit over ViV-TAVR.	ViV-TAVR shows significantly lower mortality within 30 days. This advantage disappeared between 30 days and 1 year and reversed in favour of redo-SAVR 1 year after the intervention.
Bruno et al. [24] Meta-analysis 11 studies 2022	8570	30-day all-cause and cardiovascular mortality were significantly lower in ViV-TAVR group. After a mean follow-up of 717 (180–1825) days, there was no mortality difference between the two groups. Risk of stroke, myocardial infraction, major vascular complications, and permanent pacemaker implantation at 30 days did not differ between groups. Major bleedings and new-onset atrial fibrillation were significantly lower in ViV-TAVR group.	In high- and intermediate-risk patients ViV-TAVR shows reduced short-term mortality, compared with redo-SAVR. No differences were found in all-cause and cardiovascular mortality at midterm follow-up.
Gatta et al. [25] 2023 Multi-centre retrospective propensity-score matched analysis	250	Mean age 75.2 years. In-hospital mortality was 7.2% (n = 9) for redo-SAVR vs 0 for ViV-TAVR, (p = 0.002). Redo SAVR patients suffered more post-operative complications: including IABP support, early re-operation, arrhythmias, respiratory and neurological complications and multi-organ failure. ViV-TAVR group had a shorter intensive care unit and	In elderly patients ViV-TAVR provides better early outcomes compared to redo-SAVR. However, there was no difference in mid-term survival between groups in patients successfully discharged from hospital.

DOI: http://dx.doi.org/10.5772/intechopen.112764

Study	(n)	Outcomes	Conclusions
		hospital stay. Moderate aortic regurgitation at discharge and higher post-procedural gradients were more common after ViV-TAVR. Survival probabilities in patients who were successfully discharged from hospital were similar after ViV-TAVR and redo-AVR over the 6-year follow-up period.	

Table 1.
Publications comparing ViV-TAVR with Redo-SAVR.

preventative strategy to reduce the occurrence and severity of patient prosthesis mismatch. This is particularly important in younger patients and in those with depressed left ventricular function. Patient prosthesis mismatch is defined as occurring when the effective orifice area of the implanted prosthetic valve is inadequate for the patient's body surface area and activity. Patient prosthesis mismatch is defined by indexed effective orifice area/body surface area and is graded in severity as follows: none ($>0.85\ cm^2/m^2$), moderate ($0.85–0.65\ cm^2/m^2$), and severe ($\leq 0.65\ cm^2/m^2$). The incidence of moderate to severe patient prosthesis mismatch following SAVR has been reported as high as 65% [28], and patient prosthesis mismatch post-SAVR is more common than no patient prosthesis mismatch [29, 30]. Increasing patient prosthesis mismatch grade is associated with a stepwise increase in long-term all-cause mortality [30]. The seriousness and clinical relevance of moderate patient prosthesis mismatch is unclear, controversial and still debated. Some studies propose that only severe patient prosthesis mismatch translates into clinically relevant harmful effects, with others proposing that even moderate severity is clinically damaging [28–31]. Severe patient prosthesis mismatch following SAVR has been shown to be associated with an increased risk of redo-SAVR by some [28] and not others [29, 30], but significantly raised readmission rates and decreased survival are clearly demonstrated [28–31].

1.3.3 Valve selection and surgical aortic root enlargement

Selection of bioprosthesis and accurate sizing is critical in the initial treatment of aortic valve disease. The largest valve that can be safely implanted is the general principle to be followed, and internal orifice diameter is of the primary importance. This should be identified and appreciated and differs between valve models and manufacturers for the same labelled valve size. The minimal prosthetic valve effective orifice area required to avoid patient prosthesis mismatch should be calculated and then a prosthetic valve model and size that fits into the patient's aortic annulus/root selected, which meets the minimum effective orifice area calculated.

A small aortic annulus may necessitate aortic root enlargement or root replacement during SAVR. During TAVR, the initial valve that provides the largest effective orifice area and the best haemodynamics is chosen. One advantage of TAVR planning is the detailed CT aortography and annulus assessment performed pre-intervention, thus facilitating optimum prosthesis selection. Aortic root intervention during SAVR should be guided by effective orifice area index and considered when falling below $\leq 0.85\ cm^2/m^2$, particularly in young patients. However, aortic root enlargement is performed in 10% or less of patients receiving SAVR [32].

Several surgical techniques exist to augment aortic root diameter. Detailed discussion of them is not the focus of this chapter, but more awareness of and emphasis on the principle of their use at primary aortic valve intervention. Nicks and Manouguian procedures enlarge the aortic annulus using a posterior extension of the aortotomy. The Nicks extends through the non-coronary sinus and the Manouguian through the left/non-coronary commissure with extension onto the anterior mitral leaflet [33, 34]. Closure is usually then enabled with the use of an aortic patch technique. A Konno procedure is very rarely performed in adults and involves anterior annular augmentation extending onto the right ventricle [35]. Other less common enlargement techniques are also available but are rarely used in everyday practice. Aortic root replacement during SAVR reduces rates of patient prosthesis mismatch and is safe with no added risk, but whether it improves long-term outcomes remains unproven [36, 37].

Of note, TAVR has been associated with reduced risk of patient prosthesis mismatch compared to SAVR, especially in patients with small aortic annuli, particularly in patients receiving a valve size ≤23 mm [38, 39]. SAVR with sutureless prosthesis has also shown excellent haemodynamics and similar rates of patient prosthesis mismatch to TAVR [40]. These findings and their exact future clinical relevance require further exploration and clarification. They re-highlight that valve genre/species selection as well as size, too, need careful consideration by all members of the structural heart team including the surgeon. This represents yet another critical factor when planning primary aortic valve intervention, particularly in the young and those with small aortic roots.

1.4 Technical issues associated with valve-in-valve TAVR

1.4.1 Elevated post-implantation gradients

Valve-in-Valve International Data (VIVID) Registry shows elevated post-procedural gradients and severe patient prosthesis mismatch to occur in 26.8% [41]. It is more common with balloon expandable devices compared to self-expanding devices and in surgical valves ≤21 mm. These figures apply to when the bioprosthetic valve ring fracture technique is not utilised [41]. It is suggested that only severe patient prosthesis mismatch post-ViV-TAVR may affect mortality [42]. However, it is wise to aim for as low post-procedural gradients as possible, to enhance valve durability and patient performance, particularly in patients having extended life expectancy.

Patient prosthesis mismatch is not infrequent following SAVR in patients with small anatomies and is highly relevant during the planning of reintervention for structural valve deterioration. Surgical 19 mm bioprostheses are of particular concern and display high physiological mean gradients (10–25 mmHg) [43].

ViV-TAVR is associated with haemodynamic deterioration with gradient increase ≥10 mmHg between discharge and 30-day follow-up in the STS/ACC TVT registry [44]. Understandably, patients at the greatest risk for severe patient prosthesis mismatch following ViV-TAVR were those arriving with structural valve deterioration following previous SAVR complicated by severe patient prosthesis mismatch [41, 45]. Severe patient prosthesis mismatch prior to ViV-TAVR displays higher 30-day and 1-year mortality [46]. Such clear findings again re-highlight the absolute importance of appropriate, far-sighted primary aortic valve intervention. The critical importance and complexity of post-ViV-TAVR patient prosthesis mismatch is reflected by the creation of a patient prosthesis mismatch predictive calculator by the VIVID registry [47].

Patient prosthesis mismatch following ViV-TAVR is complex and multi-factorial, and numerous contributing factors have been proposed: (A) pre-procedural—baseline patient prosthesis mismatch, stented bioprosthesis, small bioprosthesis and stenotic failure; (B) procedural—intra-annular transcatheter heart valve, deep implantation and non-fractureable valve and (C) post-procedural—structural valve deterioration, leaflets thrombosis and transcatheter heart valve-associated prosthesis-patient mismatch.

1.4.2 Positioning of valve during valve-in-valve TAVR

The choice of a supra-annular valve and a high position of implant have shown success in reducing the risk of high post-procedure gradients [48]. Better leaflet function and haemodynamic results may be achieved using transcatheter heart valve with supra-annular valve position. Experimental in-vitro study has shown that in failed surgical 19 mm stented bioprostheses, a supra-annular implantation of a transcatheter heart valve lowers post-procedural gradients and augments effective orifice area [48]. A clinical study has shown high implantation depth inside failed bioprostheses to be a strong independent predictor of lower post-procedural gradients in both self-expanding and balloon-expandable transcatheter valves [49]. The situation is complex with variations that need to be appreciated between prosthesis types. Self-expanding valves display lower post-ViV-TAVR gradients than balloon-expandable valves especially in pre-existing severe patient prosthesis mismatch [50].

In TAVR, deep implantation strongly predicts patient prosthesis mismatch, with recommended cut-offs for high positioning for CoreValve/Evolut and SAPIEN 3 being 5 mm and 20%, respectively [51, 52]. Conversely, the optimal height for deployment for ViV-TAVR prostheses remains undefined. Elevated risk of aortic regurgitation and valve embolization are concerns surrounding higher valve implantation depth, concerns that affect different prostheses to varying degrees [53, 54].

1.4.3 Bioprosthetic valve fracture

Bioprosthetic valve fracture is proposed as another technique to ameliorate or prevent high post-procedural gradients [55]. The aim is to increase the true internal orifice diameter of the transcatheter heart valve to facilitate either a (A) larger transcatheter heart valve or (B) better expanded transcatheter heart valve to be implanted, increase effective orifice area and enhance haemodynamic function.

Importantly, not all stented valves allow fracture. For example, experimental testing reveals Abbott Trifecta and Medtronic Hancock II valves cannot be fractured [56, 57]. It follows that sutureless and stentless valves are also not suitable for fracture but can be remodelled using an over-expansion technique [58].

Bioprosthetic valve fracture is performed using high-pressure, non-compliant balloons, such as the Atlas Gold (BARD Peripheral Vascular, Tempe, Arizona, USA) and TRUE balloon (BARD Peripheral Vascular). A 60 mL syringe plus an indeflator assembly connected with a high-pressure three-way stopcock is used; under rapid ventricular pacing, the syringe is quickly emptied to inflate the balloon, then switched to cranking the indeflator to achieve high-pressure inflation [59].

Bioprosthetic valve fracture can be performed prior to, or after ViV-TAVR, but the majority is performed after. The timing of bioprosthetic valve fracture, before or after ViV-TAVR, represents an important question [60, 61]. A larger-sized prosthesis can be used with bioprosthetic valve fracture before transcatheter heart valve implant, whereas further expansion of the transcatheter heart valve itself can be performed if bioprosthetic valve fracture is performed afterwards. Prior bioprosthetic valve fracture allows the implantation of a self-expanding valve reducing sizing mismatch and allows confirmation of successful fracture prior to implantation [58–61]. However, it can induce haemodynamic instability from severe acute aortic regurgitation, necessitating post-dilation in order to improve haemodynamics. Correct sizing of the balloon, a balloon slightly smaller than the constrained segment of the self-expanding transcatheter heart valve, and positioning the balloon shoulder lower, more ventricular than the leaflet anchor position, can largely avoid this state of affairs [56].

Bioprosthetic valve fracture after ViV-TAVR is likely to allow greater transcatheter heart valve expansion and reduces the risk of haemodynamic instability from acute severe aortic regurgitation. However, possible bioprosthetic valve fracture leaflet injury and unknown long-term effects on transcatheter heart valve durability are concerns. Other potential complications associated with bioprosthetic valve fracture include: transcatheter heart valve migration, annular rupture, debris embolization, coronary artery obstruction, leaflet tearing and accelerated degeneration with decreased transcatheter heart valve longevity [55, 56].

The minimum inflation pressures necessary for valve ring fracture differ according to the original surgical heart valve type. For surgical heart valve with metal ribbon ring (i.e. Magna and Magna Ease), the fracture threshold (18–24 atm) is greater than the surgical heart valve with a polymer ring (i.e. Biocor Epic, Mosaic, Mitroflow; 8–12 atm). In experimental settings, and most clinical cases, balloons sized 1 mm larger than the labelled valve size were used, although in clinical settings, smaller balloons have been used successfully. Balloons larger than the surgical heart valve internal orifice diameter are also able to fracture the valve, especially if a transcatheter heart valve is already implanted [62]. Recently, ex-vivo bench testing has shown that bioprosthetic valve fracture performed after transcatheter heart valve implantation improves residual gradients [63], but potential early and accelerated degeneration effects on the transcatheter heart valve remain unknown. Bioprosthetic valve fracture is a valid technique to be considered in avoiding and/or ameliorating high post-procedural gradients after a ViV-TAVR, but significant attention needs to be placed on balloon sizing and positioning to achieve optimal results. Improved expansion of the transcatheter heart valve leads to increased circularity of the transcatheter heart valve and therefore increased internal orifice diameter. An important mechanism thought to improve valve haemodynamic performance during higher implant, bioprosthetic valve fracture and post-implant dilatation during ViV-TAVR is the reduction of pinwheeling (**Figure 1**). Improved expansion of the transcatheter heart valve leads to increased circularity of the transcatheter heart valve and therefore increased internal orifice diameter. **Table 2** summarising the bench

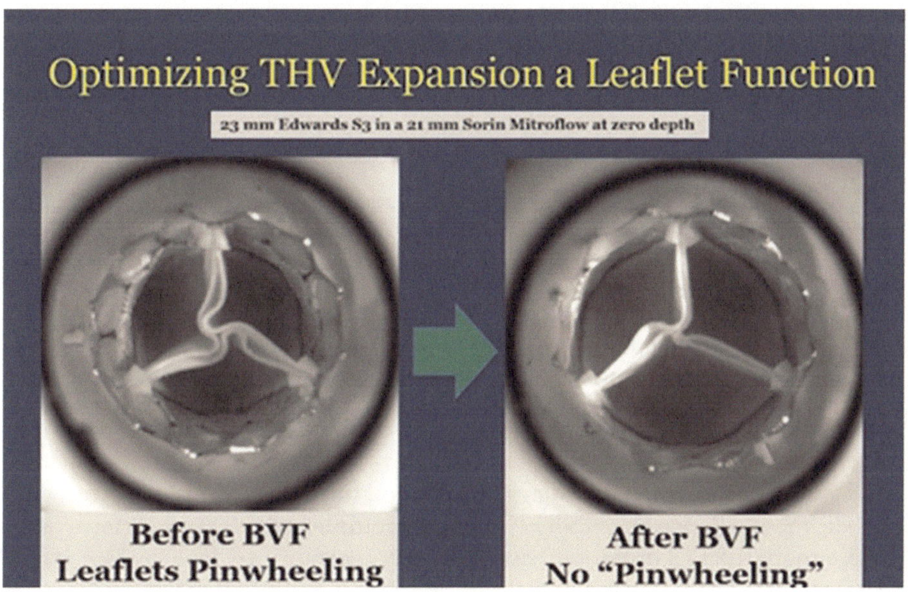

Figure 1.
Reduction of pin-wheeling effect after biological value fracture.

Manufacturer/ Brand	Valve Size	Bard TRU Balloon Fracture/Pressure	Bard Atlas Gold Balloon Fracture/Pressure	Appearance After Fracture
St. Jude Trifecta	19 mm	NO	NO	
	21 mm	NO	NO	
St. Jude Biocor Epic	21 mm	YES / 8 ATM	YES / 8 ATM	
Medtronic Mosaic	19 mm	YES / 10 ATM	YES / 10 ATM	
	21 mm	YES / 10 ATM	YES / 10 ATM	
Medtronic Hancock II	21 mm	NO	NO	
Sorin Mitroflow	19 mm	YES / 12 ATM	YES / 12 ATM	
	21 mm	YES / 12 ATM	YES / 12 ATM	
Edwards MagnaEase	19 mm	YES / 18 ATM	YES / 18 ATM	
	21 mm	YES / 18 ATM	YES / 18 ATM	
Edwards Magna	19 mm	YES / 24 ATM	YES / 24 ATM	
	21 mm	YES / 24 ATM	YES / 24 ATM	

1. Balloons sized 1 mm larger than valve size.
2. Medtronic Mosaic and Sorin Mitroflow have no metal in ring therefore appearance after fracture unchanged.

Table 2.
Summary of bench testing of high pressure balloon inflation to fracture the valve frame of commercial US surgical tissue valves (ATM 1/4 atmospheres; TRU 1/4 Tru dilation) [56].

testing of high-pressure balloon inflation to cause bioprosthetic valve fracture of several commercially available valves [56].

1.4.4 Coronary occlusion

TAVR is associated with a coronary obstruction incidence of 1% [64], and during ViV-TAVR, the incidence rises to 4% [65]. This complication is very serious, associated with a more than 15 times increase in 30-day mortality (~48% vs. 3%) [66]. The primary responsible mechanism is thought due to the displacement of native valve leaflets towards the coronary ostia. The obstruction may be partial or complete, and obstruction of the left coronary artery is more common (72%) than obstruction of both ostia (20%) or the right coronary artery alone (8%). In a third of cases, coronary obstruction has delayed onset, occurring in mainly self-expanding devices due to their continued expansion after deployment. Delayed coronary occlusion is defined as obstruction that occurs after the patient leaves the operating room. It occurs in almost two-thirds of patients within 7 days but in a third of patients beyond 60 days. Proposed mechanisms include continuous transcatheter heart valve expansion, aortic root haematoma and coronary dissection and endothelization of native or surgical bioprosthetic leaflets or thrombus embolization with delayed obstruction [67].

1.4.5 Risk factors for coronary occlusion and difficult coronary re-access

Several anatomical and valve-related risk factors have been identified for this dreaded complication. These include a low coronary ostium height and small sinus of Valsalva size. In addition, the original valve type is important, with ViV-TAVR in stented bioprostheses with leaflets mounted externally and stentless surgical bioprostheses associated with a greater incidence of coronary occlusion, compared with valves with internally mounted leaflets [68].

Other risk factors include those with small anatomies, especially narrow sinuses of Valsalva and narrow sinotubular junctions, who are likely to have received a small surgical valve.

The virtual transcatheter valve-to-coronary ostium distance predicts coronary occlusion, with a shorter distance increasing the risk. An optimal cut-off level of 4 mm has been proposed [69].

Using the VIVID registry, an anatomical classification of the aortic root and valve leaflet was designed to assess the risk of coronary obstruction [70]. Three types of patients were identified: Type I with aortic valve leaflets below the coronary ostium, Type II with leaflets above the ostium in the presence of wide (IIa) or effaced sinuses (IIb) and Type III leaflets above or very close to the sinotubular junction with wide sinotubular junction/sinuses (IIIa), with effaced sinuses (IIIb) and with narrow sinotubular junction (IIIc). According to this algorithm, some procedural strategy should be considered in case of a virtual transcatheter valve-to-coronary ostium distance <4 mm as in Types IIb, IIIb and IIIc [71].

After ViV-TAVR the leaflets of the original surgical prosthesis tilt up, creating a virtual cylinder. The height of this virtual cylinder is labelled and referred to as the neoskirt [72–74]. This forms a "barrier" to future coronary access and must be appreciated carefully during ViV-TAVR planning. The size of the sinotubular junction, the location of coronary ostia in relation to the neoskirt, the type of previous surgical prosthesis as well as the present THV all influence coronary re-access, adding to the complexity of ViV-TAVR planning [58].

1.4.6 Interventions for the prevention of coronary occlusion during ViV-TAVR

1.4.6.1 Coronary stenting

In ViV-TAVR procedures with a high risk of coronary occlusion, coronary artery stenting is valuable. It is imperative that the guide wire used to access the coronary ostia does not interfere with transcatheter heart valve implantation. Low threshold for stent deployment has been recommended in high-risk candidates even in the presence of immediate adequate coronary flow, due to the not infrequent incidence of delayed coronary occlusion [75]. Numerous sophisticated coronary stenting techniques have now evolved and are beyond the scope of this chapter [76–79]. Unfortunately, even these techniques may be associated with several complications such as the inability to withdraw the stent, mechanical stent deformation caused by bioprosthesis and inability to re-access the coronary arteries in the future. In addition, no data regarding the long-term patency of these stents are available [80].

Tarantini et al. have proposed an algorithm based on the anatomy of the aortic root and its relations with different transcatheter heart valves to predict the risk of acute coronary occlusion and feasibility of future coronary access after ViV-TAVR [72]. Using CT and coronary angiography analysis, they identified a risk plane below which the passage of a coronary catheter will be impossible after the second transcatheter heart valve and identified various situations based on a patient's anatomy and the first valve implant type, which could guide safe implantation.

1.4.6.2 Basilica procedure

Another technique developed to prevent coronary obstruction is the Bioprosthetic Aortic Scallop Intentional Laceration to prevent Iatrogenic Coronary Artery obstruction (BASILICA) procedure [81, 82]. Valve leaflets are lacerated via an electrified guidewire, thereby facilitating blood flow to the coronary artery. Excellent success rates and low mortality in high-risk patients for coronary obstruction is demonstrated during TAVR [81, 82], but results for ViV-TAVR are awaited.

1.4.7 Valve choice and implantation

The type of transcatheter heart valve is extremely relevant, and the use of a recapturable self-expanding transcatheter heart valve can be beneficial. Clinical and angiographic assessment of coronary flow after deployment can be performed prior to complete release or retrieval of transcatheter heart valve performed in the setting of coronary occlusion to restore flow. Certain newer transcatheter heart valve devices possess clipping mechanisms enabling grasping of surgical leaflets, thus preventing coronary obstruction [83]. Intentional implantation of a smaller transcatheter heart valve or under expansion of a balloon-expandable transcatheter heart valve reduces the lateral movement of surgical valve posts and leaflets, thereby decreasing chances of coronary obstruction, as does, low-depth transcatheter heart valve implantation compared to high-depth implantation, although the risk of elevated post-procedural gradients may be increased with the latter.

1.5 Valve thrombosis

Sub-clinical leaflet thrombosis is a worry that continues to surround TAVR and ViV-TAVR. The potential need for anti-coagulation is important to patient choice and lifestyle. It is defined as the presence of reduced leaflet motion associated with CT proven hypoattenuating lesions and is associated with a greater risk of transient ischemic attacks [84]. The effects on patient outcome and long-term valve performance remain unclear [85, 86]. A variety of causes are responsible for leaflet thickening and impaired leaflet motion, including leaflet thrombosis, infection and leaflet degeneration [16]. Both TAVR and SAVR are affected by a reduction in leaflet motion, and the incidence is reported as 4% and 13%, respectively [84]. Currently, no robust randomised evidence exists guiding antiplatelet versus anti-coagulation use after ViV-TAVR.

The appropriate treatment of sub-clinical leaflet thrombosis is unclear with evidence showing that it may regress spontaneously. Up to 25% of patients on antiplatelet therapy display this phenomenon, with oral anticoagulants showing efficacy in both its prevention and regression with associated improvement in valve gradients [86–88].

Whether sub-clinical leaflet thrombosis translates into an increased number of thromboembolic neurological events is unclear, but it appears to be associated with elevated valve gradients [89]. ViV-TAVR patients are likely to be at a high risk of leaflet thrombosis due to lesser haemodynamic performance and suboptimal blood flow patterns associated with low implant depth and turbulent blood flow patterns between new transcatheter heart valve leaflets and degenerated valve leaflets [90, 91]. Valve design affects propensity towards leaflet thrombosis, with certain valve types more prone than others [88]. For this reason, a more stringent anti-coagulation regimen has been recommended following ViV-TAVR particularly in patients with elevated thrombotic risk [92]. The issue of possible anti-coagulation for ViV-TAVR is hugely important especially in patents with extended life expectancy and remains unresolved. It is likely that the need for anti-coagulation will be a patient specific, bespoke decision based on anatomical and patient-related risk-factors.

1.6 Cerebral embolism

Transient ischaemic attacks and cerebrovascular accidents are a dreaded complication of any aortic valve intervention, and cerebrovascular accident remains an independent risk factor for death after TAVR [93]. Embolisation is the primary aetiopathogenic mechanism, although the pathogenesis is well known to be multifactorial. The rate of silent embolic lesions following TAVR approaches 80%, and anything that can be done to mitigate this phenomenon is welcome. Despite this, fortunately the incidence of new, persistent clinical neurological injury is only 3–6% [94, 95]. Cerebrovascular accident rates continue to decline after TAVR, but attention is still focussed on strategies to reduce this further [86]. Luckily, the incidence of major stroke following ViV-TAVR has been reported at less than 2% [41], and recent meta-analysis shows no discernible difference in 30-day stroke rate and mortality among ViV-TAVR, TAVR and redo-SAVR [96].

The main proposed factors influencing cerebrovascular accident/transient ischaemic attack risk include atrial fibrillation, acute and sub-acute thromboembolism stemming from the transcatheter heart valve, aortic debris and device instrumentation [81]. Cerebral embolic protection devices are evolving and have been mainly studied during TAVR on native valves. They have shown efficacy in reducing cerebral emboli load, without any effect on short-term cerebrovascular accident or 30-day mortality rates or hospital length of stay [97]. Despite these findings, consideration of the use of cerebral embolic protection devices during ViV-TAVR planning is important, especially where significant instrumentation or technical difficulties are anticipated.

1.7 ViV-TAVR in the young

The patient with aortic stenosis and a long life expectancy that exceeds the durability of a bioprosthesis must be managed very carefully by the heart team, as "optimal" first intervention is paramount. Future negative and positive effects of any bioprosthesis must be anticipated and the anatomy of the aortic root appreciated fully at first intervention. The heart-team approach is an integral part of valvular discussions in patients with severe aortic stenosis and will likely gain increasing importance in the future. A distinct shift of focus towards lifetime management is now occurring after the approval of low-risk TAVR.

Treatment options in younger patients is attracting considerable debate. For those that elect to undergo SAVR, the options for structural valve deterioration are ViV-TAVR or redo-SAVR. For those that undergo TAVR, the options for structural valve deterioration include TAVR explant with SAVR or TAVR-in-TAVR. Of huge importance, many patients with longer life expectancy or early valve failure may need a third valve intervention. A multitude of anatomical scenarios are likely to now be encountered and have to be adjusted for. In patients who are candidates for TAVR-first, transcatheter heart valve with a short frame and large open stent frame cells may be better within the context of large aortic roots and high coronary ostia, in patients with favourable anatomy for future TAVR-in-TAVR implantation [72, 98]. Whereas in patients with low coronary ostia and small aortic roots, TAVR-in-TAVR will be more problematic and therefore SAVR-first with bioprosthesis with as large an orifice as possible plus/minus aortic root enlargement may be better, followed by future ViV-TAVR [99].

1.7.1 SAVR-first strategy

As discussed in detail earlier, ViV-TAVR is associated with better short-term outcomes than redo-SAVR [100]. However, the long-term durability for ViV-TAVR is still unclear. Encouragingly, at mid-term follow-up, <10% of patients display clinically significant structural valve deterioration [101, 102]. Coronary obstruction, difficult re-access to coronaries, severe patient prosthesis mismatch and unclear need for anti-coagulation are residual ongoing concerns surrounding ViV-TAVR. The serious complication of coronary obstruction requires advanced techniques for coronary protection such as chimney stenting or BASILICA, both of which are not simple and increase procedural risk [103, 104]. Rates of paravalvular leak are low but significantly higher than redo-SAVR [19]. Intriguingly, after ViV-TAVR failure, the potential for repeat ViV therapy may be possible, if aortic root diameter allows [105].

1.7.2 Summary of factors favouring SAVR-first policy in young, low-risk patients

Young, low-risk patients often have high anatomical risks such as bicuspid aortic valves, severe annular calcification and low coronary heights. The long-term patient impact of increased permanent pacemaker use and paravalvular regurgitation, along with long-term transcatheter heart valve durability, remain unknown.

Leaflet thickening and coronary re-access remain significant concerns surrounding TAVR.

Valve choice in this group for SAVR also becomes important for the life-time management of aortic valve disease. The largest SAVR valve should be implanted, ideally not less than 23 mm with root enlargement if required. Implanting surgical valves which are prone to fracture for future optimisation of ViV-TAVR is also relevant for this sub-group of patients. The Edwards Inspiris Resilia valve has built-intechnology which enables easy expansion of the valve annulus, and other new generation "TAVR ready" surgical valves will no doubt follow from other manufactures.

1.7.3 Redo SAVR

Being more invasive, it is not surprising that short-term outcomes following redo-SAVR appear inferior to ViV-TAVR [102], but longer-term, major cardiovascular outcomes appear the same [102]. As discussed earlier, no randomised prospective data directly comparing the two techniques are available and are greatly needed. Redo-SAVR is much more invasive than ViV-TAVR but is considered by many as the more complete intervention. In well-selected patients, excellent outcomes with excellent freedom from intervention at 10 years is achieved [106–108], with less incidence of severe patient prosthesis mismatch, leaflet thrombosis and paravalvular leak [19]. Another perceived advantage is that redo-SAVR "resets" the clock and again facilitates the possibility of ViV-TAVR as a potential third intervention if needed.

1.7.4 TAVR-first strategy

1.7.4.1 TAVR explant and SAVR

As summarised above, the TAVR-first strategy in young patients has raised concerns from a wide group of people as doubts remain relating to permanent pacemaker rate, paravalvular leak rate, long-term durability of the TAVR valves and possible need for anti-coagulation [109]. These doubts are more striking when the excellent long-term durability, outcomes and robustness of the anatomical SAVR are used for comparison. TAVR explantation rates are increasing. Most cases have been performed due to unsuitability for the ViV-TAVR procedure and often need extensive surgery and are associated with mortality as high as 15% [110–112]. Sometimes, longer-term TAVR explants require extensive aortic endarterectomy and/or aortic root or ascending aortic replacement. Surgical explantation of SE TAVR valves is more complex and high risk than balloon-expandable TAVR valves. The self-expanding stent can be incorporated into the aortic root and require more extensive surgical procedures. Therefore, TAVR explant mortality rates have been elevated [110]. Surgical expertise is limited in this unique type of surgery and with time is likely to increase and may lead to improved mortality rates during surgical re-intervention for primary TAVR [111].

As mentioned earlier, another perceived advantage of this strategy is SAVR as the second intervention in anatomically suitable patients allows the third potential intervention if needed to be ViV-TAVR in a surgical valve.

1.7.5 TAVR-in-TAVR

TAVR-in-TAVR appears safe, but longer-term data and larger series are needed [113]. Concerns remain about durability and higher rates of paravalvular leak and valve thrombosis and the need for anti-coagulation [84]. In addition, it is believed that many patients will not be suitable for TAVR-in-TAVR because of anatomical constraints centred around the risk of coronary obstruction and coronary re-access [98]. The options for coronary protection are more limited with TAVR-in-TAVR and are a major concern if this strategy is to be employed widely in a large number of younger patients. Recent development of "balloon-assisted BASILICA" shows promise, but it is complex and requires more investigation and refinement [114].

One positive finding is that because of its greater ability to overexpand the transcatheter heart valve, a greater internal orifice diameter is achieved following

TAVR-in-TAVR than ViV-TAVR in a surgical valve, leading to less incidence of high gradients [113].

2. Conclusions

Redo-SAVR traditionally was the only treatment modality for failed bioprostheses. Many elderly patients are not good candidates for a second operation or do not desire to go through a redo-sternotomy. The arrival of transcatheter technology has transformed the landscape of therapy for aortic valve disease and structural valve deterioration. More than a decade after the first reported ViV-TAVR case, this procedure is now consistently performed worldwide in most patients with failed bioprosthetic valves. ViV-TAVR is safe and effective and now a credible, approved alternative treatment option for failed surgical bioprosthetic valves in patients deemed at a prohibitive risk for redo surgery. It is clear that ViV-TAVR is more complex than TAVR in native valves, with a greater risk of peri- and postprocedural complications. A super specialised, multi-disciplinary team with high-volume practice, precision pre-intervention planning, using multimodality imaging is required for optimum results.

With the increasing use of TAVR in younger patients and the increasing use/choice of bioprostheses for SAVR in younger patients, a future with a not inconsiderable population with failed bioprostheses is expected. A downward risk-drift for ViV-TAVR use is also anticipated. Therefore, the real future challenge is identifying what is the best lifetime treatment strategy for aortic valve disease for the individual, as primary intervention is of pre-dominant importance in dictating the individual's subsequent treatment course.

Further, improving ViV-TAVR outcomes is likely to centre around ameliorating and mitigating elevated postprocedural gradients, coronary obstruction risk and leaflet thrombosis. However, efforts focused upon (A) improving bioprosthesis durability/longevity and (B) optimising operative strategies for redo-SAVR are equally important and should be maintained. Providing a good solution for the failed SAVR and investigation into providing an acceptable technical answer for the failed TAVR and also for a potential third valve after a failed ViV-TAVR also merit consideration as part of the lifetime management of aortic valve disease.

Author details

Manoraj Navaratnarajah*, Amit Modi and Sunil Ohri
Department of Cardiac Surgery, University Hospital Southampton, Southampton, Hampshire, United Kingdom

*Address all correspondence to: manoraj.navaratnarajah@doctors.org.uk

IntechOpen

© 2023 The Author(s). Licensee IntechOpen. This chapter is distributed under the terms of the Creative Commons Attribution License (http://creativecommons.org/licenses/by/3.0), which permits unrestricted use, distribution, and reproduction in any medium, provided the original work is properly cited.

References

[1] Coffey S, Roberts-Thomson R, Brown A, Carapetis J, Chen M, Enriquez-Sarano M, et al. Global epidemiology of valvular heart disease. Nature Reviews Cardiology. 2021;**18**(12):853-864

[2] Kappetein AP, Head SJ, Généreux P, Piazza N, van Mieghem NM, Blackstone EH, et al. Updated standardized endpoint definitions for transcatheter aortic valve implantation: The valve academic research Consortium-2 consensus document. Journal of the American College of Cardiology. 2012;**60**(15):1438-1454

[3] Tarantini G, Nai Fovino L, Gersh BJ. Transcatheter aortic valve implantation in lower-risk patients: What is the perspective? European Heart Journal. 2018;**39**:658-666

[4] Leon MB, Smith CR, Mack MJ, et al. Transcatheter or surgical aortic-valve replacement in intermediate-risk patients. The New England Journal of Medicine. 2016;**374**:1609-1620

[5] Reardon MJ, Van Mieghem NM, Popma JJ, et al. Surgical or transcatheter aortic-valve replacement in intermediate-risk patients. The New England Journal of Medicine. 2017;**376**: 1321-1331

[6] Thyregod HG, Steinbruchel DA, Ihlemann N, et al. Transcatheter versus surgical aortic valve replacement in patients with severe aortic valve stenosis: 1-year results from the all-comers NOTION randomized clinical trial. Journal of the American College of Cardiology. 2015;**65**:2184-2194

[7] Mack MJ, Leon MB, Thourani VH, et al. Transcatheter aortic-valve replacement with a balloon expandable valve in low-risk patients. The New England Journal of Medicine. 2019;**380**: 1695-1705

[8] Popma JJ, Deeb GM, Yakubov SJ, et al. Transcatheter aortic-valve replacement with a self-expanding valve in low-risk patients. The New England Journal of Medicine. 2019;**380**:1706-1715

[9] Waksman R, Rogers T, Torguson R, et al. Transcatheter aortic valve replacement in low-risk patients with symptomatic severe aortic stenosis. Journal of the American College of Cardiology. 2018;**72**:2095-2105

[10] Nishimura RA, Otto CM, Bonow RO, et al. 2017 AHA/ACC focused update of the 2014 AHA/ACC guideline for the management of patients with valvular heart disease: A report of the American College of Cardiology/American Heart Association Task Force on Clinical Practice Guidelines. the American College of Cardiology. 2017;**70**(252–89):12

[11] Baumgartner H, Falk V, Bax JJ, et al. 2017 ESC/ EACTS guidelines for the management of valvular heart disease. European Heart Journal. 2017;**38**: 2739-2791

[12] Goldstone AB, Chiu P, Baiocchi M, Lingala B, Patrick WL, Fischbein MP, et al. Mechanical or biologic prostheses for aortic-valve and mitral-valve replacement. The New England Journal of Medicine. 2017;**377**:1847-1857

[13] Austin PC, Dvir D, Fremes SE. Surgical valve selection in the era of transcatheter aortic valve replacement in the Society of Thoracic Surgeons database. The Journal of Thoracic and Cardiovascular Surgery. 2020;**159**: 416-427.e8

[14] Tam DY, Rocha RV, Wijeysundera HC, Austin PC, Dvir D,

Fremes SE. Surgical valve selection in the era of transcatheter aortic valve replacement in the Society of Thoracic Surgeons database. Journal of Thoracic and Cardiovascular Surgery. 2020; **159**(2):416-427

[15] Fauvel C, Capoulade R, Durand E, et al. Durability of transcatheter aortic valve implantation: A translational review. Archives of Cardiovascular Diseases. 2020;**113**(3):209-221

[16] Généreux P, Piazza N, Alu MC, et al. Valve academic research consortium 3: Updated endpoint definitions for aortic valve clinical research. Journal of the American College of Cardiology. 2021; **77**:2717-2746

[17] Salaun E, Clavel MA, Rod'es-Cabau J, Pibarot P. Bioprosthetic aortic valve durability in the era of transcatheter aortic valve implantation. Heart. 2018; **104**(16):1323-1332

[18] Sá MPBO, Van den Eynde J, Simonato M, et al. Valve-in-valve transcatheter aortic valve replacement versus redo surgical aortic valve replacement: An updated meta-analysis. JACC. Cardiovascular Interventions. 2021;**14**:211-220

[19] Thandra A, Abusnina W, Jhand A, et al. Valve-in-valve transcatheter aortic valve replacement versus redo surgical valve replacement for degenerated bioprosthetic aortic valve: An updated meta-analysis comparing midterm outcomes. Catheterization and Cardiovascular Interventions. 2021;**97**: 1481-1488

[20] Saleem S, Ullah W, Syed MA, et al. Meta-analysis comparing valve-in-valve TAVR and redo-SAVR in patients with degenerated bioprosthetic aortic valve. Catheterization and Cardiovascular Interventions. 2021;**98**: 940-947

[21] Hirji SA, Percy ED, Zogg CK, et al. Comparison of in-hospital outcomes and readmissions for valve-in-valve transcatheter aortic valve replacement vs. re-operative surgical aortic valve replacement: A contemporary assessment of real-world outcomes. European Heart Journal. 2020;**41**: 2747-2755

[22] Raschpichler M, de Waha S, Holzhey D, Schwarzer G, Flint N, Kaewkes D, et al. Valve-in-valve transcatheter aortic valve replacement versus redo surgical aortic valve replacement for failed surgical aortic bioprostheses: A systematic review and meta-analysis. Journal of the American Heart Association. 2022;**11**:e7965

[23] Formica F, Gallingani A, Tuttolomondo D, Hernandez-Vaquero D, D'Alessandro S, Pattuzzi C, et al. Redo surgical aortic valve replacement versus valve-in-valve transcatheter aortic valve implantation: A systematic review and reconstructed time-to-event meta-analysis. Journal of Clinical Medicine. 2023;**12**:541

[24] Bruno F, Elia E, D'Ascenzo F, Marengo G, Deharo P, Kaneko T, et al. Valvein-valve transcatheter aortic valve replacement or re-surgical aortic valve replacement in degenerated bioprostheses: A systematic review and meta-analysis of short and midterm results. Catheterization and Cardiovascular Interventions. 2022;**100**: 122-130

[25] Gatta F, Haqzad Y, Gradinariu G, et al. Redo aortic valve replacement vs valve-in-valve trans-catheter aortic valve implantation: A UK propensity-matched analysis. Monaldi Archives for Chest Disease. 19 Apr 2023

[26] Ochi K, Cheng B, Zhao AA, Hardikar, Negishi K. Patient risk factors for bioprosthetic aortic valve degeneration: A systematic review and meta-analysis. Heart Lung & Circulation. 2020;**29**(5):668-678

[27] Flameng W, Herregods MC, Vercalsteren M, Herijgers P, Bogaerts K, Meuris B. Prosthesis-patient mismatch predicts structural valve degeneration in bioprosthetic heart valves. Circulation. 2010;**121**:2123-2129

[28] Fallon JM, DeSimone JP, Brennan JM, et al. The incidence and consequence of prosthesis-patient mismatch after surgical aortic valve replacement. Annals of Thoracic Surgery. 2018;**106**(1):14-22

[29] Dismorr M, Glaser N, Franco-Cereceda A, Sartipy U. Effect of prosthesis-patient mismatch on long-term clinical outcomes after bioprosthetic aortic valve replacement. Journal of the American College of Cardiology. 14 Mar 2023;**81**(10):964-975

[30] Head SJ, Mokhles MM, Osnabrugge RL, et al. The impact of prosthesis-patient mismatch on long-term survival after aortic valve replacement: A systematic review and meta-analysis of 34 observational studies comprising 27 186 patients with 133 141 patient-years. European Heart Journal. 2012;**33**(12):1518-1529

[31] Dahlbacka S, Laakso T, Kinnunen E-M, et al. Patient-prosthesis mismatch mismatch worsens long-term survival: Insights from the FinnValve registry. Annals of Thoracic Surgery. Apr 2021; **111**(4):1284-1290

[32] Norton EL, Ward AF, Greenbaum A, Grubb KJ. Management of failed bioprosthetic aortic valves: Mitigating complications and optimizing outcomes. Journal of Interventional Cardiology. 2 Sep 2022;**2022**:9737245

[33] Nicks R, Cartmill T, Bernstein L. Hypoplasia of the aortic root: The problem of aortic valve replacement. Thorax. 1970;**25**(3):339-346

[34] Manouguian S, Seybold-Epting W. Patch enlargement of the aortic valve ring by extending the aortic incision into the anterior mitral leaflet. The Journal of Thoracic and Cardiovascular Surgery. 1979;**78**(3):402-412

[35] Konno S, Imai Y, Iida Y, Nakajima M, Tatsuno K. A new method for prosthetic valve replacement in congenital aortic stenosis associated with hypoplasia of the aortic valve ring. Journal of Thoracic and Cardiovascular Surgery. 1975;**70**(5):909-917

[36] Kulik A, Al-Saigh M, Chan V, Masters RG, Bedard P, Lam BK, et al. Enlargement of the small aortic root during aortic valve replacement: Is there a benefit? The Annals of Thoracic Surgery. 2008;**85**:94-100

[37] Peterson MD, Borger MA, Feindel CM, David TE. Aortic annular enlargement during aortic valve replacement: Improving results with time. The Annals of Thoracic Surgery. 2007;**83**:2044-2049

[38] Clavel MA, Webb JG, Pibarot P, Altwegg L, Dumont E, Thompson C, et al. Comparison of the hemodynamic performance of percutaneous and surgical bioprostheses for the treatment of severe aortic stenosis. Journal of the American College of Cardiology. 2009; **53**:1883-1891

[39] Jilaihawi H, Chin D, Spyt T, Jeilan M, Vasa-Nicotera M, Bence J, et al. Prosthesis-patient mismatch after

transcatheter aortic valve implantation with the Medtronic-Corevalve bioprosthesis. European Heart Journal. 2010;**31**:857-864

[40] Sá MP, Jabagi H, Dokollari A, Awad AK, Van den Eynde J, Malin JH, et al. Early and late outcomes of surgical aortic valve replacement with sutureless and rapid-deployment valves versus transcatheter aortic valve implantation: Meta-analysis. Catheterization and Cardiovascular Interventions. 2022; **99**(6):1886-1896

[41] Dvir D, Webb JG, Bleiziffer S, Pasic M, Waksman R, Kodali S, et al. Transcatheter aortic valve implantation in failed bioprosthetic surgical valves. Journal of the American Medical Association. 2014;**312**:162-170

[42] Webb JG, Murdoch DJ, Alu MC, Cheung A, Crowley A, Dvir D, et al. 3-year outcomes after valve-in-valve transcatheter aortic valve replacement for degenerated bioprostheses: The partner 2 registry. Journal of the American College of Cardiology. 2019; **73**:2647-2655

[43] Wendt D, Thielmann M, Plicht B, et al. The new St Jude trifecta versus Carpentier-Edwards Perimount magna and magna ease aortic bioprosthesis: Is there a hemodynamic superiority? The Journal of Thoracic and Cardiovascular Surgery. 2014;**147**:1553-1560

[44] Vemulapalli S, Holmes DR Jr, Dai D, et al. Valve hemodynamic deterioration and cardiovascular outcomes in TAVR: A report from the STS/ACC TVT registry. American Heart Journal. 2018; **195**:1-13

[45] Flameng W, Herregods MC, Vercalsteren M, Herijgers P, Bogaerts K, Meuris B. Prosthesis-patient mismatch predicts structural valve degeneration in bioprosthetic heart valves. Circulation. 2010;**121**:2123-2129

[46] Jie Yao R, Simonato M, Dvir D, Department of Cardiology, St Paul's Hospital, Vancouver, Canada. Optimising the haemodynamics of aortic valve-in-valve procedures. Interventional Cardiology. 2017;**12**:40

[47] Simonato M, Dvir D. Transcatheter aortic valve replacement in failed surgical valves. Heart. 2019;**105**:s38-s43

[48] Midha PA, Raghav V, Condado JF, Arjunon S, Uceda DE, Lerakis S, et al. How can we help a patient with a small failing bioprosthesis?: An in vitro case study. JACC. Cardiovascular Interventions. 2015;**8**:2026-2033

[49] Simonato M, Webb J, Kornowski R, Vahanian A, Frerker C, Nissen H, et al. Transcatheter replacement of failed bioprosthetic valves: Large multicenter assessment of the effect of implantation depth on hemodynamics after aortic valve-in-valve. Circulation. Cardiovascular Interventions. 2016;**9**: e003651

[50] Pibarot P, Simonato M, Barbanti M, et al. Impact of pre-existing prosthesis-patient mismatch on survival following aortic valve-in valve procedures. JACC. Cardiovascular Interventions. 2018;**11**: 133-141

[51] Jilaihawi H, Chin D, Spyt T, et al. Prosthesis-patient mismatch after transcatheter aortic valve implantation with the Medtronic Corevalve bioprosthesis. European Heart Journal. 2010;**31**:857-864

[52] Simonato M, Webb J, Bleiziffer S, et al. Current generation balloon-expandable transcatheter valve positioning strategies during aortic valve-in-valve procedures and clinical

outcomes. JACC. Cardiovascular Interventions. 2019;**12**:1606-1617

[53] Azadani AN, Reardon M, Simonato M, et al. Effect of transcatheter aortic valve size and position on valve-in-valve hemodynamics: An in vitro study. The Journal of Thoracic and Cardiovascular Surgery. 2017;**153**: 1303-15.e1

[54] Zenses AS, Evin MA, Stanová V, et al. Effect of size and position of self-expanding transcatheter valve on haemodynamics following valve-in-valve procedure in small surgical bioprostheses: An in vitro study. EuroIntervention. 2018;**14**:e282-e289

[55] Aurigemma C, Burzotta F, Vergallo R, Farina P, Romagnoli E, Cangemi S, et al. Transcatether aortic valve implantation to treat degenerated surgical bioprosthesis: Focus on the specific procedural challenges. Frontiers in Cardiovascular Medicine. 2022;**9**: Article 895477

[56] Allen KB, Chhatriwalla AK, Cohen DJ, et al. Bioprosthetic valve fracture to facilitate transcatheter valve-in-valve implantation. The Annals of Thoracic Surgery. 2017;**104**:1501-1508

[57] Saxon JT, Allen KB, Cohen DJ, Chhatriwalla AK. Bioprosthetic valve fracture during valve-in-valve TAVR: Bench to bedside. Interventional Cardiology. 2018;**13**:20-26

[58] Tarantini G, Dvir D, Tang GHL. Transcatheter aortic valve implantation in degenerated surgical aortic valves. EuroIntervention. 2021;**17**:709-719

[59] Ziccardi MR, Groves EM. Bioprosthetic valve fracture for valve-in-valve transcatheter aortic valve replacement: Rationale, patient selection, technique, and outcomes. Interventional Cardiology Clinics. 2019; **8**:373-382

[60] Nielsen-Kudsk JE, Andersen A, Therkelsen CJ, et al. High-pressure balloon fracturing of small dysfunctional Mitroflow bioprostheses facilitates transcatheter aortic valve-in-valve implantation. EuroIntervention. 2017;**13**: e1020-e1025

[61] Patel JS, Krishnaswamy A, White J, et al. Optimizing hemodynamics of transcatheter aortic valve-in-valve implantation in 19-mm surgical aortic prostheses. Catheterization and Cardiovascular Interventions. 2018;**92**: 550-554

[62] Allen KB, Chhatriwalla AK, Saxon JT, Cohen DJ, Nguyen TC, Webb J, et al. Bioprosthetic valve fracture investigators. The Journal of Thoracic and Cardiovascular Surgery. 2019;**158**:1317-1328

[63] Sathananthan J, Fraser R, Hatoum H, Barlow AM, Stanová V, Allen KB, et al. A bench test study of bioprosthetic valve fracture performed before vs. after transcatheter valve-in-valve intervention. EuroIntervention. 2020;**15**: 1409-1416

[64] Ribeiro HB, Nombela-Franco L, Urena M, Mok M, Pasian S, Doyle D, et al. Coronary obstruction following transcatheter aortic valve implantation. A systematic review. JACC: Cardiovascular Intervention. 2013;**6**: 452-461

[65] Dvir D, Webb J, Brecker S, Bleiziffer S, Hildick-Smith D, Colombo A, et al. Transcatheter aortic valve replacement for degenerative bioprosthetic surgical valves: Results from the global valve-in-valve registry. Circulation. 2012;**126**:2335-2344

[66] Simonato M, Dvir D. Transcatheter aortic valve replacement in failed surgical valves. Heart. 2019;**105**:s38-s43

[67] Jabbour RJ, Tanaka A, Finkelstein A, et al. Delayed coronary obstruction after transcatheter aortic valve replacement. Journal of the American College of Cardiology. 2018;**71**:1513-1524

[68] Ribeiro HB, Rodés-Cabau J, Blanke P, Leipsic J, Kwan Park J, Bapat V, et al. Incidence, predictors, clinical outcomes of coronary obstruction following transcatheter aortic valve replacement for degenerative bioprosthetic surgical valves: Insights from the VIVID registry. European Heart Journal. 2018;**39**: 687-695

[69] Hensey M, Sellers S, Sathananthan J, Lai A, Landes U, Alkhodair A, et al. Bioprosthetic valve leaflet displacement during valve-in-valve intervention: An ex vivo bench study. JACC. Cardiovascular Interventions. 2020;**13**: 667-678

[70] Tang GHL, Komatsu I, Tzemach L, Simonato M, Wolak A, Blanke P, et al. Risk of coronary obstruction and the need to perform BASILICA: The VIVID classification. EuroIntervention. 2020; **16**:e757-e759

[71] Ziccardi MR, Groves EM. Bioprosthetic valve fracture for valve-in-valve transcatheter aortic valve replacement: Rationale, patient selection, technique, and outcomes. Interventional Cardiology Clinics. 2019; **8**:373-382

[72] Tarantini G, Fabris T, Nai FL. TAVR-in-TAVR and coronary access: Importance of preprocedural planning. EuroIntervention. 2020;**16**:e129-e132

[73] Nai Fovino L, Scotti A, Massussi M, et al. Coronary angiography after transcatheter aortic valve replacement [TAVR] to evaluate the risk of coronary access impairment after TAVR-in-TAVR. Journal of the American Heart Association. 2020;**9**:016446

[74] Tang GHL, Zaid S, Gupta E, et al. Feasibility of repeat tavr after SAPIEN 3 TAVR: A novel classification scheme and pilot angiographic study. JACC. Cardiovascular Interventions. 2019;**12**: 1290-1292

[75] Palmerini T, Chakravarty T, Saia F, Bruno AG, Bacchi-Reggiani ML, Marrozzini C, et al. Coronary protection to prevent coronary obstruction during TAVR: A multicenter international registry. JACC. Cardiovascular Interventions. 2020;**13**:739-747

[76] Fetahovic T, Hayman S, Cox S, Cole C, Rafter T, Camuglia A. The prophylactic chimney snorkel technique for the prevention of acute coronary occlusion in high risk for coronary obstruction transcatheter aortic valve replacement/implantation cases. Heart, Lung & Circulation. 2019;**28**:e126-e130

[77] Burzotta F, Kovacevic M, Aurigemma C, Shoeib O, Bruno P, Cangemi S, et al. An "orthotopic" snorkel-stenting technique to maintain coronary patency during transcatheter aortic valve replacement. Cardiovascular Revascularization Medicine. 2021;**28S**: 94-97

[78] Mercanti F, Rosseel L, Neylon A, et al. Chimney stenting for coronary occlusion during TAVR: Insights from the chimney registry. JACC. Cardiovascular Interventions. 2020;**13**: 751-761

[79] Romano V, Buzzatti N, Latib A, Colombo A, Montorfano M. Chimney technique for coronary obstruction after

aortic valve in valve: Pros and cons. European Heart Journal Cardiovascular Imaging. 2018;**19**:1194

[80] Edelman JJ, Khan JM, Rogers T, et al. Valve-in-valve TAVR: State-of-the-art review. Innovations [Phila]. 2019;**14**: 299-310

[81] Khan JM, Greenbaum AB, Babaliaros VC, et al. The BASILICA trial: Prospective multicenter investigation of intentional leaflet laceration to prevent TAVR coronary obstruction. JACC. Cardiovascular Interventions. 2019;**12**: 1240-1252

[82] De Backer O, Søndergaard L. Is BASILICA the standard for preventing coronary obstruction in high-risk transcatheter aortic valve replacement? JACC. Cardiovascular Interventions. 2021;**14**:949-951

[83] Hensey M, Sellers S, Sathananthan J, Lai A, Landes U, Alkhodair A, et al. Bioprosthetic valve leaflet displacement during valve-in-valve intervention: An ex vivo bench study. JACC. Cardiovascular Interventions. 2020;**13**: 667-678

[84] Chakravarty T, Søndergaard L, Friedman J, et al. Subclinical leaflet thrombosis in surgical and transcatheter bioprosthetic aortic valves: An observational study. Lancet. 2017;**389**: 2383-2392

[85] Blanke P, Leipsic JA, Popma JJ, et al. Bioprosthetic aortic valve leaflet thickening in the evolut low risk sub-study. Journal of the American College of Cardiology. 2020;**75**:2430-2442

[86] De Backer O, Dangas GD, Jilaihawi H, et al. Reduced leaflet motion after transcatheter aortic-valve replacement. The New England Journal of Medicine. 2020;**382**:130-139

[87] Makkar RR, Blanke P, Leipsic J, et al. Subclinical leaflet thrombosis in transcatheter and surgical bioprosthetic valves: PARTNER 3 cardiac computed tomography substudy. Journal of the American College of Cardiology. 2020; **75**:3003-3015

[88] Abdel-Wahab M, Simonato M, Latib A, et al. Clinical valve thrombosis after transcatheter aortic valve-in-valve implantation. Circulation. Cardiovascular Interventions. 2018;**11**: e006730

[89] Ten Berg J, Sibbing D, Rocca B, et al. Management of antithrombotic therapy in patients undergoing transcatheter aortic valve implantation: A consensus document of the ESC Working Group on Thrombosis and the European Association of Percutaneous Cardiovascular Interventions [EAPCI], in collaboration with the ESC Council on Valvular Heart Disease. European Heart Journal. 2021;**42**:2265-2269

[90] Jose J, Sulimov DS, El-Mawardy M, et al. Clinical bioprosthetic heart valve thrombosis after transcatheter aortic valve replacement: Incidence, characteristics, and treatment outcomes. JACC. Cardiovascular Interventions. 2017;**10**:686-697

[91] Vahidkhah K, Javani S, Abbasi M, et al. Blood stasis on transcatheter valve leaflets and implications for valve-in-valve leaflet thrombosis. The Annals of Thoracic Surgery. 2017;**104**:751-759

[92] Otto CM, Nishimura RA, Bonow RO, et al. ACC/AHA guideline for the management of patients with valvular heart disease: Executive summary: A report of the American College of Cardiology/American Heart Association Joint Committee on Clinical Practice Guidelines. Journal of the American

College of Cardiology. 2020;**2021**(77): 450-500

[93] Eggebrecht H, Schmermund A, Voigtländer T, Kahlert P, Erbel R, Mehta RH. Risk of stroke after transcatheter aortic valve implantation [TAVI]: A meta-analysis of 10,037 published patients. EuroIntervention. 2012;**8**:129-138

[94] Altisent OAJ, Rishi Puri R, Rodés-Cabau J. Embolic protection devices during TAVI: Current evidence and uncertainties. Revista Española de Cardiología (English ed.). 2016;**69**: 962-972

[95] Kahlert P, Knipp SC, Schlamann M, et al. Silent and apparent cerebral ischemia after percutaneous transfemoral aortic valve implantation: A diffusion-weighted magnetic resonance imaging study. Circulation. 2010;**121**:870

[96] Macherey S, Meertens M, Mauri V, et al. Meta-analysis of stroke and mortality rates in patients undergoing valve-in-valve transcatheter aortic valve replacement. Journal of the American Heart Association. 2021;**10**:e019512

[97] Teitelbaum M, Kotronias RA, Sposato LA, Bagur R. Cerebral embolic protection in TAVI: Friend or foe. Interventional Cardiology. 2019;**14**:22-25

[98] De Backer O, Landes U, Fuchs A, et al. Coronary access after TAVR-in-TAVR as evaluated by multidetector computed tomography. JACC. Cardiovascular Interventions. 2020;**13**: 2528-2538

[99] Tarantini G, Nai FL. Lifetime strategy of patients with aortic stenosis: The first cut is the deepest. JACC. Cardiovascular Interventions. 2021;**14**: 1727-1730

[100] Deharo P et al. Transcatheter valve-in-valve aortic valve replacement as an alternative to surgical re-replacement. Journal of the American College of Cardiology. 2020;**76**:489-499

[101] Webb JG et al. 3-year outcomes after valve-in-valve transcatheter aortic valve replacement for degenerated bioprostheses: The PARTNER 2 registry. Journal of the American College of Cardiology. 2019;**73**:2647-2655

[102] Campos et al. Long-term outcomes after transcatheter aortic valve-in-valve replacement. Circulation, Cardiovasc Interventions. Sep 2018;**11**(9):e007038

[103] Khan JM, Dvir D, Greenbaum AB, Babaliaros VC, Rogers T, Aldea G, et al. Transcatheter laceration of aortic leaflets to prevent coronary obstruction during transcatheter aortic valve replacement: Concept to first-in-human. JACC. Cardiovascular Interventions. 2018;**11**: 677-689

[104] Mercanti F, Rosseel L, Neylon A, Bagur R, Sinning JM, Nickenig G, et al. Chimney stenting for coronary occlusion during TAVR. JACC: Cardiovascular Interventions. 2020;**13**:751-761

[105] Basman C, Seetharam K, Pirelli L, Kliger CA. Transcatheter aortic valve-in–Valve-in-valve implantation with three-dimensional printing guidance: A case report. Journal of Cardiac Surgery. 2020; **35**:1676-1680

[106] Onorati F, Biancari F, De Feo M, Mariscalco G, Messina A, Santarpino G, et al. Outcome of redo surgical aortic valve replacement in patients 80 years and older: Results from the multicenter RECORD initiative. The Annals of Thoracic Surgery. 2014;**97**:537-543

[107] Maganti M, Rao V, Armstrong S, Feindel CM, Scully HE, David TE.

Redo valvular surgery in elderly patients. The Annals of Thoracic Surgery. 2009; **87**:521-525

[108] Onorati F, Biancari F, De Feo M, Mariscalco G, Messina A, Santarpino G, et al. Mid-term results of aortic valve surgery in redo scenarios in the current practice: Results from the multicentre European RECORD [REdo cardiac operation research database] initiative. European Journal of Cardio-Thoracic Surgery. 2015;**47**:2

[109] Navaratnarajah M, Luthra S, Ohri S. Transcatheter aortic valve implantation in low-risk patients: A case of rational over exuberance. The time is not now. Asian Cardiovascular & Thoracic Annals. 2021;**29**(8):836-847

[110] Hirji SA, Percy ED, McGurk S, Malarczyk A, Harloff MT, Yazdchi F, et al. Incidence, characteristics, predictors, and outcomes of surgical explantation after transcatheter aortic valve replacement. Journal of the American College of Cardiology. 2020; **76**:1848-1859

[111] Fukuhara S, Brescia AA, Shiomi S, Rosati CM, Yang B, Kim KM, et al. Surgical explantation of transcatheter aortic bioprostheses: Results and clinical implications. The Journal of Thoracic and Cardiovascular Surgery. 2021;**162**: 539-547

[112] Fukuhara S, Tanaka D, Brescia AA, Wai Sang SL, Grossman PM, Sukul D, et al. Aortic valve reintervention in patients with failing transcatheter aortic bioprostheses: Z statewide experience. The Journal of Thoracic and Cardiovascular Surgery. Jun 2023;**165** (6):2011-2020.e5

[113] Landes U, Sathananthan J, Witberg G, De Backer O, Sondergaard L, Abdel-Wahab M, et al. Transcatheter replacement of transcatheter versus surgically implanted aortic valve bioprostheses. Journal of the American College of Cardiology. 2021;**77**:1-14

[114] Greenbaum AB, Kamioka N, Vavalle JP, Lisko JC, Gleason PT, Paone G, et al. Balloon-assisted BASILICA to facilitate redo TAVR. JACC. Cardiovascular Interventions. 2021;**14**:578-580

Chapter 8

Stroke Risk during TAVR: Is Prevention Better than Cure?

Gianluca Di Pietro, Improta Riccardo, Marco Tocci, Lucia Ilaria Birtolo, Emanuele Bruno, Colantonio Riccardo, Massimo Mancone and Gennaro Sardella

Abstract

Periprocedural stroke is an uncommon but feared complication in patients undergoing transcatheter aortic valve replacement (TAVR). Typically embolic, it occurs more frequent in the first days (within seven days) after the procedure and it is secondary to procedural factors. It has a wide clinical spectrum and it is associated with increased mortality and a controversial worse impact on cognitive functions. Capture of the debris by different cerebral embolic protection devices (CEPDs) during the TAVR were thought to be a safe and effective preventive strategy to reduce the risk of stroke. A lot of trials were conducted to demonstrate a benefit of CEPDs, but the current evidence is not conclusive on their impact on periprocedural strokes.

Keywords: periprocedural stroke, transcatheter aortic valve replacement, mortality, cognitive functions, neurocognitive, cerebral embolic protection devices

1. Introduction

Transcatheter aortic valve replacement (TAVR) is a rapidly growing minimally invasive alternative in patients with symptomatic severe aortic stenosis and intermediate or greater pre-operative surgical risk [1–3]. While TAVR is associated with a lower risk of complications, shorter recovery and overall effectiveness, periprocedural stroke remains a significant concern [4] with a relevant impact on mortality, cognitive decline and quality of life (QoL) [5–8]. The progressively expanded recommendation of TAVR for younger or low-risk patients [9–11] makes it necessary to consider preventive strategies to reduce the incidence of this devasting complication for TAVR patients. Over the years, several studies have investigated the safety and effectiveness of different protection devices whose temporary positioning during percutaneous biological valve implantation is still controversial.

2. The risk of stroke in the early phase after TAVR: Why to prevent?

Periprocedural stroke is defined as a neurological dysfunction of at least 24 hours and/or visible on imaging within seven days after TAVR [7, 12–15]. In particular, less than half of postoperative strokes occur within the first day after the index procedure [16, 17]. The cerebral embolization of debris during manipulation of the catheters, the calcified native valve and the aortic wall is supposed to be the main pathogenetic mechanism. The impact of sedation and anesthesia on cerebral blood flow has a considerable additional impact [18]. The debris types comprised arterial wall tissue, native valve tissue, calcifications and foreign body material detached from percutaneous devices [19, 20]. Neuroimaging in stroke revealed more frequent supratentorial cerebral left-side lesions [21, 22]. The middle cerebral anterior (MCA) is the most commonly involved artery [22].

Over the years, the impact of vascular access on periprocedural stroke during TAVR was not wholly verified. The Transfemoral (TF) approach is the route of choice for TAVR. Initially, it was associated with a higher risk of periprocedural stroke than transapical (TA) one, supposing that TA-TAVR could allow an accessible and direct implantation and avoid the manipulation of catheters and devices in the aortic arch [23–25]. However, recent studies did not observe worse outcomes in TF-TAVR than in TA-TAVR [26, 27]. Other vascular approaches (trans-carotid, TC; trans-subclavian TS; direct trans-aortic, TAO) were compared to the gold standard. However, neither TC-/TS [28] nor TAO [29] were associated to lower risk of periprocedural stroke.

The choice of a self-expandable valve (SEV) or a balloon-expandable valve (BEV) is another challenging procedural aspect. SEV-related strokes occur during slow stepwise implantation, while BEV-related strokes occur during valve positioning [30]. The CHOICE trial [31], the REPRISE III trial [32] and the randomized SOLVE-TAVI trial [33] were inconclusive because of the cohorts of patients selected, the frequency of the follow-up and the neurological assessment. However, recent stronger evidences registered that patients who underwent BEV implantation have lower rates of strokes or less silent cerebral lesions detected by DWI-MRI [20, 22, 34–37].

During the biological valve implantation, the role of pre- (BAV) and post- (BPD) dilatation is also crucial. Pre-dilatation was initially thought mandatory to cross the stenosed valve, to prepare the prosthesis, and to decrease the radial counterforces. However, the DIRECT and DIRECTAVI trials demonstrated the feasibility of direct-TAVI approaches without increasing rates of periprocedural strokes [38, 39]. Instead, post-dilatation guarantees an optimal frame expansion, reduces paravalvular leak (PVL) and avoids the patient-prosthesis mismatch (PPM). This aspect is not irrelevant, considering that small aortic valvular areas (AVA) after TAVR or malposition predispose to ischemic cerebral embolism due to subclinical leaflet thrombus [40]. Despite this, in several studies, BPD seems to double the risk of periprocedural strokes [41–44] and nowadays it is considered an independent risk factor of early stroke after TAVR [45]. In conclusion, BAV has no apparent impact on stroke rates, but reduced pre-dilatation is not justified if BPD increases in a direct-TAVR approach. On the contrary, BPD should be minimized more and more, improving the sizing of the annulus by cardiac tomography (CT).

The "intrinsic" thromboembolic risk of the patient should also be considered. Several factors, including age, female sex, prior stroke or TIA, obesity, diabetes, chronic renal failure, and atrial fibrillation, are independent predictors of TAVR postoperative stroke [17]. Recent data showed that carotid artery disease is not associated with increased rates of early stroke [46].

The incidence of periprocedural stroke is still debated (**Figure 1**). Initially, in the high-risk patients-PARTNER 1 trial [7], neurological events were higher in TAVR-group compared to the open-surgery standard of care at one year (8.3% vs. 4.3%, p = 0.04). The cross-clamping of the aorta was supposed to allow the debris removal. However, the selection bias of the high risk group eligible for TAVR seems to be related to these results. Conversely, the PARTNER trial 2 [3] and the SURTAVI [47] selected non-high risk patients showing a significant lower rate of strokes in the TAVR-group. Nevertheless, observational registries are frequently based on self-reporting events without a strict neurological assessment or monitoring and a central adjudication of events. The ADVANCE trial [48] first tried to evaluate the neurological outcomes after TAVR thanks to an Independent Clinical Events Committee. It showed an incidence of about 1.4% from zero to one postoperative day. Additionally, the CoreValve US Extreme Risk and High Pivotal Trials were studied by Kleiman et al. with a particular issue about cerebrovascular events (CVEs) [14]. The paper was drawn from trials (and not registries or prospective studies) that involved a rigorous method of neurological assessment of patients after TAVR. In the early phase (0–10 days after the procedure), the incidence of stroke was found to be at 4%, higher compared to previous registries.

However, the real world rate of periprocedural cerebral events (CVEs) may be underestimated. The phenomenon of silent cerebral embolism (SCE) may be a partial explanation. Silent brain lesions were detected in at least 70% of patients underwent DWI-MRI after TAVR [22, 49, 50], but only 27% of lesions evolved into gliotic scars at the follow-up [22]. Other reasons for under-reporting are: (a) sedating drugs and anesthesia; (b) lack of understanding of symptoms; (c) formation of thrombus after depositing of embolus.

In 2020, an STS/ACC TVT Registry analysis [51] included over 276,316 patients undergoing TAVR between 2011 and 2019. The authors found that the incidence of in-hospital stroke or transient ischemic attack (TIA) has decreased from 2011 (2.1%)

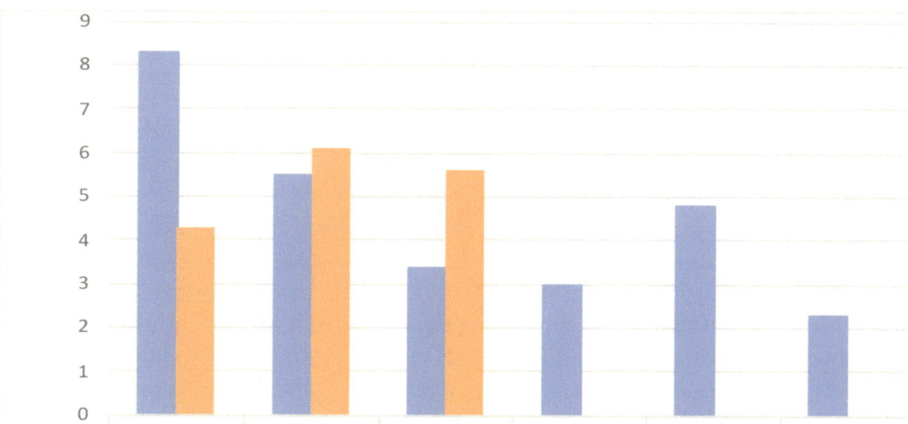

	PARTNER TRIAL 1	PARTNER TRIAL 2	SURTAVI TRIAL	ADVANCE TRIAL	CoreValve US Extreme Risk and High Pivotal Trials	STS/ACC TVT Registry
TAVR	8,3	5,5	3,4	3	4,8	2,3
SAVR	4,3	6,1	5,6			

Figure 1.
Thromboembolic incidence in larger studies about TAVR.

to 2019 (1.6%), as well as 30-day stroke rates (2.75% vs. 2.3%). It could be partly influenced by the operator experience improved over time. Salemi et al. high-lightened that procedures performed by more experienced operators are associated with significantly lower risks for post-procedural stroke [52].

The occurrence of significant strokes after TAVR has a meaningful clinical impact on mortality and neurocognition. The PARTNER trial [13] was the first to demonstrate that patients with stroke after TAVR had a higher mortality rate at 30 days and one year than those without. Subsequently, either Huded et al. [16] or Kleiman et al. [14] confirmed these results. In addition, in 2023, Castelo et al. affirmed more precisely that patients with stroke after TAVR have longer intensive unit care (ICU) stay (12 vs. 4 days) and higher rates of intra-hospital mortality (21.1% vs. 4.3%) especially cardiovascular 30-days mortality (15,8% vs. 4,1%) [45].

A large body of evidence indicated adverse cognitive consequences of cerebral brain lesions (clinically silent or overt), either in atrial fibrillation [53] or after cardiac surgery [54]. The impact of SCE on cognitive decline has been debated for a long time because several studies were controversial. In 2010, Khalert et al. reported that cerebral lesions are not associated with the deterioration of cognitive functions [55]. On the contrary, in the subsequent Neuro-TAVI trial, Lansky et al. confirmed that one in three patients after TAVI had a cognitive decline assessed by the Montreal Cognitive Assessment score (MoCA) [49]. In the SENTINEL trial, Kapadia reported a correlation between changes in cognition and median silent cerebral lesions volume ($p < 0.002$, 21]. Similarly, De Carlo et al. observed that patients developing SCILs had a significant worsening in neurocognitive function at discharge with incomplete recovery at the follow-up [22]. However, the small numbers enrolled, the attrition rate, the shorter time of reassessment after discharge and the modest magnitude change in Mini-Mental State Examination (MMSE) or MOCA at the follow-up do not allow a robust conclusion on neurocognitive effects of the early phase stroke after TAVR. More extended studies with longer reassessment are needed for conclusive findings.

3. Embolic protection devices

TAVR is nowadays going to address even low-risk and younger population [56]: widespread and frequent use of embolic protection devices (EPDs) is necessary to improve outcomes (such as in-hospital mortality and stroke).

EPDs have been projected to hinder the embolization of different kinds of material, released during valve implantation to the brain; the two main classes of EPDs allow to deflect or to filter potential debris thus avoiding cerebrovascular events (**Table 1**). They are usually positioned along the aortic arch or into the anonymous branch and left common carotid before the valve advancement and release from different peripheric vascular access (both femoral and radial routes are viable alternatives, depending on the device) with dedicated catheters; finally, they are retrieved at the end of the procedure before vascular closure.

3.1 Deflectors

The first type of devices consists of large porous webs on top of the aortic arch and/or descending aorta, enabling embolic material to be deflected down in the

Device	Fr – Access – protected vessels	Latest evidence
TriGUARD Deflector	8 Fr Femoral Contralateral 3 Vessels	REFLECT II (2021) **No difference** with unprotected procedures for: • All-cause mortality or any stroke at 30 days • Worsening NIHSS score at 2 to 5 days • Freedom from any cerebral ischemic lesions detected on DW MRI at 2 to 5 days. • Total volume of cerebral ischemic lesions detected on DW MRI at 2 to 5 days
Embrella Deflector	6 Fr Right Brachial or Radial 2 Vessels	PROTAVI C (2014) **No difference** with unprotected procedures for: • Stroke, TIA Major vascular complications life-threatening bleeding, AKI, Mortality at 30 days **Increased** high-intensity transient signals (HITS) at each step of the transcatheter aortic valve replacement procedure
Point Guard Deflector Filter	10 Fr Femoral 3 Vessels	Point Guard CENTER Trial (2018) Ongoing
ProtEmbo Deflector	6 Fr Left Radial 3 Vessels	PROTEMBO SF Trial (2022) New DW-MRI **lesion volumes** with ProtEmbo **were smaller** than in historical data.
Sentinel Filter	6 Fr Right Radial 2 Vessels	PROTECTED TAVR (2022) **No difference** with unprotected procedures for: • All-cause mortality or any stroke at 72 hours • TIA • Delirium
Emboliner Filter	6 Fr Femoral Pigtail Catheter Access 3 Vessels and subdiaphragmatic vessels	SAFEPASS 2 Trial (2020) • The overall major adverse cardiac and cerebrovascular rate was 6.5% for the Embroliner device, a 46% reduction compared with the historical performance goal • One hundred percent of subjects resulted m debris captured in the Emboliner filter.
Embolk Filter	11 Fr Femoral Access 3 Vessels and subdiaphragmatic vessels	First-in-Man Study Evaluating the Emblok Embolic Protection System During TAVR or 20 patients (2020) • The Emblok embolic protection system appears to be feasible and safe during TAVR. • The device was successfully placed and retrieved in all cases and no neurological events were observed

Table 1.
Main EPDs, technical features and supporting evidences.

thoracic descending aorta thus protecting the brain from ischemic injury. Some devices cover just the first two collateral vessels from the arch, whereas others are also developed for the left subclavian artery.

3.1.1 TriGUARD

TriGUARD (Keystone Heart) is one of the most studied EPDs and the first deflector device to receive a CE mark. At the moment, the newest technology available is the TriGUARD 3 that guarantees an improved device visualization and more precise positioning and stability. Through an On The Wire, 8 French delivery system the device is introduced in the contralateral femoral artery and accommodates a 5 Fr pigtail catheter into the lumen; it does not require an additional access site. The deflection filter consists of a nitinol frame (74 mm x 98 mm) with a dome-shaped web designed to allow adequate blood flow to the brain. It enables the covering of all three aortic arch branches ostia.

The older generation devices (TriGUARD and TriGUARD HDH) safety and efficacy (defined as decreased lesion volume as compared to unprotected TAVR) were explored through two randomized controlled trials, the DEFLECT I and DEFLECT II [57, 58].

The DEFLECT III trial was a multicentre, randomized controlled trial testing TriGUARD HDH device against unprotected TAVR in a group of 85 patients. In this exploratory study, subjects undergoing protected TAVI had significantly more freedom from ischaemic brain lesions, numerically reduced single and maximum lesion volumes and better cognitive function in some domains [36]. No statistically significant difference was observed for what concerns rates of stroke.

These results were partially confirmed from the prospective, multicentre, single-blind randomized REFLECT II trial [59] that compared TriGUARD 3 protected procedures with unprotected procedures (for a total of 220 patients), finding no significant differences between treatment and control arm regarding rates of stroke, brain lesions volume and neurological impairment at discharge.

3.1.2 Embrella

This device from Edwards Lifescience is designed to cover all three cerebral vessels and it has the advantage of being delivered from a right radial or brachial access through a 6 Fr sheath. However, the main study (PROTAVI-C) [60] comparing unprotected and device-protected TAVR failed to show a reduction in cerebral ischemic events in EPD treated population, reporting, on the contrary, an increased rate of micro-embolization to the brain.

On the other side, the use of the Embrella system was associated with lower lesion volume than the control group. Furthermore, every new cerebral lesion disappeared on the MRI performed 30 days after TAVR.

3.1.3 Other devices

There are a large number of EPDs that are undergoing testing and safety/efficacy studies. We herein mention:

- The Point-Guard (Transverse Medical) provides complete cerebral protection by covering all supra-aortic arteries via an embolic material deflection, capture and removal. Like similar devices, it consists of a flexible nitinol frame with a filter web covering the aortic arch, positioned by a femoral route. It also has a supporting extension basket at the distal end: by sealing and conforming the arch anatomy, it addresses the challenge of devices with non-sealing edges. The Point

Guard CENTER trial started in 2018 and will be the main multicentre trial across the EU evaluating the safety and efficacy of the device.

- ProtEmbo (Protembi) is delivered via a 6 Fr sheath through left radial/brachial artery; it provides protection for all three cerebral vessels and has the smallest pores between the EPDs. Safety and efficacy were assessed through the PROTEMBO C trial showing encouraging results: fewer MACEs and smaller volume brain MRI lesions were observed in comparison to pre-specified performance goals [61].

3.2 Filters

The second class gathers systems of different sizes, positions and access; the entrapment of the embolic material and its removal represents the common denominator between the different devices.

3.2.1 Sentinel

Sentinel was the first capture system to obtain the CE mark and FDA approval, respectively in 2013 and 2017. Two sequential mesh develop on a single 6 Fr catheter and are positioned into the left common carotid artery (the distal one) and into the brachiocephalic artery (the proximal one) from right radial access. The webs are connected by an articulating positioning sheath that allows good manipulation and rapid delivery (less than 10 minutes) during the procedure. The device comes in only one size, thus may not be adequate for some particular aortic and arterial anatomies; moreover, the vertebral artery is not protected.

The three main randomized controlled trials evaluating the efficacy of the Sentinel system highlighted different and controversial results. In almost every patient in the treatment group, embolic debris was captured by the filter.

The MISTRAL-C [37] showed statistically significant reduction in neurocognitive deterioration in the EPD group. The CLEAN-TAVI [62] trial randomized 100 patients to protected vs. unprotected procedures and demonstrated that the EPD group had a decrement in the new-onset brain lesions and reduced volume lesions. The SENTINEL [20] trial failed to demonstrate a significant reduction in stroke rates and lesion volume.

The last and largest randomized trial about Sentinel efficacy is the PROTECTED TAVR [63] study: 3000 patients were randomized in 1:1 fashion to unprotected and protected procedure. The rate of disabling stroke was significantly lower in the Sentinel group with a relative risk reduction of 60%, although this trial was not powered to assess disabling stroke.

3.2.2 Emboliner

Emboliner (Emboline) consist of a cylindrical nitinol mesh filter that circumferentially conforms to the aortic anatomy, covering all three cerebral vessels and, through a downstream filter end captures embolic debris directed to kidneys, abdomen and lower body. Plus, the Emboliner shares the transfemoral access site used for the pigtail catheter, so no additional access or closure is required. After valve advancement and deployement (passing the downstream filter with the prosthesis delivery device), the EPD and the materials entrapped between the mesh are removed. The

SAFEPASS 2 [64] study analyzed the safety and efficacy of the device between 31 patients undergoing TAVR compared with an historical performance goal, demonstrating encouraging results. A larger ongoing study will evaluate if the benefit in terms of reduction of stroke and systemic embolism rates is consistent when a protected procedure is compared to an unprotected one.

3.2.3 Emblok

The Emblok (Innovative Medical Solutions) is the only capture device including a radiopaque 4 Fr pigtail catheter, that aids in identifying the non-coronary cusp and favoring correct alignment and positioning of the valve. It is deployed in a single 11 Fr femoral route and covers the ascending aorta and aortic arch [65]. The first 20 patients that underwent TAVR protected procedure with the device were totally free from MACCE at 30 days even if post-procedural MRI showed that 95% of the group developed new silent ischemic brain lesions.

4. Summary of evidence

The safety of embolic protection devices in TAVR has been extensively demonstrated in many trials and studies. However, CEPDs' efficacy and impact on hard clinical outcomes remains a controversial argument of debate. Some of the most recent meta-analyses showed indeed conflictual results. Woldendrop et al. on the European Heart Journal stated that using CEPDs did not result in a significant decrease in the occurrence of silent brain infarcts [50]. In two reviews and meta-analyses [66, 67] reporting results from randomized controlled trials (RCTs) and observational studies, the use of EPDs was effectively associated to fewer short-term stroke events. In contrast, other ones [68–70] (predominantly based on RCTs) did not show any difference on clinical outcomes or neuroimaging parameters. One of the most recent and updated summaries of evidence by Baloch et al. [71] comprehended 128,471 patients from RCTs and observational studies and highlighted the benefit of CEPD in reducing incidence of 30 day disabling stroke in patients undergoing TAVR; the majority of studies was based on TriGUARD and Sentinel devices.

5. Conclusions

Stroke is a major concern in patients undergoing TAVR that can affect mortality and morbidity. TAVR expanding indication to low risk young patients raises issues on prevent or reduce the incidence of cerebrovascular ischaemic events that could be pursued through embolic protection devices. Clear univocal evidence does not support the routine use of cerebral embolic protection devices during TAVR to prevent stroke and improve outcomes. However, it may be useful in patients judged at high risk of neurological events; further studies about the ideal patient selection are warranted.

Conflict of interest

The authors declare no conflict of interest.

Author details

Gianluca Di Pietro, Improta Riccardo, Marco Tocci, Lucia Ilaria Birtolo, Emanuele Bruno, Colantonio Riccardo, Massimo Mancone* and Gennaro Sardella
Department of Clinical Internal, Anesthesiologic and Cardiovascular Sciences, Sapienza University of Rome, Rome, Italy

*Address all correspondence to: massimo.mancone@uniroma1.it

IntechOpen

© 2023 The Author(s). Licensee IntechOpen. This chapter is distributed under the terms of the Creative Commons Attribution License (http://creativecommons.org/licenses/by/3.0), which permits unrestricted use, distribution, and reproduction in any medium, provided the original work is properly cited.

References

[1] Leon MB, Smith CR, Mack M, Miller DC, Moses JW, Svensson LG, et al. Transcatheter aortic-valve implantation for aortic stenosis in patients who cannot undergo surgery. The New England Journal of Medicine. 2010;**363**(17):1597-1607

[2] Makkar RR, Fontana GP, Jilaihawi H, Kapadia S, Pichard AD, Douglas PS, et al. Transcatheter aortic-valve replacement for inoperable severe aortic stenosis. The New England Journal of Medicine. 2012;**366**(18):1696-1704

[3] Leon MB, Smith CR, Mack MJ, Makkar RR, Svensson LG, Kodali SK, et al. Transcatheter or surgical aortic-valve replacement in intermediate-risk patients. The New England Journal of Medicine. 2016;**374**(17):1609-1620

[4] Alqahtani F, Sengupta PP, Badhwar V, McCarthy P, Alkhouli M. Clinical and economic burden of acute ischemic stroke following transcatheter aortic valve replacement. Structural Heart. 2019;**3**(1):72-73

[5] Muralidharan A, Thiagarajan K, Van Ham R, Gleason TG, Mulukutla S, Schindler JT, et al. Meta-analysis of perioperative stroke and mortality in transcatheter aortic valve implantation. The American Journal of Cardiology. 2016;**118**(7):1031-1045

[6] Vermeer SE, Prins ND, den Heijer T, Hofman A, Koudstaal PJ, Breteler MMB. Silent brain infarcts and the risk of dementia and cognitive decline. The New England Journal of Medicine. 2003;**348**(13):1215-1222

[7] Miller DC, Blackstone EH, Mack MJ, Svensson LG, Kodali SK, Kapadia S, et al. Transcatheter (TAVR) versus surgical (AVR) aortic valve replacement: Occurrence, hazard, risk factors, and consequences of neurologic events in the PARTNER trial. The Journal of Thoracic and Cardiovascular Surgery. 2012;**143**(4):832-843.e13

[8] Arnold SV, Zhang Y, Baron SJ, McAndrew TC, Alu MC, Kodali SK, et al. Impact of short-term complications on mortality and quality of life after transcatheter aortic valve replacement. JACC. Cardiovascular Interventions. 2019;**12**(4):362-369

[9] Spears J, Al-Saiegh Y, Goldberg D, Manthey S, Goldberg S. TAVR: A review of current practices and considerations in low-risk patients. Journal of Interventional Cardiology. 2020;**2020**:2582938

[10] Mack MJ, Leon MB, Thourani VH, Makkar R, Kodali SK, Russo M, et al. Transcatheter aortic-valve replacement with a balloon-expandable valve in low-risk patients. The New England Journal of Medicine. 2019;**380**(18):1695-1705

[11] Thyregod HGH, Steinbrüchel DA, Ihlemann N, Nissen H, Kjeldsen BJ, Petursson P, et al. Transcatheter versus surgical aortic valve replacement in patients with severe aortic valve stenosis: 1-Year Results From the All-Comers NOTION Randomized Clinical Trial. Journal of the American College of Cardiology. 2015;**65**(20):2184-2194

[12] Kappetein AP, Head SJ, Généreux P, Piazza N, van Mieghem NM, Blackstone EH, et al. Updated standardized endpoint definitions for transcatheter aortic valve implantation: The Valve Academic Research Consortium-2 consensus document (VARC-2). European

Journal of Cardio-Thoracic Surgery. 2012;**42**(5):S45-S60

[13] Kapadia S, Agarwal S, Miller DC, Webb JG, Mack M, Ellis S, et al. Insights into timing, risk factors, and outcomes of stroke and transient ischemic attack after transcatheter aortic valve replacement in the PARTNER Trial (Placement of Aortic Transcatheter Valves). Circulation Cardiovascular Intervention. 2016;**9**:9

[14] Kleiman NS, Maini BJ, Reardon MJ, Conte J, Katz S, Rajagopal V, et al. Neurological events following transcatheter aortic valve replacement and their predictors: A report from the CoreValve Trials. Circulation Cardiovascular Interventions. 2016;**9**:e003551

[15] Davlouros PA, Mplani VC, Koniari I, Tsigkas G, Hahalis G. Transcatheter aortic valve replacement and stroke: A comprehensive review. Journal of Geriatric Cardiology. 2018;**15**(1):95-104

[16] Huded CP, Tuzcu EM, Krishnaswamy A, Mick SL, Kleiman NS, Svensson LG, et al. Association between transcatheter aortic valve replacement and early postprocedural stroke. Journal of the American Medical Association. 2019;**321**(23):2306-2315

[17] Linder M, Higgen FL, Voigtländer L, Weimann J, Ludwig S, Waldschmidt L, et al. Stroke events after transcatheter aortic valve implantation: Temporal relationships and affected brain regions. American Heart Journal. 2022;**247**:112-122

[18] Alassar A, Soppa G, Edsell M, Rich P, Roy D, Chis Ster I, et al. Incidence and mechanisms of cerebral ischemia after transcatheter aortic valve implantation compared with surgical aortic valve replacement. The Annals of Thoracic Surgery. 2015;**99**(3):802-808

[19] Van Mieghem NM, El Faquir N, Rahhab Z, Rodríguez-Olivares R, Wilschut J, Ouhlous M, et al. Incidence and predictors of debris embolizing to the brain during transcatheter aortic valve implantation. JACC. Cardiovascular Interventions. 2015;**8**(5):718-724

[20] Kapadia SR, Kodali S, Makkar R, Mehran R, Lazar RM, Zivadinov R, et al. Protection against cerebral embolism during transcatheter aortic valve replacement. Journal of the American College of Cardiology. 2017;**69**(4):367-377

[21] Eschenbach LK, Erlebach M, Deutsch MA, Ruge H, Bleiziffer S, Holzer L, et al. Stroke after transcatheter aortic valve replacement: A severe complication with low predictability. Catheterization and Cardiovascular Interventions. 2022;**99**(6):1897-1905

[22] De Carlo M, Liga R, Migaleddu G, Scatturin M, Spaccarotella C, Fiorina C, et al. Evolution, predictors, and neurocognitive effects of silent cerebral embolism during transcatheter aortic valve replacement. JACC. Cardiovascular Interventions. 2020;**13**(11):1291-1300

[23] Eggebrecht H, Schmermund A, Voigtländer T, Kahlert P, Erbel R, Mehta RH. Risk of stroke after transcatheter aortic valve implantation (TAVI): A meta-analysis of 10,037 published patients. EuroIntervention. 2012;**8**(1):129-138

[24] Walther T, Schuler G, Borger MA, Kempfert J, Seeburger J, Rückert Y, et al. Transapical aortic valve implantation in 100 consecutive patients: Comparison to propensity-matched conventional aortic valve replacement. European Heart Journal. 2010;**31**(11):1398-1403

[25] Biancari F, Rosato S, D'Errigo P, Ranucci M, Onorati F, Barbanti M, et al.

Immediate and intermediate outcome after transapical versus transfemoral transcatheter aortic valve replacement. The American Journal of Cardiology. 2016;**117**(2):245-251

[26] Ferrari E, Eeckhout E, Keller S, Muller O, Tozzi P, Berdajs D, et al. Transfemoral versus transapical approach for transcatheter aortic valve implantation: Hospital outcome and risk factor analysis. Journal of Cardiothoracic Surgery. 2017;**12**(1):78

[27] Elbadawi A, Naqvi SY, Saad M, Elgendy IY, Mahmoud AA, Zainal A, et al. In-hospital outcomes with transfemoral versus transapical access for transcatheter aortic valve replacement in patients with peripheral arterial disease. Cardiovascular Revascularization Medicine. 2020;**21**(5):604-609

[28] Villecourt A, Faroux L, Muneaux A, Tassan-Mangina S, Heroguelle V, Poncet A, et al. Comparison of clinical outcomes after transcarotid and transsubclavian versus transfemoral transcatheter aortic valve implantation: A propensity-matched analysis. Archives of Cardiovascular Diseases. 2020;**113**(3):189-198

[29] Ferrari E, Pozzoli A, Klersy C, Toto F, Torre T, Cassina T, et al. Ten-year experience with transapical and direct transaortic transcatheter aortic valve replacement to address patients with aortic stenosis and peripheral vascular disease. Journal of Cardiovascular Developmental Diseases. 2022;**9**(12)

[30] Kahlert P, Al-Rashid F, Döttger P, Mori K, Plicht B, Wendt D, et al. Cerebral embolization during transcatheter aortic valve implantation: A transcranial Doppler study. Circulation. 2012;**126**(10):1245-1255

[31] Abdel-Wahab M, Mehilli J, Frerker C, Neumann FJ, Kurz T, Tölg R, et al. Comparison of balloon-expandable vs self-expandable valves in patients undergoing transcatheter aortic valve replacement: The CHOICE randomized clinical trial. Journal of the American Medical Association. 2014;**311**(15):1503-1514

[32] Feldman TE, Reardon MJ, Rajagopal V, Makkar RR, Bajwa TK, Kleiman NS, et al. Effect of mechanically expanded vs self-expanding transcatheter aortic valve replacement on mortality and major adverse clinical events in high-risk patients with aortic stenosis: The REPRISE III Randomized Clinical Trial. Journal of the American Medical Association. 2018;**319**(1):27-37

[33] Thiele H, Kurz T, Feistritzer HJ, Stachel G, Hartung P, Eitel I, et al. Comparison of newer generation self-expandable vs. balloon-expandable valves in transcatheter aortic valve implantation: The randomized SOLVE-TAVI trial. European Heart Journal. 2020;**41**(20):1890-1899

[34] Vlastra W, Chandrasekhar J, Muñoz-Garcia AJ, Tchétché D, de Brito FS, Barbanti M, et al. Comparison of balloon-expandable vs. self-expandable valves in patients undergoing transfemoral transcatheter aortic valve implantation: From the CENTER-collaboration. European Heart Journal. 2019;**40**(5):456-465

[35] Kajio K, Mizutani K, Hara M, Nakao M, Okai T, Ito A, et al. Self-expandable transcatheter aortic valve replacement is associated with frequent periprocedural stroke detected by diffusion-weighted magnetic resonance imaging. Journal of Cardiology. 2019;**74**(1):27-33

[36] Lansky AJ, Schofer J, Tchetche D, Stella P, Pietras CG, Parise H, et al. A prospective randomized evaluation

of the TriGuardTM HDH embolic DEFLECTion device during transcatheter aortic valve implantation: Results from the DEFLECT III trial. European Heart Journal. 2015;**36**(31):2070-2078

[37] Van Mieghem NM, van Gils L, Ahmad H, van Kesteren F, van der Werf HW, Brueren G, et al. Filter-based cerebral embolic protection with transcatheter aortic valve implantation: The randomised MISTRAL-C trial. EuroIntervention. 2016;**12**(4):499-507

[38] Toutouzas K, Benetos G, Voudris V, Drakopoulou M, Stathogiannis K, Latsios G, et al. Pre-dilatation versus no pre-dilatation for implantation of a self-expanding valve in all comers undergoing TAVR: The DIRECT Trial. JACC. Cardiovascular Interventions. 2019;**12**(8):767-777

[39] Leclercq F, Robert P, Akodad M, Macia JC, Gandet T, Delseny D, et al. Prior balloon valvuloplasty versus direct transcatheter aortic valve replacement: Results from the DIRECTAVI Trial. JACC. Cardiovascular Interventions. 2020;**13**(5):594-602

[40] Takagi K, Naganuma T, Tada N, Yamanaka F, Araki M, Shirai S, et al. The predictors of peri-procedural and sub-acute cerebrovascular events following TAVR from OCEAN-TAVI Registry. Cardiovascular Revascularization Medicine. 2020;**21**(6):732-738

[41] Nombela-Franco L, Webb JG, de Jaegere PP, Toggweiler S, Nuis RJ, Dager AE, et al. Timing, predictive factors, and prognostic value of cerebrovascular events in a large cohort of patients undergoing transcatheter aortic valve implantation. Circulation. 2012;**126**(25):3041-3053

[42] Jochheim D, Zadrozny M, Ricard I, Sadry TM, Theiss H, Baquet M, et al. Predictors of cerebrovascular events at mid-term after transcatheter aortic valve implantation - Results from EVERY-TAVI registry. International Journal of Cardiology. 2017;**244**:106-111

[43] Hahn RT, Pibarot P, Webb J, Rodes-Cabau J, Herrmann HC, Williams M, et al. Outcomes with post-dilation following transcatheter aortic valve replacement: The PARTNER I trial (placement of aortic transcatheter valve). JACC. Cardiovascular Interventions. 2014;7(7):781-789

[44] Goel K, Nkomo VT, Slusser JP, Lennon R, Brown RD, Greason KL, et al. Relationship between procedural characteristics and cerebrovascular events after transcatheter aortic valve replacement. Open Heart. 2018;**5**(2):e000816

[45] Castelo A, Grazina A, Teixeira B, Mendonça T, Rodrigues I, Garcia Brás P, et al. Outcomes and predictors of periprocedural stroke after transcatheter aortic valve implantation. Journal of Stroke and Cerebrovascular Diseases. 2023;**32**(5):107054

[46] Kochar A, Li Z, Harrison JK, Hughes GC, Thourani VH, Mack MJ, et al. Stroke and cardiovascular outcomes in patients with carotid disease undergoing transcatheter aortic valve replacement. Circulation. Cardiovascular Interventions. 2018;**11**(6):e006322

[47] Reardon MJ, Van Mieghem NM, Popma JJ, Kleiman NS, Søndergaard L, Mumtaz M, et al. Surgical or transcatheter aortic-valve replacement in intermediate-risk patients. The New England Journal of Medicine. 2017;**376**(14):1321-1331

[48] Bosmans J, Bleiziffer S, Gerckens U, Wenaweser P, Brecker S, Tamburino C, et al. The incidence and predictors of

early- and mid-term clinically relevant neurological events after transcatheter aortic valve replacement in real-world patients. Journal of the American College of Cardiology. 2015;**66**(3):209-217

[49] Lansky AJ, Brown D, Pena C, Pietras CG, Parise H, Ng VG, et al. Neurologic complications of unprotected transcatheter aortic valve implantation (from the Neuro-TAVI Trial). The American Journal of Cardiology. 2016;**118**(10):1519-1526

[50] Woldendorp K, Indja B, Bannon PG, Fanning JP, Plunkett BT, Grieve SM. Silent brain infarcts and early cognitive outcomes after transcatheter aortic valve implantation: A systematic review and meta-analysis. European Heart Journal. 2021;**42**(10):1004-1015

[51] Carroll JD, Mack MJ, Vemulapalli S, Herrmann HC, Gleason TG, Hanzel G, et al. STS-ACC TVT Registry of Transcatheter Aortic Valve Replacement. Journal of the American College of Cardiology. 2020;**76**(21):2492-2516

[52] Salemi A, Sedrakyan A, Mao J, Elmously A, Wijeysundera H, Tam DY, et al. Individual operator experience and outcomes in transcatheter aortic valve replacement. JACC. Cardiovascular Interventions. 2019;**12**(1):90-97

[53] Kühne M, Krisai P, Coslovsky M, Rodondi N, Müller A, Beer JH, et al. Silent brain infarcts impact on cognitive function in atrial fibrillation. European Heart Journal. 2022;**43**(22):2127-2135

[54] Schwarz N, Kastaun S, Schoenburg M, Kaps M, Gerriets T. Subjective impairment after cardiac surgeries: The relevance of postoperative cognitive decline in daily living. European Journal of Cardio-Thoracic Surgery. 2013;**43**(6):e162-e166

[55] Kahlert P, Knipp SC, Schlamann M, Thielmann M, Al-Rashid F, Weber M, et al. Silent and apparent cerebral ischemia after percutaneous transfemoral aortic valve implantation: A diffusion-weighted magnetic resonance imaging study. Circulation. 2010;**121**(7):870-878

[56] Pibarot P, Salaun E, Dahou A, Avenatti E, Guzzetti E, Annabi MS, et al. Echocardiographic results of transcatheter versus surgical aortic valve replacement in low-risk patients: The PARTNER 3 Trial. Circulation. 2020;**141**(19):1527-1537

[57] Baumbach A, Mullen M, Brickman AM, Aggarwal SK, Pietras CG, Forrest JK, et al. Safety and performance of a novel embolic deflection device in patients undergoing transcatheter aortic valve replacement: Results from the DEFLECT I study. EuroIntervention. 2015;**11**(1):75-84

[58] Samim M, van der Worp B, Agostoni P, Hendrikse J, Budde RPJ, Nijhoff F, et al. TriGuard(TM) HDH embolic deflection device for cerebral protection during transcatheter aortic valve replacement. Catheterization and Cardiovascular Interventions. 2017;**89**(3):470-477

[59] Nazif TM, Moses J, Sharma R, Dhoble A, Rovin J, Brown D, et al. Randomized evaluation of TriGuard 3 cerebral embolic protection after transcatheter aortic valve replacement: REFLECT II. JACC. Cardiovascular Interventions. 2021;**14**(5):515-527

[60] Rodés-Cabau J, Kahlert P, Neumann FJ, Schymik G, Webb JG, Amarenco P, et al. Feasibility and exploratory efficacy evaluation of the Embrella Embolic Deflector system for the prevention of cerebral emboli in patients undergoing transcatheter aortic valve replacement: The PROTAVI-C

pilot study. JACC. Cardiovascular Interventions. 2014;**7**(10):1146-1155

[61] Jagielak D, Targonski R, Frerker C, Abdel-Wahab M, Wilde J, Werner N, et al. Safety and performance of a novel cerebral embolic protection device for transcatheter aortic valve implantation: The PROTEMBO C Trial. EuroIntervention. 2022;**18**(7):590-597

[62] Haussig S, Mangner N, Dwyer MG, Lehmkuhl L, Lücke C, Woitek F, et al. Effect of a cerebral protection device on brain lesions following transcatheter aortic valve implantation in patients with severe aortic stenosis: The CLEAN-TAVI Randomized Clinical Trial. Journal of the American Medical Association. 2016;**316**(6):592-601

[63] Kapadia SR, Makkar R, Leon M, Abdel-Wahab M, Waggoner T, Massberg S, et al. Cerebral embolic protection during transcatheter aortic-valve replacement. The New England Journal of Medicine. 2022;**387**(14):1253-1263

[64] Sanjeevan P. TCT CONNECT-458 clinical performance of a total embolic protection device: Results of the Emboliner SafePass 2 Study. Journal of the American College of Cardiology. 2020;**76**(17 Supplement S):B196-B196

[65] Latib A, Mangieri A, Vezzulli P, Spagnolo P, Sardanelli F, Fellegara G, et al. First-in-Man Study Evaluating the Emblok embolic protection system during transcatheter aortic valve replacement. JACC. Cardiovascular Interventions. 2020;**13**(7):860-868

[66] Zahid S, Ullah W, Zia Khan M, Faisal Uddin M, Rai D, Abbas S, et al. Cerebral embolic protection during transcatheter aortic valve implantation: Updated systematic review and meta-analysis. Current Problems in Cardiology. 2023;**48**(6):101127

[67] Shimamura J, Kuno T, Malik A, Yokoyama Y, Gupta R, Ahmad H, et al. Safety and efficacy of cerebral embolic protection devices in patients undergoing transcatheter aortic valve replacement: A meta-analysis of in-hospital outcomes. Cardiovascular Intervention and Therapeutics. 2022;**37**(3):549-557

[68] Nazir S, Zafrullah F, Virk HUH, Sandhu CS, Ameen M, Ahuja KR. Meta-analysis of cerebral embolic protection during transcatheter aortic valve replacement. The American Journal of Cardiology. 2021;**139**:138-139

[69] Ahmad Y, Howard JP. Meta-analysis of usefulness of cerebral embolic protection during transcatheter aortic valve implantation. The American Journal of Cardiology. 2021;**146**:69-73

[70] Pérez-Camargo D, Travieso A, Carnero-Alcázar M, Taramasso M, Cobiella-Carnicer J, Maroto-Castellanos LC. Neurological outcomes of transcatheter aortic valve implantation with or without cerebral embolic protection devices: A meta-analysis. Journal of Stroke and Cerebrovascular Diseases. 2022;**31**(9):106605

[71] Baloch ZQ, Haider SJ, Siddiqui HF, Shaikh FN, Shah BUD, Ansari MM, et al. Utility of cerebral embolic protection devices in transcatheter procedures: A systematic review and meta-analysis. Current Problems in Cardiology. 2023;**48**(7):101675

Chapter 9

Cerebral Protection Devices in Transcatheter Aortic-Valve Replacement

Gian-Manuel Jiménez-Rodríguez, José-Luis Elizalde-Silva, Mariana Chaire-Hernandez, Jesus Diaz-Marin, Guering Eid Lidt and Gustavo Rojas Velasco

Abstract

Transcatheter aortic valve replacement (TAVR) is a common procedure used in the treatment of severe aortic stenosis and other cardiac valve diseases. Although this procedure has been shown to be effective and safe in improving cardiac function and life expectancy in this population, there is an inherent risk of neurological complications such as stroke and cognitive impairment. In the last years, there has been a breakthrough in the development of brain protection devices that minimize the risk of brain embolism during the procedure. These devices are designed to capture clots and calcium debris that could become dislodged during the valve implant, therefore keeping the embolus from entering the nervous system *via* the supra-aortic vessels. Some studies indicate that using brain protection devices during an aortic valve replacement could substantially decrease the burden of stroke and other associated neurological complications. However, despite the promising expected results, further studies are required to sustain the benefit of using these devices, besides with the ongoing development in this area it would be fundamental a face-to-face interaction between the devices in the current development. Furthermore, although the experience with these devices is limited and the recent experience indicates they are safe, it would be fundamental to identify and take in consideration possible risks and complications related to these devices.

Keywords: cerebral embolic protection devices, cerebrovascular events, transcatheter aortic valve replacement, stroke, brain injuries

1. Introduction

Aortic stenosis is the most prevalent valve disease in the developed countries. Its prevalence increases in the elderly; in this population, transcatheter aortic valve replacement (TAVR) is a viable option for subjects with intermediate or high risk of cardiac surgery. Despite the development of new generations of TAVR, cerebrovascular events are one of the most severe and scary complications because of the increase in morbidity and mortality, the risk of stroke at 30 days ranges from 2.7 to 10% [1, 2]. Apart from clinical strokes, subclinical strokes, defined by the appearance of new ischemic cerebral lesions by MRI, appear in 90% of patients undergoing TAVR [3]; however, their clinical significance is still unknown.

TAVR implantation-related strokes are divided into acute or periprocedural and late. For prevention, various methods have been identified. In the first group (acute), the main factors to take into consideration include optimization of the TAVR technique with reduction of embolization of calcified fragments and atheroma, and adequate anticoagulation during the procedure. For late strokes, the main factor is the use of an optimal antithrombotic regimen after implantation.

The greatest risk of embolization to the brain occurs during the procedure, during the positioning or implantation phase of the valve, as a result of manipulation of highly calcified structures or atheromatous embolization of thrombi or material [4]. Up to 70% of patients experience a stroke in the first 24 hours [5–7] with a considerable deterioration in quality of life and a 3–5-fold increase in mortality [8]. Cerebral protection devices (CPDs) have the potential to reduce stroke and ischemic brain injury associated with percutaneous aortic valve replacement. The results of a recent study that analyzed a database with 36,220 patients (525 of them with CPD systems and 35,695 without them) found that the use of a CPD was associated with a lower incidence of ischemic stroke (1.0% vs. 3.8%, $p < 0.002$) and lower in-hospital mortality. Importantly, silent strokes account for a significant proportion of these complications and are associated with a threefold increased risk of having a stroke, a further decline in cognitive function, and a twofold increased risk of developing dementia after follow-up for 4 years [9].

Until March 2023, only two authorized devices were identified as DPC, the Sentinel device, which is designed to capture emboli or debris detached during TAVI. It consists of a dual filter into the left common carotid and brachycephalic artery; inside a 6Fr catheter that is accessed through the radial artery, the proximal filter is placed in the brachiocephalic artery and the distal filter in the common carotid artery (available in United States and Europe) [1] and the TriGUARD 3 (available in Europe) is the only device that covers all the arteries of the aortic arch. Being a deflector device, it rejects emboli during TAVR placement. This device is advanced *via* femoral contralateral access to TAVI placement and is deployed to protect the supra-aortic vessels [10].

2. Risk factors for cerebrovascular events

The risk factors for post-TAVR stroke are divided into early (acute and subacute) and late (**Table 1**).

Indicators of an early stroke encompass features of the patient and the procedure itself. Procedure features associated with early stroke risk include a greater number of dilations of the aortic valve annulus, a greater degree of valve acceleration velocity before implantation (reflecting more severe plaques with more calcium deposits, or the need for additional instrumentation to cross the aortic valve and complete the procedure), and a greater number of pacing events [11].

In a study carried out in more than 20,000 patients from Europe and Canada, the predictors of post-TAVR stroke were evaluated. Age, previous stroke and peripheral arterial disease, chronic kidney disease, atrial fibrillation, and diabetes were identified as risk factors [9].

• Multiple dilations of the aortic annulus or post-dilatation of the valve.
• Pacing stimulation in multiple times.
• Higher acceleration speed of the native aortic valve (greater calcification).
• Non-femoral vascular access (axillary, transaortic, carotid, transapical).
• Chronic kidney disease.
• Female gender.
• Decreased ejection fraction of the left ventricle.
• Atrial fibrillation.

Table 1.
Risk factors for stroke in TAVR implantation.

In a recent analysis of the Transcatheter Valve Therapy (TVT) registry by Thourani et al., which included 97,600 patients, the approach with an alternative access for TAVR (i.e., use of an access other than transfemoral or direct aortic access) was identified to had the highest relative risk for TAVR intrahospital stroke [12].

In the CoreValve studies, factors such as reduced body surface area, severe aortic calcification, and frequent falls in the past 6 months were found to be indicators of increased risk of subsequent stroke [13].

3. Current evidence on the use of cerebral protection devices (CPD) in TAVR

An analysis of 108,315 patients undergoing TAVR examined the use of CPD in 4380 patients (4.0%). The results revealed that adjusted mortality was lower in those patients who underwent TAVR with CPD compared with those without CPD (0.5% vs. 1.3%, $p < 0.01$).

In addition, neurological complications, including hemorrhagic stroke and ischemic stroke, were also lower in the CPD group compared with the non-CPD group (1.4% vs. 2.2%, $p < 0.01$). Likewise, patients who experienced a stroke after TAVR and used CPD were found to have a significantly lower in-hospital mortality rate compared with those without CPD (6.3% vs. 11.8%; $p = 0.023$). These findings suggest the possibility that CPDs may prevent more severe and debilitating strokes, which in turn could reduce stroke-related morbidity and mortality [14].

A recent meta-analysis demonstrated that the use of CPD was associated with a lower risk of mortality related to stroke (odds ratio 0.47; 95% CI, 0.28–0.80), lower risk of stroke (odds ratio 0.54; 95% CI, 0.39–0.75), transient ischemic attack (odds ratio 0.47; 95% CI, 0.31–0.71), and adverse cardiovascular and cerebrovascular events (odds ratio 0.70; 95% CI, 0.56–0.87). These data suggest that CPD should be considered during TAVR procedures to reduce the risk of stroke-related mortality and other complications [15].

An observational study was conducted in 2023 using the TriGUARD 3 ™ (**Figure 1**) device to assess the incidence of stroke and transient ischemic attacks (TIA) within 72 hours or at discharge after TAVR implantation. The results revealed stroke incidence of 0.8%, suggesting that the use of this device is associated with a low frequency of clinically detectable strokes and device-related adverse events [11].

The PROTECTED TAVR study evaluated the effectiveness of cerebral embolic protection (CEP) during TAVR in reducing the risk of stroke. The study involved 3000 patients, the primary endpoint being the identification of clinical stroke within

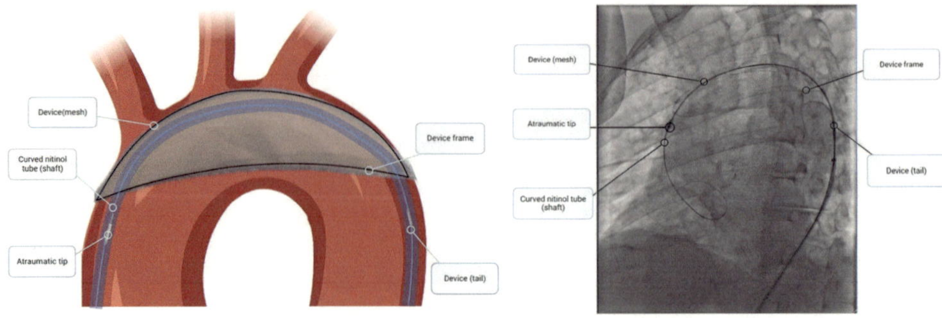

Figure 1.
TriGUARD ™ device.

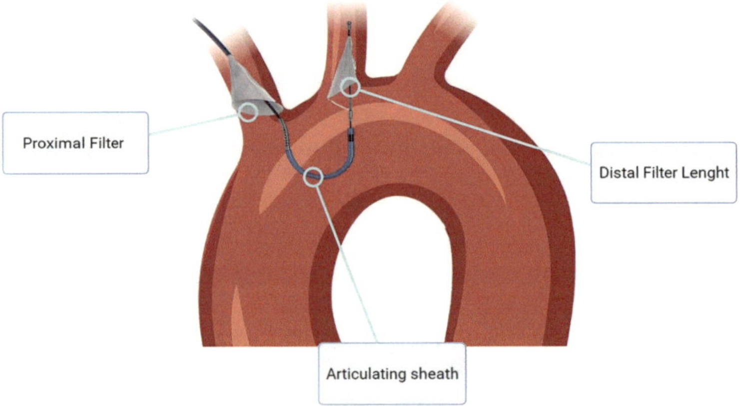

Figure 2.
Sentinel ™ device.

72 hours of TAVR or before discharge. The study found that the use of CEP did not have a significant effect on the incidence of periprocedural stroke; however, it reduced the incidence of disabling stroke. The study concluded that among patients with aortic stenosis undergoing transfemoral TAVR, the use of CEP had no significant effect on the incidence of periprocedural stroke [14] using Sentinel ™ (**Figure 2**).

4. Conclusions

Stroke related to TAVR represents one of the most common and scary complications and is an independent risk factor that predicts morbidity and mortality; therefore, new strategies have been implemented to reduce its appearance. CPDs represent a novel strategy in stroke protection in patients undergoing TAVR. This evidence suggests that the use of CPD reduces the number and size of ischemic lesions identified on magnetic resonance; however, they are not yet established as a protective measure in the appearance of embolic phenomena and the reduction of ischemic lesions in TAVR patients. None of the devices we mainly studied managed to reduce the appearance of stroke; however, there was a reduction in the number of disabling strokes, which has an impact ultimately in a possible better quality of life.

Author details

Gian-Manuel Jiménez-Rodríguez[1*], José-Luis Elizalde-Silva[2], Mariana Chaire-Hernandez[3], Jesus Diaz-Marin[1], Guering Eid Lidt[1] and Gustavo Rojas Velasco[4]

1 Interventional Cardiac Departement, Instituto Nacional de Cardiología Ignacio Chávez, Mexico City, Mexico

2 Cardiovascular Critical Care Unit, Instituto Nacional de Cardiología Ignacio Chávez, Mexico City, Mexico

3 Regional Hospital ISSSTE León, Mexico

4 Intensive Cardiovascular Care, Instituto Nacional de Cardiología Ignacio Chávez, Mexico City, Mexico

*Address all correspondence to: gianma21@hotmail.com

IntechOpen

© 2023 The Author(s). Licensee IntechOpen. This chapter is distributed under the terms of the Creative Commons Attribution License (http://creativecommons.org/licenses/by/3.0), which permits unrestricted use, distribution, and reproduction in any medium, provided the original work is properly cited.

References

[1] Gasior T, Mangner N, Bijoch J, Wojakowski W. Cerebral embolic protection systems for transcatheter aortic valve replacement. Journal of Interventional Cardiology. 2018;**31**(6):891-898

[2] Kapadia SR, Kodali S, Makkar R, Mehran R, Lazar RM, Zivadinov R, et al. Protection against cerebral embolism during transcatheter aortic valve replacement. Journal of the American College of Cardiology. 2017;**69**(4):367-377

[3] Kahlert P, Knipp SC, Schlamann M, Thielmann M, Al-Rashid F, Weber M, et al. Silent and apparent cerebral ischemia after percutaneous transfemoral aortic valve implantation: A diffusion-weighted magnetic resonance imaging study. Circulation. 2010;**121**(7):870-878

[4] Richter I, Abdel-Wahab M, Desch S, Thiele H. Cerebral embolic protection in patients undergoing transcatheter aortic valve implantation: Recent advances. Kardiologia Polska. 2022;**80**(6):644-650

[5] Adams DH, Popma JJ, Reardon MJ, Yakubov SJ, Coselli JS, Deeb GM, et al. Transcatheter aortic-valve replacement with a self-expanding prosthesis. The New England Journal of Medicine. 2014;**370**(19):1790-1798

[6] Miller DC, Blackstone EH, Mack MJ, Svensson LG, Kodali SK, Kapadia S, et al. Transcatheter (TAVR) versus surgical (AVR) aortic valve replacement: Occurrence, hazard, risk factors, and consequences of neurologic events in the PARTNER trial. The Journal of Thoracic and Cardiovascular Surgery. 2012;**143**(4):832-843.e13

[7] Nombela-Franco L, Webb JG, De Jaegere PP, Toggweiler S, Nuis RJ, Dager AE, et al. Timing, predictive factors, and prognostic value of cerebrovascular events in a large cohort of patients undergoing transcatheter aortic valve implantation. Circulation. 2012;**126**(25):3041-3053

[8] Eggebrecht H, Schmermund A, Voigtländer T, Kahlert P, Erbel R, Mehta RH. Risk of stroke after transcatheter aortic valve implantation (TAVI): A meta-analysis of 10,037 published patients. EuroIntervention. 2012;**8**(1):129-138

[9] Vlastra W, Jimenez-Quevedo P, Tchétché D, Chandrasekhar J, De Brito FS, Barbanti M, et al. Predictors, incidence, and outcomes of patients undergoing transfemoral transcatheter aortic valve implantation complicated by stroke: From the CENTER-collaboration. Circulation. Cardiovascular Interventions. 2019;**12**(3):e007546

[10] Demir OM, Iannopollo G, Mangieri A, Ancona MB, Regazzoli D, Mitomo S, et al. The role of cerebral embolic protection devices during transcatheter aortic valve replacement. Frontiers in Cardiovascular Medicine. 2018;**5**:150

[11] Daal SM, Jimenez-Rodriguez GMJ, Voskuil M, et al. Clinical outcome of transcatheter aortic valve replacement with TriGUARD 3™ cerebral embolic protection device. Cardiovascular Revascularization Medicine. 2023;**50**:8-12. DOI: 10.1016/j.carrev.2023.01.008

[12] Thourani VH, O'Brien SM, Kelly JJ, Cohen DJ, Peterson ED, Mack MJ, et al. Development and application of a risk prediction model for In-hospital

stroke after transcatheter aortic valve replacement: A report from the society of thoracic surgeons/American college of cardiology transcatheter valve therapy registry. The Annals of Thoracic Surgery. 2019;**107**(4):1097-1103

[13] Kleiman NS, Maini BJ, Reardon MJ, Conte J, Katz S, Rajagopal V, et al. Neurological events following transcatheter aortic valve replacement and their predictors: A report from the CoreValve trials. Circulation: Cardiovascular Interventions. 2016;**9**(9):e003551

[14] Kapadia SR, Makkar R, Leon M, Abdel-Wahab M, Waggoner T, Massberg S, et al. Cerebral embolic protection during transcatheter aortic-valve replacement. The New England Journal of Medicine. 2022;**387**(14):1253-1263

[15] Al-Abdouh A, Mhanna M, Jabri A, Ahmed T, Altibi AM, Ghanem F, et al. Meta-analysis of cerebral embolic protection during transcatheter aortic valve replacement. The American Journal of Cardiology. 2023;**192**:255-257

Chapter 10

Surgical Treatment of Patients with Aortic Valve Disease in Association with Atrial Fibrillation

Alexandr Zotov, Oleg Shelest, Emil Sakharov, Robert Khabazov and Alexandr Troitsky

Abstract

The frequency of atrial fibrillation development in patients with severe aortic valve stenosis ranges from 4 to 30%. This arrhythmia significantly worsens patients' long-term survival. Currently, it is considered that performing ablation of arrhythmogenic myocardial areas during valve surgery does not impact in-hospital mortality and does not lead to prolonged hospital stay. According to modern recommendations, this procedure should be performed in all patients diagnosed with atrial fibrillation if the pericardium is opened. There are numerous ablation protocols available. For patients with isolated aortic valve disease, there is no need to open the atria during ablation. For the majority of patients with persistent atrial fibrillation, isolating the posterior wall of the left atrium, including the pulmonary vein areas, is sufficient. This article proposes an original approach to the combined treatment of valve disease and arrhythmia using the Perceval-S sutureless valve and the Gemini-S clamp-ablator. This approach reduces the time of cardiopulmonary bypass, which can benefit high-risk surgical patients.

Keywords: aortic valve, atrial fibrillation, aortic stenosis, sutureless, radio frequency ablation, Gemini-S, bicuspid valve

1. Introduction

Atrial fibrillation (AF) is a common arrhythmia, affecting around 1–2% of the general population. The prevalence increases with age, reaching approximately 5–15% in individuals over 80 years [1]. Aortic valve disease, including aortic stenosis and aortic regurgitation, has reported a prevalence of around 0.5–1% in developed countries, increasing with age [2].

Aortic stenosis narrows the aortic valve opening, limiting blood flow from the left ventricle to the aorta. It is primarily a disease of aging caused by calcific degeneration, and it is the most common valvular heart disease in developed countries. The prevalence of AS in the elderly population (≥75 years) is estimated to be between 2.8 and 4.6% [3]. On the other hand, aortic regurgitation, the leaking or backflow of blood through the aortic valve, can be caused by various conditions, including aging, hypertension and endocarditis. The prevalence of moderate to severe AR in the general population is estimated to be around 0.5% [4].

The co-occurrence of AF and aortic valve disease is not uncommon because there are shared risk factors [5]. Research suggests that AF occurs in approximately 4–30% of patients with severe aortic stenosis, depending on the study population and diagnostic methods [6]. AF is also associated with poorer outcomes in patients with aortic valve disease, including increased mortality and morbidity [7]. AF in the context of AS is associated with a higher risk of stroke and systemic embolism, which significantly complicates the management of these patients [7]. The epidemiology of AF in patients with AR is less researched. However, given the shared risk factors, it is not uncommon to see these conditions together. AF in AR patients is also associated with worse outcomes, similar to AS patients [8].

However, specific epidemiological data for the combination of AF and aortic valve disease is limited and further research is needed to understand this patient population better.

Managing patients with AF and aortic valve disease is complex and requires a multidisciplinary approach. Therapeutic strategies often involve a combination of rate or rhythm control, anticoagulation and valve intervention [8].

In the 1980s, several scientists developed surgical methods for treating atrial fibrillation. Williams proposed a procedure for isolating the left atrium [9]. However, this method showed its effectiveness mainly in the "left atrial" form of atrial fibrillation, leaving other forms less responsive to the procedure [10]. Guiraudon introduced the "Corridor" procedure, which involved the surgeon isolating the impulse conduction path from the sinoatrial node to the atrioventricular [11]. Despite its promise, the procedure was limited in restoring an adequate ventricular response to the sinus node's operation, while the atrial myocardium continued to contract asynchronously [12]. Both procedures could not comprehensively address three main challenges of arrhythmia: asynchronous contractions of the atria and ventricles, an inadequate ventricular response to stimulation, and blood stagnation in the atria [13]. Consequently, patients remained in the high-risk group for thromboembolic complications.

In 1987, Cox, based on electrophysiological studies and animal experiments, identified "macro-reentry" waves and established their size and the duration of circulation in a specific place of the atria [14]. This discovery led to the development of the "Labyrinth" procedure, which created a single path for the impulse from the sinus node to the atrioventricular by cutting and sewing the atria, thereby interrupting the circulation of the "macro-reentry" wave while preserving the activation of atrial tissues by the sinus node [15]. The first operation on a human heart took place on September 25, 1987, ultimately allowing the patient to avoid arrhythmia and the intake of antiarrhythmic drugs for 20 years [16].

The maze procedure had its drawbacks due to a high risk of complications. One of the lines in the surgical schema was situated near the sinus node, disrupting fibers responsible for the stress-induced response [17]. Another line blocked the Bachmann's bundle, significantly impairing interatrial conduction [18]. The procedure was carried out exclusively under conditions of artificial circulation, accompanied by a corresponding amount of complications [19].

For these reasons, the procedure was modified and technically simplified over the following decade. At a median observation period of 5.4 years, sinus rhythm was maintained in 97% of patients' post-surgery [20]. However, the procedure remained technically challenging, not easily accessible for mastering, and still accompanied by high perioperative risk [21]. These factors laid the groundwork for exploring energy sources that would allow the creation of ablation lines without cutting atrial tissue and for seeking ways to minimize surgical access [22]. In 1996, after accumulating experience from over 200 variously modified maze procedures, the authors performed the first operation on isolated AF, utilizing cryoablation technology to create patterns that disrupted the circulating "macro-reentry" waves [23]. The operation time was significantly reduced, and cryoenergy simplified the procedure [24]. Around the same time, experiments were conducted with other energy sources, such as radiofrequency and microwave [25]. These various energy sources used to achieve transmural lesions of the atrial myocardium following the original procedures pattern formed the basis for creating its fourth modification, the "Maze-IV" [26]. Radiofrequency energy gained the most widespread adoption [27].

Currently, according to guidelines from the European Association for Cardiothoracic Surgery (EACTS), cardiac procedures, including ablation, are divided into two categories: primary open atrial operations and primary closed atrial operations. Aortic valve replacement surgery and coronary artery bypass surgery are classified as the second type [28].

The optimal protocol for radiofrequency ablation (RFA) during aortic valve surgery is a subject of ongoing research debate. There are multiple approaches to consider, each with its benefits and drawbacks. The decision to perform an entire maze-IV operation or a non-maze procedure pulmonary vein isolation (PVI), Box-Lesion and variations (PVI) without atrial incision depends on patient-specific factors.

The maze-IV procedure is the most complex form of surgical ablation for AF. It involves creating a "maze" of lesions in the atria, effectively interrupting the abnormal electrical pathways. The reported success rates are high, with up to approximately 80% of patients free from AF 1 year post-operatively. However, the procedure is time-consuming, and it carries risks of complications such as bleeding and pacemaker dependency [29]. The limitation of this procedure is using two types of ablation devices to achieve the full line protocol of the original procedure [30]. Ablation requires the use of monopolar devices, which cannot always create a homogeneous lesion line. If the mitral line of the maze procedure is incomplete, these partial lines can result in peri-mitral atrial flutter. Performing a complete maze procedure is only possible by using cryosurgery [31]. On the other hand, a PVI procedure without atrial incision is a less invasive procedure that involves using the radiofrequency bipolar clamp to create lesions around the pulmonary veins, thereby isolating them electrically and preventing AF. The significant advantage of this procedure is its simplicity and shorter operative time, which translates into less surgical risk. However, the success rate is generally lower than the full maze procedure, particularly in patients with persistent AF [32]. Oral et al. demonstrated that complete PVI might not be sufficient in all AF patients, suggesting that non-PV foci can contribute to AF in these individuals [33]. Other studies have extended these findings and identified additional trigger sites within the left atrium, including the posterior wall, the left atrial appendage, and the coronary sinus [34]. For these reasons, all patients with persistent atrial fibrillation should undergo isolation of the posterior wall of the left atrium (BOX-Lesion), including the orifices of the pulmonary veins. Resection of the left atrial appendage makes it possible to form an additional line passing from the ridge zone to the collector of the left pulmonary veins [35].

The decision between the three procedures should consider the patient's individual characteristics, including the type and duration of AF, left atrium volume index (LAVI), the patient's overall health status, and the risk of surgical complications. For example, in younger, healthier patients or those with persistent AF, an entire maze-IV operation may be more beneficial despite its invasiveness. On the other hand, for older patients, those with significant comorbidities or those with paroxysmal AF, a PVI procedure without atrial incision may be preferable due to its lower surgical risk.

The optimal protocol for RFA during aortic valve surgery with AF is a tailored approach that considers the patient's characteristics and balances the potential benefits of AF elimination against the procedure's risks. Maze-III and non-maze procedures (PVI, Box-Lesion) without atrial incision have their place in the treatment of AF, and the choice between them should be made on a case-by-case basis.

2. Aortic valve replacement and radiofrequency isolation of the posterior wall of the left atrium in a high surgical risk patient: How we do it

Patients with aortic stenosis and atrial fibrillation who are considered to be at high surgical risk typically exhibit a range of clinical features and comorbidities. Here are some of the key factors that are often considered when determining surgical risk:

1. Advanced age: Older patients are often considered at a higher surgical risk due to the increased likelihood of comorbidities and reduced physiological reserve [36].

2. Severe comorbidities: Conditions such as severe pulmonary disease, chronic kidney disease, and liver disease [37].

3. Frailty: This includes factors such as cognitive impairment, reduced mobility, malnutrition, and dependency in activities of daily living [38].

4. Left ventricular dysfunction: A reduced left ventricular ejection fraction (LVEF) can increase surgical risk [39].

Cardiopulmonary bypass (CPB) duration plays a significant role in the outcomes in this group. The length of CPB has been linked with several potential complications, including organ dysfunction, postoperative bleeding and increased mortality. A study by Ranucci et al. demonstrated that CPB duration is an independent predictor of overall mortality and major complications following cardiothoracic surgeries [40]. According to their analysis, every additional 10 minutes of CPB increases the risk of overall mortality by 16%, the risk of significant complications by 18%, and the risk of postoperative bleeding by 12%. An article by Gansera and colleagues (2007) emphasized that CPB duration is associated with the risk of postoperative renal dysfunction and thrombocytopenia [41]. This finding reinforces the importance of minimizing CPB time in aortic valve replacement surgeries. In another study by Raja and co-authors (2005), CPB duration was an independent risk factor for developing postoperative acute lung injury [42].

In order to reduce the duration of cardiopulmonary bypass in such patients, we employ the Perceval-S sutureless valve, Box-Lesion radiofrequency ablation protocol with an additional line in the Ridge zone, and Marshall ligament destruction. The Perceval-S valve is an artificial valve made from bovine pericardium, implanted within a self-expanding nitinol frame that secures the valve in the implantation site. The valve is stored in an antibacterial solution, eliminating the need for pre-rinsing. The valve implantation involves three guiding sutures, which are subsequently removed. These factors combined allow us to achieve a myocardial ischaemic time of 15–18 minutes.

Along with ablation and left atrial appendage occlusion, the total duration of cardiopulmonary bypass in our clinic for such procedures averages around 40 minutes.

Indications for the implantation of the Perceval-S prosthesis:

1. Age over 65 years.

2. Aortic valvular stenosis or a combination of stenosis with insufficiency with a fibrous ring size of 19–27 mm.

3. Aortic valvular insufficiency with fibrous ring size 19–27 mm.

4. Infective endocarditis without violation of the integrity of the fibrous ring and the configuration of the aortic root.

It should be noted that the main contraindications for using the valve are aortic root dilation and disruption of the fibrous annulus integrity. Many surgical teams have successfully used Perceval-S in cases of bicuspid aortic valve.

3. Operation

The first step involves the Box-Lesion ablation procedure. For RFA, we used a Cardioblate Gemini-S ablative device. The procedure is performed under parallel cardiopulmonary bypass due to hemodynamic instability during pulmonary vein occlusion. The right atrium is cannulated with a two-stage cannula. The aorta is cannulated as high as possible from the sinotubular ridge. After initiation of cardiopulmonary bypass using a dissector and forceps, the connective tissue in the area of the transverse sinus is separated by a blunt manoeuvre between the superior right pulmonary vein and the superior vena cava, and the inferior vena cava is mobilized. For the convenience and safety of bipolar clamp-ablator placement, we utilize specialized guides that minimize the risk of damaging surrounding anatomical structures. The guides are inserted similarly to the "Galaxy" procedure (**Figure 1**) [43]. The first guide is passed through the transverse sinus and removed behind the left atrial appendage. The second guide is passed through the oblique sinus of the pericardium between the inferior vena cava and the right inferior pulmonary vein. Since the ablation clamp and guidewires have a flexible structure, there is no need to rotate the heart at this stage. Next, the Cardioblate Gemini-S electrode is attached to the guidewires, and the electrode branches are introduced into the oblique and transverse sinuses of the pericardium on the left side to perform ablation of the left pulmonary veins and the posterior wall of the left atrium (**Figure 2**). The ablation of the right pulmonary vein orifices and the posterior wall of the left atrium is performed similarly (**Figure 3**). To create complete lines, we perform about 10 applications lasting about 10 minutes on each side. After completion of the ablation of the left atrium posterior wall, it is mandatory to perform an Exit-block test. Gemini-S electrodes allow ablation of the entire posterior wall of the left atrium as a single block according to the "box-lesion" scheme in the minimum amount of time (**Figure 4**). Additionally, the infusion of physiological solution into the clamp branches enables conducting ablation without charring the myocardium.

The second step involves a prosthetic implantation. Carbon dioxide gas insufflation is carried out into the surgical wound to prevent air embolism. Valve implantation is typically performed in a single session of blood cardioplegia. During the implantation of a sutureless valve, the aortotomy should be performed approximately

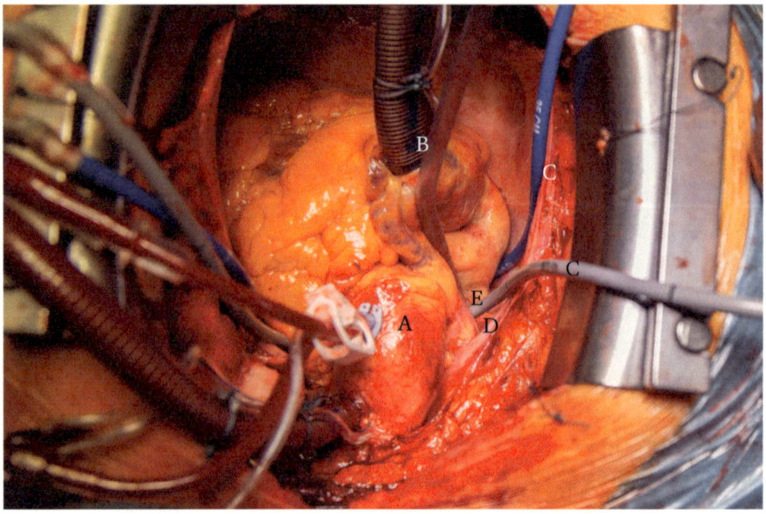

Figure 1.
Flexible guides in pericardial cavity. (A) Ascendence part of the aorta, (B) right atrium canula, (C) flexible guides, (D) superior right pulmonary vein, and (E) inferior right pulmonary vein.

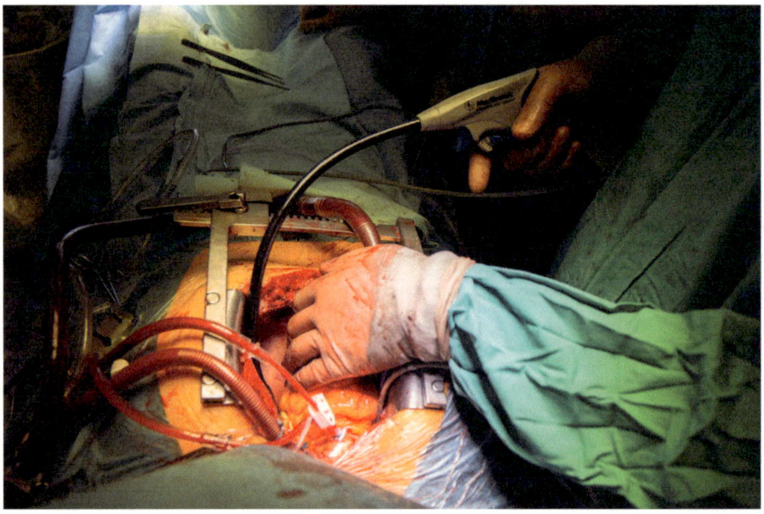

Figure 2.
Performing left-side ablation.

3–3.5 cm above the coronary artery ostia to ensure a safe aortotomy closure at the end of the procedure without interfering with the upper edge of the valve frame. After decalcification, we leave a rim of approximately 3 mm and provide valve sizing. We do not open the specific size of the prosthesis until we evaluate the patient's valve and measure its fibrous annulus. It is worth noting that a fibrous annulus larger than 27 mm is a contraindication for valve implantation.

After valve sizing, the prosthesis is prepared on a separate surgical table. The valve must be loaded into the delivery system to accomplish this. A valve holder and a collapser are set up on the stand (**Figure 5**). The collapser compresses the valve on the holder. In this state, the valve is presented to the operating surgeon (**Figure 6**).

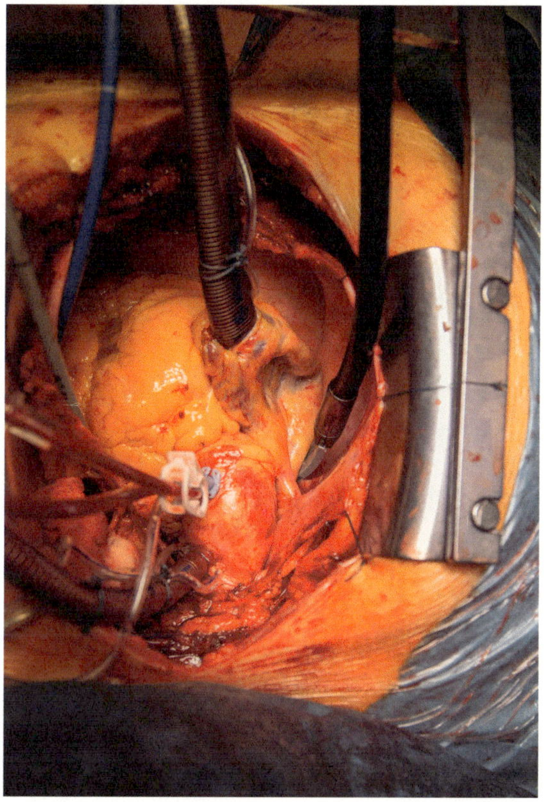

Figure 3.
Performing right-side ablation.

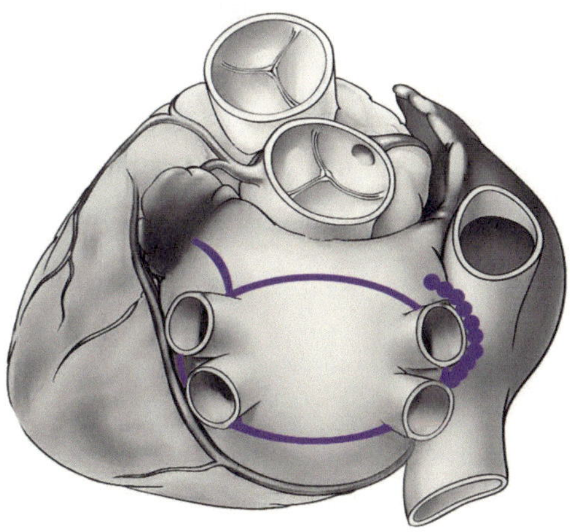

Figure 4.
Final ablation scheme. Trasmural injury marked with a blue line.

Following decalcification of the valve and preparation of the prosthesis for implantation, we proceed with suture occlusion of the left atrial appendage. At this point in the operation, creating an additional ablation line connecting the Ridge zone and the left pulmonary vein collector is possible. In patients with persistent atrial

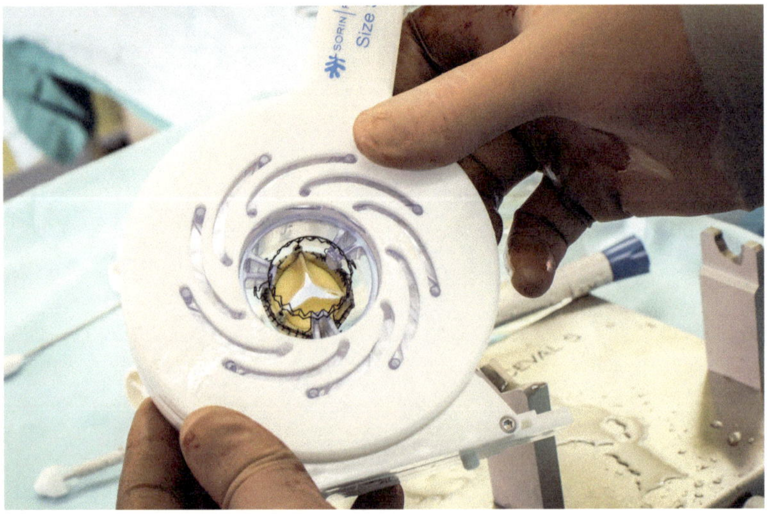

Figure 5.
Perceval-S fixed in collapser.

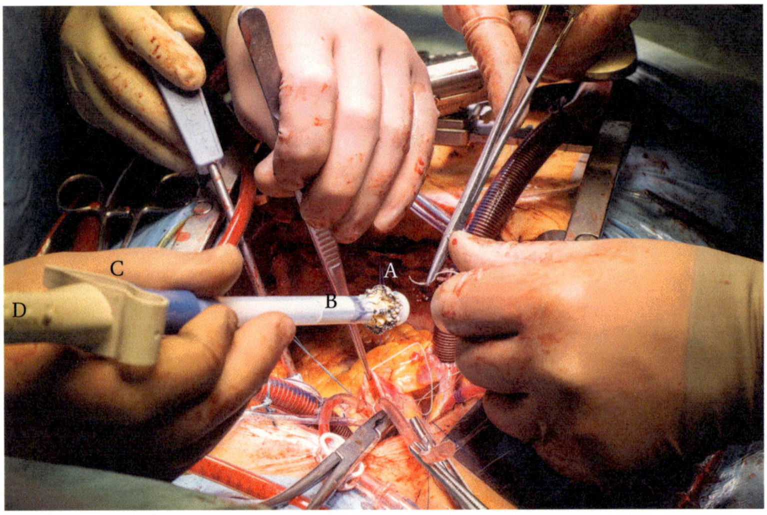

Figure 6.
Perceval-S prepared for implantation. (A) Valve prosthesis, (B) sheath, (C) smart clip, and (D) handle of the holder.

fibrillation, we disrupt the adipose tissue in the Waterston's groove area and perform ablation of this zone with a Cardioblate MAPS monopolar electrode. Then we proceed with aortic valve implantation. Guiding sutures are sewn in the nadir of the leaflets. Incorrect distribution of guiding sutures can lead to the formation of paravalvular fistulas.

The sutures are passed through the valve ears (**Figure 7**). The valve is positioned at the fibrous annulus. The lower portion of the valve is opened first, followed by the upper portion. This sequence of unfolding allows us to verify the correct positioning of the lower part while it is still visually accessible. After unfolding the upper part,

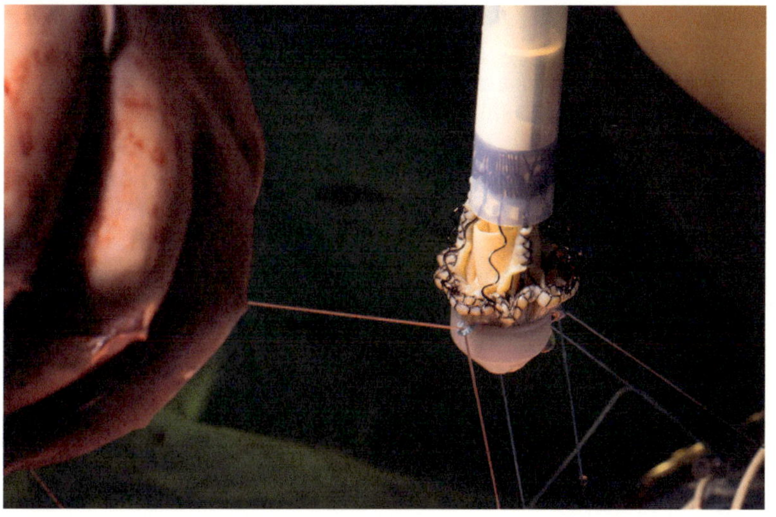

Figure 7.
Fixation of the guide sutures.

any changes in the prosthesis position can only be made through explanation of the prosthesis. After removing the holder, the position of the prosthesis relative to the fibrous ring and coronary artery ostia is visually evaluated (**Figure 8**). The final step of the implantation is balloon dilation, inserted into the valve lumen to a pressure of 4 ATM for 40–60 seconds. During this process, warm physiological saline is used to irrigate the valve frame for complete expansion of the nitinol frame. The main stage of the operation concludes with the formation of a double-row suture on the aortotomy. At this stage, it is critically important to visualize each suture to avoid capturing the prosthesis frame in the suture.

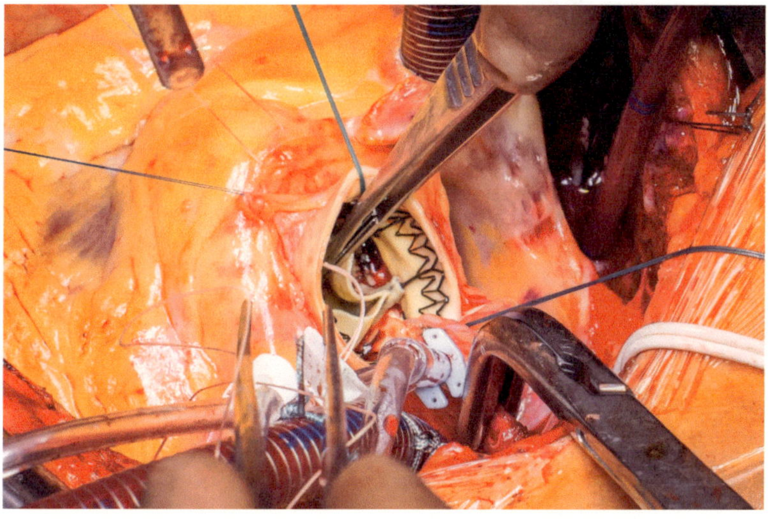

Figure 8.
Perceval-S implanted in aortic root.

4. Features of perceval-S prosthesis implantation in bicuspid aortic valve

Bicuspid aortic valve can pose a significant challenge during the implantation of a sutureless valve. The most common variants encountered are Sievers 1 or 2. Abnormal distribution of leaflets and commissures around the fibrous annulus circumference may lead to improper positioning of guiding sutures. Improper positioning of the valve frame can result in the formation of paravalvular fistulas. It is also essential to pay attention to the coronary artery ostia, which may have non-standard origins.

For correct valve seating, it is necessary to create guiding sutures around the circumference at points of 120–120-120 degrees and pre-calculate the position of the valve struts relative to the coronary artery ostia. The valve should not be implanted in case of aortic root dilatation. Isolated dilation of the ascending aorta above the sinotubular ridge is not a contraindication for implantation.

5. Conclusion

Performing ablation in patients with a concomitant correction of aortic valve disease is not associated with increased in-hospital mortality, more frequent pacemaker implantation or neurological complications and is indicated for all patients diagnosed with arrhythmia. Combined open procedures show significantly better long-term outcomes than isolated transcatheter aortic valve implantation in elderly patients with low surgical risk and persistent atrial fibrillation. An analysis conducted by William L Patrick et al. demonstrates reduced mortality, pacemaker implantation rates, and hospitalizations due to decompensated heart failure in the long-term period for patients who underwent arrhythmia correction and prosthetic valve replacement under cardiopulmonary bypass, compared to the transcatheter aortic valve implantation group (TAVI) group where ablation was not performed [44].

We again emphasize that the choice of ablation protocol depends on the form of atrial fibrillation, the patient's atrial size, and concomitant pathology. According to the authors, the ablation protocol presented in this chapter is appropriate for most clinical situations.

Author details

Alexandr Zotov, Oleg Shelest*, Emil Sakharov, Robert Khabazov
and Alexandr Troitsky
Federal Scientific and Clinical Center for Specialized Medical Assistance and Medical Technologies of the Federal Medical Biological Agency, Moscow, Russian Federation

*Address all correspondence to: toshelest@gmail.com

IntechOpen

© 2023 The Author(s). Licensee IntechOpen. This chapter is distributed under the terms of the Creative Commons Attribution License (http://creativecommons.org/licenses/by/3.0), which permits unrestricted use, distribution, and reproduction in any medium, provided the original work is properly cited.

References

[1] Cox JL, Schuessler RB, D'Agostino HJ Jr, Stone CM, Chang BC, Cain ME, et al. Worldwide epidemiology of atrial fibrillation: A global burden of disease 2010 study. Circulation. 2014;**129**(8):837-847

[2] Nkomo VT, Gardin JM, Skelton TN, Gottdiener JS, Scott CG, Enriquez-Sarano M. Burden of valvular heart diseases: A population-based study. The Lancet. 2006;**368**(9540):1005-1011

[3] Osnabrugge RL, Mylotte D, Head SJ, Van Mieghem NM, Nkomo VT, LeReun CM, et al. Aortic stenosis in the elderly: Disease prevalence and number of candidates for transcatheter aortic valve replacement: A meta-analysis and modeling study. Journal of the American College of Cardiology. 2013;**62**(11):1002-1012

[4] Singh JP, Evans JC, Levy D, Larson MG, Freed LA, Fuller DL, et al. Prevalence and clinical determinants of mitral, tricuspid, and aortic regurgitation (the Framingham heart study). The American Journal of Cardiology. 1999;**83**(6):897-902

[5] Benjamin EJ, Levy D. Why is left ventricular hypertrophy so predictive of morbidity and mortality? The American Journal of Medicine. 1999;**106**(5):554-556

[6] Roselli EE, Murthy SC, Rice TW, Houghtaling PL, Pierce CD, Karchmer DP, et al. Atrial fibrillation complicating the course of degenerative aortic stenosis: The need for a guideline-driven approach. The Journal of Thoracic and Cardiovascular Surgery. 2010;**140**(3):659-664

[7] Baumgartner H, Falk V, Bax JJ, De Bonis M, Hamm C, Holm PJ, et al. 2017 ESC/EACTS guidelines for the management of valvular heart disease. European Heart Journal. 2017;**38**(36):2739-2791

[8] January CT, Wann LS, Calkins H, Chen LY, Cigarroa JE, Cleveland JC, et al. 2019 AHA/ACC/HRS focused update of the 2014 AHA/ACC/HRS guideline for the Management of Patients with Atrial Fibrillation: A report of the American College of Cardiology/American Heart Association task force on clinical practice guidelines and the Heart Rhythm Society in collaboration with the Society of Thoracic Surgeons. Circulation. 2019;**140**(2):e125-e151

[9] Williams JM, Ungerleider RM, Lofland GK, Cox JL. Left atrial isolation: New technique for the treatment of supraventricular arrhythmias. The Journal of Thoracic and Cardiovascular Surgery. 1980;**80**(3):373-380

[10] Gallagher JJ, Svenson RH, Kasell JH, German LD, Bardy GH, Broughton A, et al. Catheter technique for closed-chest ablation of the atrioventricular junction. The New England Journal of Medicine. 1982;**306**(4):194-200

[11] Guiraudon GM, Klein GJ, Sharma AD, Yee R, McLellan DG. The coronary sinus diverticulum: A pathologic entity associated with the Wolff-Parkinson-white syndrome. The American Journal of Cardiology. 1989;**64**(17):1216-1219

[12] Guiraudon G, Fontaine G, Frank R, Escande G, Etievent P, Cabrol C, et al. Encircling endocardial ventriculotomy: A new surgical treatment for life-threatening ventricular tachycardias resistant to medical treatment following myocardial infarction. The Annals of Thoracic Surgery. 1977;**24**(5):451-459

[13] Cox JL, Schuessler RB, D'Agostino HJ Jr, Stone CM, Chang BC, Cain ME, et al. The surgical treatment of atrial fibrillation. III. Development of a definitive surgical procedure. The Journal of Thoracic and Cardiovascular Surgery. 1991;**101**(4):569-583

[14] Cox JL, Canavan TE, Schuessler RB, Cain ME, Lindsay BD, Stone C, et al. The surgical treatment of atrial fibrillation. II. Intraoperative electrophysiologic mapping and description of the electrophysiologic basis of atrial flutter and atrial fibrillation. The Journal of Thoracic and Cardiovascular Surgery. 1991;**101**(3):406-426

[15] Cox JL, Boineau JP, Schuessler RB, Jaquiss RD, Lappas DG. Modification of the maze procedure for atrial flutter and atrial fibrillation. II. Surgical technique of the maze III procedure. The Journal of Thoracic and Cardiovascular Surgery. 1995;**110**(2):485-495

[16] Cox JL, Ad N, Palazzo T, Fitzpatrick S, Suyderhoud JP, DeGroot KW, et al. Current status of the maze procedure for the treatment of atrial fibrillation. Seminars in Thoracic and Cardiovascular Surgery. 1999;**11**(1):15-19

[17] Cox JL, Schuessler RB. The surgical treatment of atrial fibrillation. The Journal of Thoracic and Cardiovascular Surgery. 1991;**101**(4):584-592

[18] Schuessler RB, Kay MW, Melby SJ, Branham BH, Boineau JP, Cox JL. Spatial and temporal stability of the dominant frequency of activation in human atrial fibrillation. The Journal of Thoracic and Cardiovascular Surgery. 2010;**140**(6):1303-1308

[19] Ad N, Henry L, Hunt S, Holmes SD, Halpin L. The Cox-maze III procedure success rate: Comparison by electrocardiogram, 24-hour holter monitoring and long-term monitoring. The Annals of Thoracic Surgery. 2012;**94**(1):101-106

[20] Ad N, Holmes SD, Massimiano PS, Rongione AJ, Fornaresio LM, Fitzgerald D. Long-term outcome following concomitant mitral valve surgery and Cox maze procedure for atrial fibrillation. The Journal of Thoracic and Cardiovascular Surgery. 2013;**145**(2):468-475

[21] Calkins H, Kuck KH, Cappato R, Brugada J, Camm AJ, Chen SA, et al. 2012 HRS/EHRA/ECAS expert consensus statement on catheter and surgical ablation of atrial fibrillation: Recommendations for patient selection, procedural techniques, patient management and follow-up, definitions, endpoints, and research trial design. Journal of Interventional Cardiac Electrophysiology. 2012;**33**(2):171-257

[22] Gaynor SL, Diodato MD, Prasad SM, Ishii Y, Schuessler RB, Bailey MS, et al. A prospective, single-center clinical trial of a modified Cox maze procedure with bipolar radiofrequency ablation. The Journal of Thoracic and Cardiovascular Surgery. 2004;**128**(4):535-542

[23] Cox JL. The surgical treatment of atrial fibrillation. IV. Surgical technique. The Journal of Thoracic and Cardiovascular Surgery. 2003;**125**(3):632-635

[24] Cox JL, Ad N, Palazzo T. Impact of the maze procedure on the stroke rate in patients with atrial fibrillation. The Journal of Thoracic and Cardiovascular Surgery. 2000;**120**(4):833-840

[25] Khargi K, Hutten BA, Lemke B, Deneke T. Surgical treatment of atrial fibrillation; a systematic review. European Journal of Cardio-Thoracic Surgery. 2005;**27**(2):258-265

[26] Prasad SM, Maniar HS, Camillo CJ, Schuessler RB, Boineau JP, Sundt TM III, et al. The Cox maze III procedure for atrial fibrillation: Long-term efficacy in patients undergoing lone versus concomitant procedures. The Journal of Thoracic and Cardiovascular Surgery. 2003;**126**(6):1822-1828

[27] McCarthy PM, Kruse J, Shalli S, Ilkhanoff L, Goldberger JJ, Kadish AH, et al. Where does atrial fibrillation surgery fail? Implications for increasing effectiveness of ablation. The Journal of Thoracic and Cardiovascular Surgery. 2008;**135**(4):860-867

[28] Badhwar V, Rankin JS, Damiano RJ Jr, Gillinov AM, Bakaeen FG, Edgerton JR, et al. The society of thoracic surgeons 2017 clinical practice guidelines for the surgical treatment of atrial fibrillation. The Annals of Thoracic Surgery. 2017;**103**(1):329-341

[29] Izumoto H, Kawazoe K, Eishi K, Kamata J. Medium-term results after the modified Cox/maze procedure combined with other cardiac surgery. European Journal of Cardio-Thoracic Surgery. 2000;**17**(1):25-29

[30] McCarthy PM. The maze IV operation is not always the best choice: Matching the procedure to the patient. JTCVS Techniques. 2021;**17**:79-83

[31] Cox JL, Malaisrie SC, Kislitsina ON, McCarthy PM. The electrophysiologic basis for lesions of the contemporary maze operation. The Journal of Thoracic and Cardiovascular Surgery. 2019;**157**(2):584-590

[32] Sasaki K, Kunihara T, Suzuki S, Matsumiya G, Fukuda H, Shiiya N, et al. Multicenter study of surgical ablation for atrial fibrillation in aortic valve replacement. ASAIO Journal. 2023;**69**(5):483-489

[33] Oral H, Knight BP, Tada H, et al. Pulmonary vein isolation for paroxysmal and persistent atrial fibrillation. Circulation. 2002;**105**(9):1077-1081

[34] O'Neill MD, Wright M, Knecht S, et al. Long-term follow-up of persistent atrial fibrillation ablation using termination as a procedural endpoint. European Heart Journal. 2009;**30**(9):1105-1112

[35] Kumar P, Bamimore AM, Schwartz JD, Chung EH, Gehi AK, Kiser AC, et al. Challenges and outcomes of Posterior Wall isolation for ablation of atrial fibrillation. Journal of the American Heart Association. 2016;**5**(9):e003885

[36] Brown JM, O'Brien SM, Wu C, Sikora JA, Griffith BP, Gammie JS. Isolated aortic valve replacement in North America comprising 108,687 patients in 10 years: Changes in risks, valve types, and outcomes in the society of thoracic surgeons national database. The Journal of Thoracic and Cardiovascular Surgery. 2009;**137**(1):82-90

[37] Thourani VH, Kodali S, Makkar RR, Herrmann HC, Williams M, Babaliaros V, et al. Transcatheter aortic valve replacement versus surgical valve replacement in intermediate-risk patients: A propensity score analysis. The Lancet. 2016;**387**(10034):2218-2225

[38] Afilalo J, Lauck S, Kim DH, Lefèvre T, Piazza N, Lachapelle K, et al. Frailty in older adults undergoing aortic valve replacement: The FRAILTY-AVR study. Journal of the American College of Cardiology. 2017;**70**(6):689-700

[39] Herrmann HC, Pibarot P, Hueter I, Gertz ZM, Stewart WJ, Kapadia S, et al. Predictors of mortality and outcomes of therapy in low-flow severe aortic

stenosis: A placement of aortic Transcatheter valves (PARTNER) trial analysis. Circulation. 2013;**127**(23):2316-2326

[40] Ranucci M, Castelvecchio S, Menicanti L, Frigiola A, Pelissero G. Risk of assessing mortality risk in elective cardiac operations: Age, creatinine, ejection fraction, and the law of parsimony. Circulation. 2009;**119**(24):3053-3061

[41] Gansera B, Schmidtler F, Spiliopoulos K, Angelis I, Neumaier-Prauser P, Kemkes BM. Does the duration of cardiopulmonary bypass or aortic cross-clamp in coronary artery bypass surgery affect survival? European Journal of Cardio-Thoracic Surgery. 2007;**32**(4):654-658

[42] Raja SG, Dreyfus GD. Impact of off-pump coronary artery bypass surgery on postoperative renal dysfunction and systemic inflammatory response: A randomised controlled study. Heart, Lung & Circulation. 2005;**14**(1):25-31

[43] Doty JR, Clayson SE. Surgical treatment of isolated (lone) atrial fibrillation with Gemini-S ablation and left atrial appendage excision (GALAXY procedure). Innovations (Phila). 2012;**7**(1):33-38

[44] Patrick WL, Chen Z, Han JJ, Smood B, Rao A, Khurshan F, et al. Patients with atrial fibrillation benefit from SAVR with surgical ablation compared to TAVR alone. Cardiology and Therapy. 2022;**11**(2):283-296

Section 5

Management of Aortic Regurgitation

Chapter 11

Transcatheter Therapies for Aortic Regurgitation: Where Are We in 2023?

Muhammad Asim Shabbir, Nidhish Tiwari and Poonam Velagapudi

Abstract

Aortic regurgitation (AR) is retrograde flow across the aortic valve in diastole and is classified from stage A to D based on severity and symptoms. Severe symptomatic AR (stage D) is a class I indication for surgical aortic valve replacement per the 2020 American College of Cardiology/American Heart Association guidelines. Though off-label, patients with prohibitive surgical risk may benefit from transcatheter aortic valve replacement (TAVR) in appropriately selected patients. However, TAVR is challenging in AR due to a lack of leaflet and annular calcification and dilation of the perivalvular apparatus, compromising the optimal anchorage of the bioprosthesis with a risk of prosthetic valve leak and embolization. Valve oversizing by 10–15% is frequently required, with caution not to oversize beyond 20%. Multimodality imaging, including echocardiography, magnetic resonance imaging, and computerized tomography, is essential for procedural planning. Registry data shows acceptable results for off-label TAVR with newer generation valves such as Medtronic Evolut and Edwards Sapien 3 for native AR. The JenaValve designed especially for TAVR for native AR is currently undergoing clinical trial. Until the results of randomized clinical trials are available, careful selection of native AR patients for TAVR is paramount to procedural and clinical success.

Keywords: aortic regurgitation, aortic insufficiency, aortic valve replacement, TAVR, transcatheter therapy, bioprosthetic valve, valvular heart disease, valvular leak, paravalvular leak, valve-in-valve

1. Introduction

Aortic regurgitation (AR) is defined as retrograde blood flow across the aortic valve (AV) during diastole. A normal AV is tricuspid, whereas a bicuspid aortic valve could accelerate the degenerative process leading to aortic stenosis (AS) or AR. According to Framingham Heart study, AR was observed in 13% of men (n = 1326) and 8.5% of women (n = 1539) using echocardiography data [1].

IntechOpen

AR may be acute or chronic. While acute severe AR (e.g., with type A aortic dissection) is a surgical emergency, chronic AR progresses gradually, requiring serial imaging and appropriate therapy when it becomes severe. There are several etiologies of AR. Diseases of aortic valve leaflets, aortic root, annulus, or ascending aorta may result in AR. AR is subdivided into four clinical stages (A to D) elaborated in **Table 1** [2–4]. Stage D signifies severe symptomatic AR, and surgical aortic valve replacement (SAVR) is a class I indication per 2020 American College of Cardiology (ACC)/American Heart Association (AHA) [3]. Asymptomatic patients

Aortic regurgitation stage	Clinical Description	Echocardiography criteria	NYHA class
Stage A	**Patients at risk:** bicuspid AV, aortic root or ascending aorta dilation, aortic valve sclerosis, history of rheumatic valve disease	None to trace AR	I
Stage B	**Progressive AR:** Mild to moderate AR due to any cause	Mild AR: Central Jet with width < 25% of LVOT, VCW <0.3 cm, RVol <30 mL/beat; RF < 30%, PHT > 500 ms, soft or incomplete jet by CW, EROA <0.10 cm^2, LV size normal (AR grade I) Moderate AR: Central Jet width 25–64% of LVOT, VCW 0.3–0.6 cm, RVol 30–59 mL/beat, RF 30–49%, PHT 500-200 ms, dense CW jet, EROA 0.10–0.29 cm^2, normal or dilated LV (AR grade II-III)	I
Stage C1	Severe asymptomatic AR	Severe AR: Central Jet width ≥ 65% of LVOT, VCW >0.6 cm, large flow convergence, prominent holo-diastolic flow reversal in descending aorta, RVol ≥60 mL/beat, RF ≥ 50%, PHT < 200 ms, dense CW jet, EROA ≥0.3 cm^2, LVEF ≥55% and mild-to-moderate LV dilation (LVESD ≤50 mm) (AR grade Grade III-IV)	I
Stage C2	Severe asymptomatic AR	Same as stage C1 except with LVEF <55% or severe LV dilation (LVESD >50 mm or LVESD index >25 mm/m^2 (Grade III-IV) Exercise testing is reasonable to confirm symptoms.	I
Stage D	Severe symptomatic AR	Same as stage C1–2 with normal or abnormal LV size and LVEF	II-IV

AR = aortic regurgitation, AV = aortic valve, CW = continuous wave, EROA = effective regurgitant orifice area, LV = left ventricle, LVEF = left ventricle ejection fraction, LVOT = left ventricle outflow tract, PHT = pressure half time, RF = regurgitant fraction, RVol = regurgitant volume, VCW = vena contracta width.

Table 1.
Clinical stages of chronic aortic regurgitation.

with severe AR and left ventricular ejection function (LVEF) < 55% (stage C2) also qualify for SAVR if no other cause of left ventricle (LV) dysfunction is identified [3]. Symptomatic patients with severe AR have 10–20% annual mortality if left untreated. A study by Dujardin et al. demonstrated a mortality rate of 34 ± 5% at ten years in patients (n = 246) with moderate to severe AR [5]. They also had higher morbidity at ten years follow-up (47 ± 6% heart failure and 62 ± 4% AV surgery). A prospective study of valvular heart disease in Europe demonstrated that 7.8% of patients with severe AR qualifying for aortic valve replacement (AVR) had no intervention due to high peri-operative risk [6, 7]. Such patients may benefit from transcatheter aortic valve replacement (TAVR) after carefully assessing procedural safety and feasibility. In contrast to AS, TAVR is challenging in AR due to the dilation of the perivalvular apparatus and lack of annular/leaflet calcification, compromising the optimal anchorage of the bioprosthesis. The potential complications include improper valve seal, paravalvular leak (PVL), valve embolization, and malalignment or malposition of the bioprosthetic valve [8, 9]. This chapter discusses transcatheter therapies for chronic native valvular AR.

2. Imaging for aortic regurgitation

The incompetence of aortic valve leaflets during diastole results in the backflow of blood into the left ventricle. The regurgitation leads to increased blood volume at the end of diastole and elevated stress on the ventricular walls, eventually causing compensatory eccentric hypertrophy due to excessive volume.

Transthoracic echocardiography (TTE) is the primary tool to assess the mechanism, severity, secondary impact on LV remodeling, and hemodynamic consequences of AR. Moreover, TTE and computerized tomography (CT) are valuable in assessing aortic root size. Wenzel et al. demonstrated a proportional relationship between the degree of aortic root dilation and AR severity [10]. Even with nondilated aortic roots, pure AR is associated with degeneration of aortic walls as evidenced by histological and immunohistochemical analyses by Balint et al [11]. According to the 2020 ACC/AHA valvular heart disease guidelines [3], severe AR is defined by specific criteria: Doppler jet width of ≥65% of the left ventricular outflow tract (LVOT), vena contracta width >0.6 cm, regurgitant volume of ≥60 mL/beat, regurgitant fraction of ≥50%, and effective orifice area of ≥0.3 cm. However, identifying subtle LV dysfunction in the early stages of the disease is desirable, as severe dilation and reduced LVEF indicate a late stage of the disease.

2.1 Speckle tracking echocardiography in aortic regurgitation

With chronic AR, speckle tracking echocardiography reveals that the eccentric changes in the LV predominantly affect the circumferentially arranged fibers, leading to more severe impairment in global circumferential strain (GCS) compared to global longitudinal strain (GLS). Therefore, circumferential strain is a more sensitive marker for AR and volume overload compared to longitudinal strain for AS and pressure overload [12]. A retrospective study of 314 patients with chronic moderate to severe AR demonstrated that reduced GLS independently predicted mortality, with a threshold of −12.5% [13]. Patients with progressive AR and symptoms had significantly lower longitudinal strain compared to those with stable disease, despite similar LVEF.

In a longitudinal study of 64 patients, reduced GLS, strain rate, and early diastolic strain were associated with progressive disease and worse outcomes following surgery [14]. Impaired LV radial systolic strain rate was predictive of LVEF post-surgery, and decreased baseline GLS or GCS predicted the need for surgery in asymptomatic patients [15].

2.2 3-dimensional echocardiography

3-Dimensional (3D) echocardiography is crucial in assessing AR severity. While numerous 2-Dimensional (2D) echocardiography parameters can be used to quantify AR, it remains challenging due to variations in the scan plane and irregularities in the shape of the vena contracta jet. 3D echocardiography, specifically measuring the vena contracta area (3D-VCA), provides a direct and accurate evaluation. Studies have shown that severe AR can be detected with a sensitivity of 89% and specificity of 98% using a 3D-VCA cutoff of 32 mm^2 [16]. 2D-derived parameters such as proximal iso-velocity surface area (PISA) and regurgitant volume (RVol) affected by geometric assumptions, angle correction limitations, and difficulty assessing multiple jets. Full-volume color Doppler echocardiography in 3D has been reported to be more accurate than 2D-PISA, especially for eccentric or multiple jets [17]. Moreover, 3D color Doppler echocardiography has demonstrated high accuracy and reproducibility for AR evaluation, exhibiting a strong correlation with cardiac magnetic resonance (CMR) imaging, considered the gold standard [18].

2.3 Cardiac magnetic resonance imaging

CMR has emerged as a valuable tool for assessing AR patients. It is the current reference standard for evaluating cardiac volumes, mass, and systolic function. Furthermore, CMR provides insights into myocardial tissue characterization, offering additional prognostic information. It enables both anatomical and functional assessment of the aortic valve and the entire thoracic aorta.

2.4 Computed tomography

In preprocedural evaluations of patients with AR, ECG-gated CT is indispensable because it provides precise information about the aortic size and valve morphology, among other vital details, for optimal procedural planning. Additionally, CT can help exclude the presence of associated coronary artery disease. It is worth noting that the asymmetrical nature of the aortic root, especially in cases of a bicuspid aortic valve, can lead to underestimation of the actual size of the aortic valve when measured using single-plane echocardiography.

3. Transcatheter aortic valve replacement (TAVR) for native aortic regurgitation

TAVR has evolved as a treatment for AS in the United States (U.S.) across all risk categories [19, 20]. More recently, TAVR has been increasingly used for off-label indications such as bicuspid AV stenosis, subaortic stenosis, and severe AR [21]. Off-label TAVR has shown similar 1-year mortality (25.6%) compared to on-label TAVR in a study using STS/TVT data [21].

According to 2020 ACC/AHA valvular heart disease guidelines, SAVR is a class I indication for pure native AR stage C2-D [3]. However, TAVR has been performed as an off-label treatment for AR in patients with prohibitive surgical risk [22]. TAVR poses unique technical challenges in pure AR due to lack of annular/leaflet calcification and, in some cases, aortic root dilation. Current data suggests oversizing the prosthetic valve by 10–15% with caution and not exceeding 20% due to the risk of annular rupture and conduction abnormalities [23–25]. Severe aortic root dilation with large annuli may exceed the size of commercially approved bioprosthetic valves and make the TAVR riskier and unsuccessful due to the risk of valve embolization. Additionally, it may cause more than mild residual PVL due to a lack of proper seal. The maximum size of the commercially available self-expanding valve is 34 mm (Evolut FX by Medtronic), providing a maximal annular area of 940 mm^2 [26]. It is larger than the area of the largest commercially available balloon-expandable valve, e.g., 29 mm Edwards SAPIEN 3 Ultra or RESILIA valve provides an annular area of 683 mm^2 [27].

Alharbi et al. compared TAVR (n = 912) vs. SAVR (n = 13,808) for pure native AR using the US national inpatient sample database from 2016 to 2017 and found no difference in in-hospital mortality between both groups. Although the need for a permanent pacemaker (PPM) was higher in the TAVR group, these patients had lower acute renal injury, cardiogenic shock, respiratory complications, and length of hospital stay despite having worse baseline characteristics compared to the SAVR group [28]. Another large-scale study by Arora et al [29] demonstrated 3.3% 30-day all-cause mortality with TAVR for AR compared with 3.4% in the PARTNER trial for AS in high-risk population [30]. Newer-generation devices depicted lower mortality with higher procedural success of TAVR in pure AR when compared with first-generation devices across observational studies [31–33].

Examples of first-generation TAVR devices include Edwards Sapien XT and Medtronic CoreValve. Second-generation valves have an improved design to provide better anchoring mechanisms, optimal seal, and superior hemodynamic results. Examples of second-generation valves include Edwards Sapien 3, Medtronic Evolut R, Evolut PRO, Evolut FX, Acurate Neo, Acurate TA, Direct Flow Valve, J-valve, JenaValve, and Portico valves.

3.1 Edwards Sapien 3

The Edwards Sapien 3 valve by Edwards Lifesciences comprises bovine pericardial tissue with a balloon expandable cobalt-chromium frame and an inner and outer skirt. The outer skirt provides more durability and prevents PVL without excessive overexpanding [34]. The valve is designed to be delivered by transfemoral approach via 14 or 16 F sheath, depending on valve size, and is available in sizes 20 mm, 23 mm, 26 mm, and 29 mm. It is not approved for AR but has been used as an off-label indication in selected high-risk patients [35]. A recent observational study showed a 94.6% (n = 35) device success rate and 8.1% all-cause mortality at 30 days using Sapien 3 valve for pure AR with non-calcified leaflets. The valve migration occurred in 10.8% of cases (n = 4) (**Figures 1** and **2**) [36].

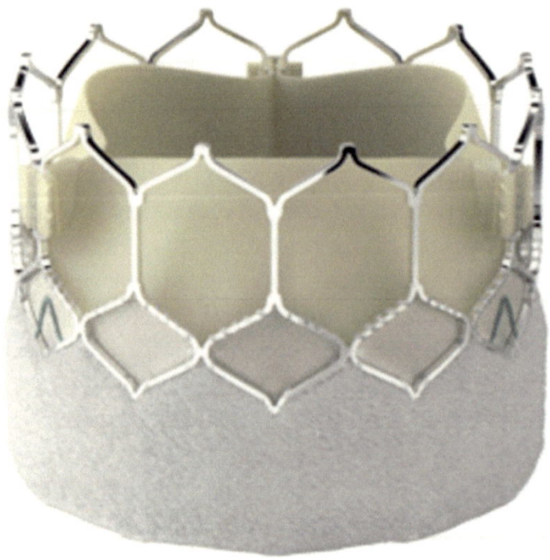

Figure 1.
Edwards Sapien 3 ultra valve comprises bovine pericardium tissue polyethylene terephthalate outer skirt (credit: Edwards Lifesciences).

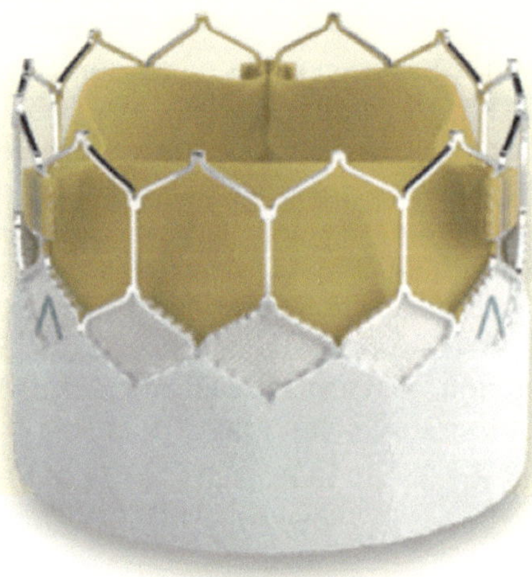

Figure 2.
Newer generation Edwards Sapien 3 RESILIA tissue valve with anti-calcification technology (credit: Edwards Lifesciences).

3.2 Medtronic Evolut

Medtronic Evolut valve consists of a porcine tissue pericardial valve with a self-expanding nitinol frame. The latest iteration is the Evolut FX system. It is delivered transfemorally via 14 F or 16 F inline sheath, and available sizes are 23 mm, 26 mm, 29 mm, and 34 mm. The delivery system is designed to fully retrieve the valve for

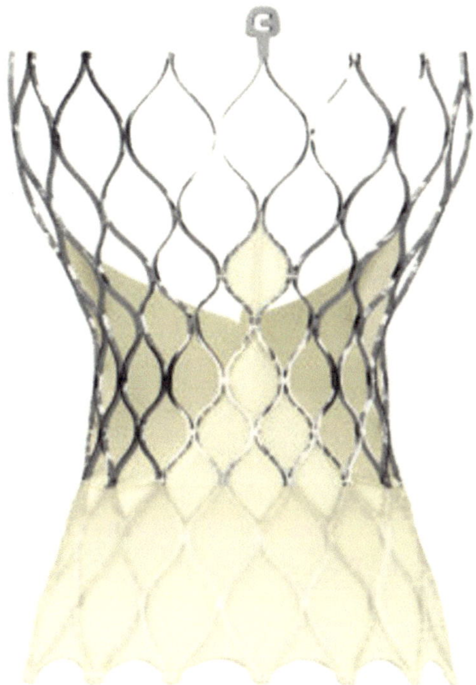

Figure 3.
Evolut FX 34 mm self-expanding nitinol frame with bovine tissue (credit: Medtronic).

repositioning. Federal Drug Administration (FDA) has not yet approved it for AR. However, it has been used off-label in patients with AR who are not eligible for surgery with acceptable results (**Figure 3**) [32, 37].

3.3 ACURATE valve Neo2

The ACURATE Neo2 valve by Boston Scientific is a porcine tissue pericardial valve with a self-expanding nitinol frame. It is available in 23 mm, 25 mm, and 27 mm sizes and is inserted transfemorally. In a multicenter European study, [38] the ACURATE Neo valve demonstrated good feasibility and early safety in 24 patients with native AR. The device success rate was 87.5%, with 4.1% all-cause mortality at 30 days. Two patients had moderate PVL and three required implantation of a second device for severe PVL and device displacement. The need for new PPM was 21.1% which is higher than the other commercially available TAVR valves. Acurate Neo2 is an investigational device restricted to experimental use in the United States (**Figure 4**) [39].

3.4 ACURATE TA

The ACCURATE TA device by Symetis, Switzerland, is composed of a self-expanding nitinol frame and is delivered trans-apically (**Figure 5**). It was explored as a treatment for severe native AR in patients with high surgical risk. A small single-center German case center series demonstrates the feasibility of transapical TAVR with the self-expandable ACURATE TA device in high-risk patients with 100%

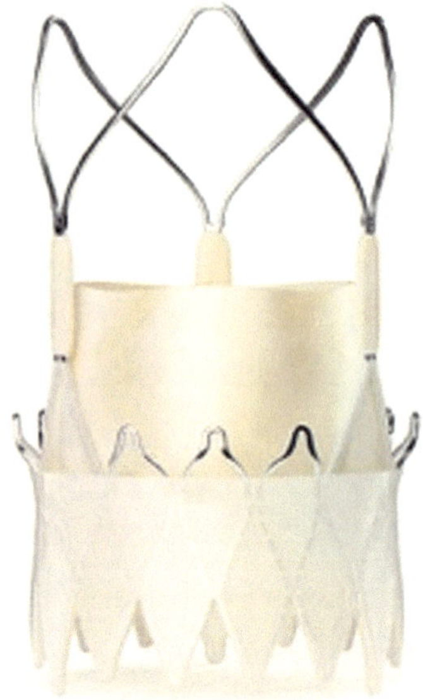

Figure 4.
ACURATE Neo2 valve with self-expanding nitinol frame (credit: Boston Scientific).

procedural success and 0% all-cause mortality at 30 days. However, in the current era of transfemoral TAVR, the transapical approach may be considered too invasive [40].

3.5 Portico valve system

The Portico valve by Abbot comprises bovine pericardial tissue with a self-expandable nitinol frame. It comes in 23 mm, 25 mm, 27 mm, and 29 mm sizes (**Figure 6**). It provides a fully retrievable system.

3.6 J-valve Ausper system

J-valve Ausper system by Jiecheng Medical Technology has been certified by China FDA for AR. It consists of bovine pericardial leaflets with nitinol stent frame within three U-shaped anchor rings (**Figure 7**). The earlier device was designed to be delivered via transapical access. A large-scale single-center Chinese study for severe AS and severe AR showed acceptable safety with 3% and 3.7% mortality at 30 days and 6 months, respectively [41]. The newer device can be delivered by a transfemoral approach using an 18 F sheath. Available sizes are 21 mm, 23 mm, 25 mm, 27 mm, and 29 mm.

3.7 JenaValve system

The JenaValve system by JenaValve technology is designed for patients with severe AS, AR, and both [42]. The valve comprises porcine leaflets with a self-expanding framework for transfemoral delivery. Sizes in development include 65–92 mm (**Figure 8**). It provides the advantage of calcium-independent anchorage by grasping

DOI: http://dx.doi.org/10.5772/intechopen.112679

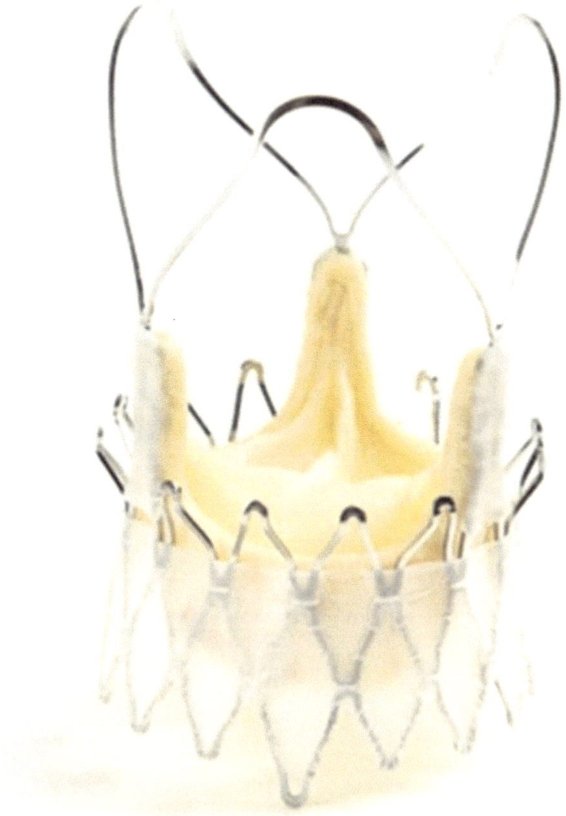

Figure 5.
ACURATE TA valve with self-expanding nitinol frame (credit: Symetis).

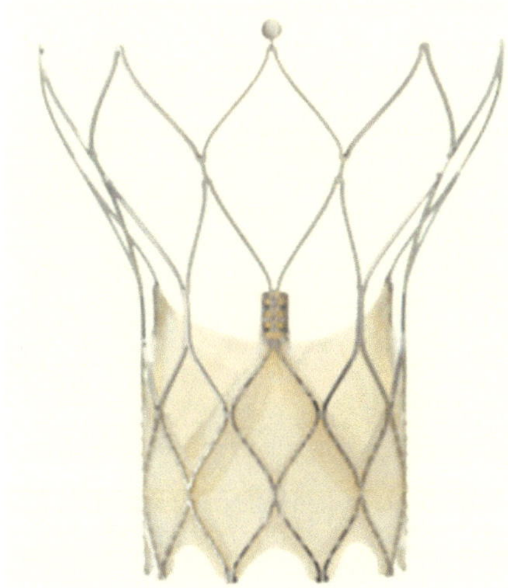

Figure 6.
Portico valve with self-expandable nitinol frame (credit: Abbot).

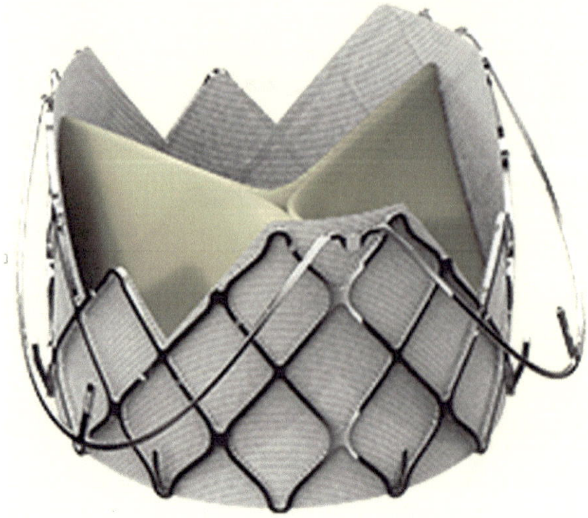

Figure 7.
J-valve Ausper with nitinol stent frame (credit: Jiecheng medical technology).

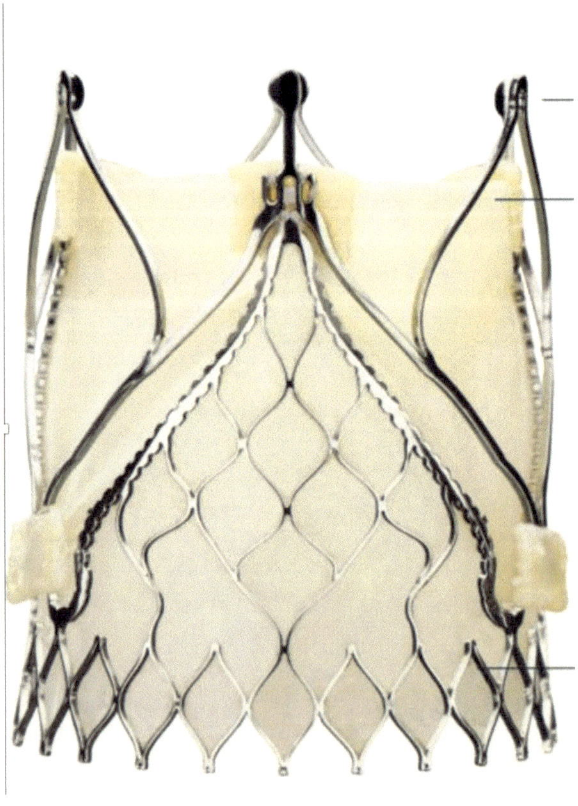

Figure 8.
Jena valve with self-expanding calcium-independent anchorage frame.

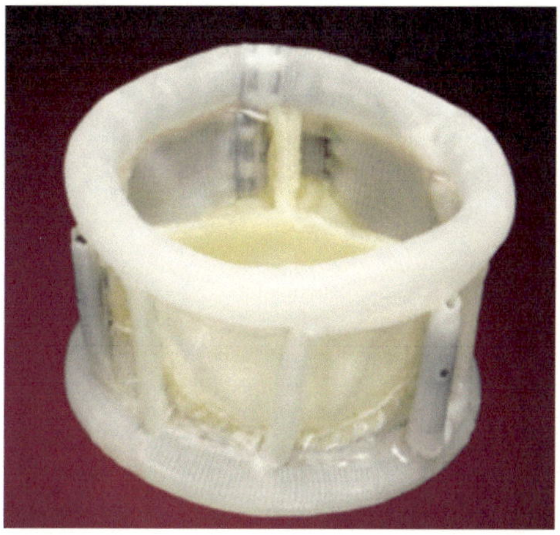

Figure 9.
Direct flow medical valve with two rings and polyester fabric skirt (credit: Direct flow medical).

the native leaflets and moving them towards the periphery, forming a natural seal (paper clip-like anchorage) [43]. The prosthetic leaflets are supra-annular. Large cells provide easy access for coronary engagement post-procedure. JenaValve is currently explored in ALIGN-AR pivotal, multicenter trial (NCT04415047) for severe AR in the USA. Key inclusion criteria include severe AR, high surgical risk, and NYHA class ≥ II. Exclusion factors are previous prosthetic valves, hemodynamic instability, endocarditis, unicuspid or bicuspid valve, and severe mitral regurgitation.

3.8 Direct flow medical

Direct Flow Medical (DFM) valve by Direct Flow Medical, California, comprises three bovine pericardial leaflets attached to a frame covered with polyester fabric (**Figure 9**). The frame comprises aortic (upper) and ventricular (lower) rings [44]. The size chart includes 25 mm, 27 mm, and 29 mm valves. It is delivered via an 18 F transfemoral approach and is commercially available in Europe. A small multicenter retrospective European study of 11 patients showed the feasibility of DFM valve for severe non-calcific native AR [45]. The device success rate was 100%, with one patient requiring SAVR after the downward dislocation of the prosthesis by TAVR. All patients had a reduction in NYHA class, and 30-day all-cause mortality was 9% (n = 1 due to pneumonia).

4. Procedural technique

Appropriate valve sizing is crucial in TAVR for pure AR to allow optimal valve anchorage and prevent complications such as annular rupture from oversizing or prosthetic valve embolization from under-sizing. Pre-procedural multimodality imaging (i.e., TTE, transesophageal echocardiogram (TEE), CT, and CMR) can help understand the size of the aortic annulus and aortic root [46, 47]. Fluoroscopy and TEE are important intra-operative tools for deploying the prosthetic valve at the appropriate position. Valve oversizing is frequently required for optimal apposition of the valve to dilated annulus and prevent PVL. Oversizing by 10–15% is recommended

Clinical trial	Valve	Trial description and location	Outcomes of interest	Inclusion criteria	Exclusion criteria
ALIGN-AR (NCT02732704)	JenaValve by JenaValve technology	Safety and effectiveness of TAVR by JenaValve for symptomatic severe AR (single arm) **Location**: USA, Germany, Netherlands	**Primary**: All-Cause Mortality at 30 days **Secondary**: Peri-Procedural AMI within 72 hr., stroke-free Survival at 30 days, bleeding & vascular complications	Severe AR, NYHA≥II, high surgical risk	History of AVR, hemodynamic instability, endocarditis, unicuspid or bicuspid valve, and severe MR.
SENSE-AR (NCT05737264)	Unspecified	Safety and effectiveness of TAVR for severe native AR with self-expandable valve implantation (single arm) **Location**: China	**Primary**: 12-month all-cause mortality, 12-month disabling stroke, 12-month heart failure hospitalization **Secondary**: Device success, new PPM, new LBBB, valve dysfunction, periprocedural complications (life-threatening bleeding, AKI, vascular complications, repeat procedure for valve-related dysfunction), NYHA class III or IV	Age > 60, severe AR	History of AVR, mod-severe MR, acute endocarditis
SEASON-AR (NCT04864145)	Unspecified	Safety and effectiveness of TAVR for severe native AR with self-expandable valve implantation (compared with medical therapy) **Location**: China	**Primary**: 12-month composite of all-cause death, disabling stroke, or heart failure rehospitalization **Secondary**: (all within 12 months) procedural complications (aortic, coronary, or vascular complications, new ppm), 6-minute walk distance, NYHA class, stroke, mortality, bleeding complications, prosthetic valve dysfunction, rehospitalization for valve-related symptoms or worsening congestive heart failure.	Symptomatic severe AR, asymptomatic AR with LVEF<55%, LVEDD>65 mm or LVESD>50 mm, AV mean pressure gradient <20 mmHg; annular perimeter ≤85 mm, LVOT: AV annulus perimeter 0.95–1.05, STS score ≥ 8.	Age < 60, ascending aorta >45 mm, multivessel CAD, life expectancy <1 year, LVEF <30%, AMI within 30 days.

AMI = acute myocardial infarction, AKI = acute kidney injury, AR = aortic regurgitation, AV = aortic valve, AVR = aortic valve replacement, CAD = coronary artery disease, LBBB = left bundle branch block, LVEF = left ventricular ejection fraction, LVEDD = left ventricular end-diastolic dimension, LVESD = left ventricular end-systolic dimension, LVOT = left ventricular outflow tract, MR = mitral regurgitation, NYHA = New York Heart Association, STS = Society of Thoracic Surgeons, TAVR = transcatheter aortic valve replacement.

Table 2.
Comparison of ongoing TAVR clinical trials.

with caution not to oversize beyond 20% [23–25]. The newer generation valve, JenaValve, is designed for pure AR grasps onto native leaflets and can be beneficial in the absence of leaflet calcium [43].

5. Future directions

The newer generation valves are undergoing clinical trials for TAVR for treating pure AR. As with any procedure, patient selection is key to procedural and clinical success. Ongoing prospective trials are listed in **Table 2**.

6. Conclusion

Symptomatic AR carries a high mortality if left untreated. Patients at high or prohibitive surgical risk may be candidates for off-label TAVR on a case-by-case basis, as determined by the heart team. The off-label use of TAVR for AR has shown promising results from registry data. The challenges of TAVR for AR include improper valvular seal, PVL, valve embolization, and malalignment or malposition of the bioprosthetic valve due to lack of calcification and enlarged aortic annuli. Valve oversizing can help overcome technical issues but carries the risk of annular rupture. The newer generation transcatheter valves designed especially for the treatment of pure native AR are undergoing clinical trials. Until the results of randomized clinical trials are available, careful selection of patients is paramount to procedural and clinical success.

Conflict of interest

Poonam Velagapudi received speaking fees from Medtronic, Abiomed, Opsens, and Shockwave and participated in advisory boards for Abiomed and Sanofi.

Muhammad Asim Shabbir and Nidhish Tiwari have nothing to disclose.

Author details

Muhammad Asim Shabbir, Nidhish Tiwari and Poonam Velagapudi*
Division of Cardiovascular Medicine, University of Nebraska Medical Center, Omaha, NE, USA

*Address all correspondence to: poonamchou@gmail.com

IntechOpen

© 2023 The Author(s). Licensee IntechOpen. This chapter is distributed under the terms of the Creative Commons Attribution License (http://creativecommons.org/licenses/by/3.0), which permits unrestricted use, distribution, and reproduction in any medium, provided the original work is properly cited. (cc) BY

References

[1] Singh JP et al. Prevalence and clinical determinants of mitral, tricuspid, and aortic regurgitation (the Framingham heart study). The American Journal of Cardiology. 1999;**83**(6):897-902

[2] Akinseye OA, Pathak A, Ibebuogu UN. Aortic valve regurgitation: A comprehensive review. Current Problems in Cardiology. 2018;**43**(8):315-334

[3] Otto CM et al. 2020 ACC/AHA guideline for the Management of Patients with Valvular Heart Disease: Executive summary. Journal of the American College of Cardiology. 2021;**77**(4):450-500

[4] Zoghbi WA et al. Recommendations for noninvasive evaluation of native Valvular regurgitation: A report from the American Society of Echocardiography developed in collaboration with the Society for Cardiovascular Magnetic Resonance. Journal of the American Society of Echocardiography. 2017;**30**(4):303-371

[5] Dujardin KS et al. Mortality and morbidity of aortic regurgitation in clinical practice. A long-term follow-up study. Circulation. 1999;**99**(14):1851-1857

[6] Anna Franzone MTP. TAVR for Aortic Regurgitation. 2017. Available from: https://www.acc.org/latest-in-cardiology/articles/2017/12/21/08/16/tavr-for-aortic-regurgitation

[7] Iung B et al. A prospective survey of patients with valvular heart disease in Europe: The euro heart survey on Valvular heart disease. European Heart Journal. 2003;**24**(13):1231-1243

[8] Sawaya FJ et al. Safety and efficacy of Transcatheter aortic valve replacement in the treatment of pure aortic regurgitation in native valves and failing surgical bioprostheses: Results from an international registry study. JACC: Cardiovascular Interventions. 2017;**10**(10):1048-1056

[9] Roy DA et al. Transcatheter aortic valve implantation for pure severe native aortic valve regurgitation. Journal of the American College of Cardiology. 2013;**61**(15):1577-1584

[10] Wenzel JP et al. Aortic root dimensions as a correlate for aortic regurgitation's severity. The International Journal of Cardiovascular Imaging. 2021;**37**(12):3439-3449

[11] Balint B et al. Aortic regurgitation is associated with ascending aortic Remodeling in the nondilated aorta. Arteriosclerosis, Thrombosis, and Vascular Biology. 2021;**41**(3):1179-1190

[12] Tiwari N, Patel K. Newer echocardiographic techniques for aortic-valve imaging: Clinical aids today, clinical practice tomorrow. World Journal of Cardiology. 2018;**10**(8):62-73

[13] Park SH et al. Left ventricular strain as predictor of chronic aortic regurgitation. Journal of Cardiovascular Ultrasound. 2015;**23**(2):78-85

[14] Olsen NT et al. Speckle-tracking echocardiography for predicting outcome in chronic aortic regurgitation during conservative management and after surgery. JACC: Cardiovascular Imaging. 2011;**4**(3):223-230

[15] Onishi T et al. Preoperative systolic strain rate predicts postoperative left ventricular dysfunction in patients with chronic aortic regurgitation.

Circulation. Cardiovascular Imaging. 2010;**3**(2):134-141

[16] Sato H et al. Severity of aortic regurgitation assessed by area of vena contracta: A clinical two-dimensional and three-dimensional color Doppler imaging study. Cardiovascular Ultrasound. 2015;**13**:24

[17] Choi J et al. Automatic quantification of aortic regurgitation using 3D full volume color doppler echocardiography: A validation study with cardiac magnetic resonance imaging. The International Journal of Cardiovascular Imaging. 2015;**31**(7):1379-1389

[18] Perez de Isla L et al. 3D color-Doppler echocardiography and chronic aortic regurgitation: A novel approach for severity assessment. International Journal of Cardiology. 2013;**166**(3):640-645

[19] Popma JJ et al. Transcatheter aortic-valve replacement with a self-expanding valve in low-risk patients. New England Journal of Medicine. 2019;**380**(18):1706-1715

[20] Carroll John D et al. STS-ACC TVT registry of Transcatheter aortic valve replacement. Journal of the American College of Cardiology. 2020;**76**(21):2492-2516

[21] Hira RS et al. Trends and outcomes of off-label use of Transcatheter aortic valve replacement: Insights from the NCDR STS/ACC TVT registry. JAMA Cardiology. 2017;**2**(8):846-854

[22] Franzone A et al. Transcatheter aortic valve replacement for the treatment of pure native aortic valve regurgitation: A systematic review. JACC: Cardiovascular Interventions. 2016;**9**(22):2308-2317

[23] Dvir D et al. Multicenter evaluation of transcatheter aortic valve replacement using either SAPIEN XT or CoreValve: Degree of device oversizing by computed-tomography and clinical outcomes. Catheterization and Cardiovascular Interventions. 2015;**86**(3):508-515

[24] Alkhouli M, Sengupta P, Badhwar V. Toward precision in balloon-expandable TAVR. JACC: Cardiovascular Interventions. 2017;**10**(8):821-823

[25] Arias EA et al. TAVI for pure native aortic regurgitation: Are we there yet? Interventional Cardiology. 2019;**14**(1):26-30

[26] Medtronic Evolut R System. https://www.medtronic.com/us-en/healthcare-professionals/products/cardiovascular/transcatheter-aortic-heart-valves/evolut-r.html

[27] Edwards SAPIEN 3 Transcatheter Heart Valve with the Edwards Commander Delivery System. https://www.accessdata.fda.gov/cdrh_docs/pdf14/P140031c.pdf

[28] Alharbi AA et al. Transcatheter aortic valve replacement vs surgical replacement in patients with pure aortic insufficiency. Mayo Clinic Proceedings. 2020;**95**(12):2655-2664

[29] Arora S et al. Transcatheter aortic valve replacement in aortic regurgitation: The U.S. experience. Catheterization and Cardiovascular Interventions. 2021;**98**(1):E153-e162

[30] Smith CR et al. Transcatheter versus surgical aortic-valve replacement in high-risk patients. The New England Journal of Medicine. 2011;**364**(23):2187-2198

[31] Wernly B et al. Transcatheter aortic valve replacement for pure

aortic valve regurgitation: "On-label" versus "off-label" use of TAVR devices. Clinical Research in Cardiology. 2019;**108**(8):921-930

[32] Yin W-H et al. Outcomes of transcatheter aortic valve replacement for pure native aortic regurgitation with the use of newer- vs . Early-generation devices. Annals of Translational Medicine. 2022;**10**(1):24

[33] Yoon S-H et al. Transcatheter aortic valve replacement in pure native aortic valve regurgitation. Journal of the American College of Cardiology. 2017;**70**(22):2752-2763

[34] Denise, Todaro AP, Barbanti M. Current TAVR devices. Cardiac Interventions Today. 2017. Available from: https://citoday.com/articles/2017-mar-apr/current-tavr-devices [Last accessed: August 16, 2023]

[35] Urena M et al. Transcatheter aortic valve replacement to treat pure aortic regurgitation on noncalcified native valves. Journal of the American College of Cardiology. 2016;**68**(15):1705-1706

[36] Delhomme C et al. Transcatheter aortic valve implantation using the SAPIEN 3 valve to treat aortic regurgitation: The French multicentre S3AR study. Archives of Cardiovascular Diseases. 2023;**116**(2):98-105

[37] Bruschi G et al. Evolut R implantation to treat severe pure aortic regurgitation in a patient with mitral bioprosthesis. The Annals of Thoracic Surgery. 2016;**102**(6):e521-e524

[38] Purita PAM et al. Transcatheter treatment of native aortic valve regurgitation: Results from an international registry using the transfemoral ACURATE neo valve. International Journal of Cardiology: Heart & Vasculature. 2020;**27**:100480

[39] Boston Scientific's. Acurate Neo2 TAVR device evaluated for hemodynamic performance and clinical outcomes. Cardiac Interventions Today. 2022. Available from: https://citoday.com/news/boston-scientifics-acurate-neo2-tavr-device-evaluated-for-hemodynamic-performance-and-clinical-outcomes [Last accessed: August 16, 2023]

[40] Wendt D et al. Transapical Transcatheter aortic valve for severe aortic regurgitation. JACC: Cardiovascular Interventions. 2014;**7**(10):1159-1167

[41] Liu L et al. Transcatheter aortic valve replacement in aortic regurgitation. The Annals of Thoracic Surgery. 2020;**110**(6):1959-1965

[42] Costanzo P et al. Transcatheter aortic valve implantation for severe pure aortic regurgitation with dedicated devices. Interventional Cardiology. 2022;**17**(e11):2022

[43] Poschner T et al. The JenaValve pericardial transcatheter aortic valve replacement system to treat aortic valve disease. Future Cardiology. 2022;**18**(2):101-113

[44] Jeffrey Southard RL. Direct flow valve. Cardiac Interventions Today. 2012. Available from: https://citoday.com/articles/2012-july-aug/direct-flow-valve [Last accessed: August 16, 2023]

[45] Schofer J et al. Transfemoral implantation of a fully repositionable and retrievable Transcatheter valve for noncalcified pure aortic regurgitation. JACC: Cardiovascular Interventions. 2015;**8**(14):1842-1849

[46] Saadi RP et al. Preoperative TAVR planning: How to do it. Journal of Clinical Medicine. 2022;**11**(9):2582

[47] Perry TE et al. A guide for pre-procedural imaging for transcatheter aortic valve replacement patients. Perioperative Medicine. 2020;**9**(1):36

Section 6

Surgical Therapy for Bicuspid Aortic Valve Syndrome

Chapter 12

Bicuspid Aortic Valve: Current Therapeutic Strategies

Syed Usman Bin Mahmood, Prashanth Vallabhajosyula and Rita Milewski

Abstract

Bicuspid aortic valve (BAV) is the most common congenital valvular pathology with an incidence of 1–2% in the general population. It is associated with an ascending aortic aneurysm phenotype in 26–50%, and aortic root (+/− ascending aneurysm) phenotype in up to 20–32% of patients. Bicuspid aortic valve patients present with a spectrum of valvular, ascending, and aortic root aneurysmal pathophysiologies. This variable spectrum has mandated the development of an array of surgical procedures to be able to tailor an individualized approach to BAV syndrome for a typically younger BAV population in which long-term outcomes are especially relevant . This chapter will delineate the current evidence-based surgical therapeutic strategies for patients with a BAV syndrome of aortic valve stenosis or insufficiency phenotype and aortic phenotype pathophysiology and include aortic valve replacement, aortic valve repair, aortic valve and supracoronary ascending aorta replacement (AVRSCAAR), Bentall procedure, and valve-sparing root reimplantation.

Keywords: bicuspid aortic valve, aortic valve replacement, aortic valve repair, aortic root replacement, valve sparing root reimplantation, Bentall, supracoronary ascending aorta replacement

1. Introduction

Bicuspid aortic valve (BAV) is the most common congenital anomaly of the cardiac valves. It occurs in approximately 1–2% of the general population [1–5]. Its incidence is known to be higher in Caucasian males and lower in female or non-Caucasian populations [6]. BAV syndrome is a heterogeneous disease that can manifest with various valvular, ascending aortic, and aortic root pathophysiologies. The bicuspid aortic valve can be functionally normal, or it may be insufficient or stenotic. Asymptomatic BAV patients with no other hemodynamic deficiencies have good long-term survival; however, valvular degeneration, either aortic stenosis or insufficiency, may develop with time and require close surveillance [7]. This heterogeneity of BAV syndrome has mandated the development of varied surgical procedures to address the valvular/aortic root pathophysiologies as delineated in **Figure 1** [4]. Therefore, definitive management of BAV syndrome requires a personalized approach according to patient-specific pathophysiology. Therapeutic management strategies for valvular

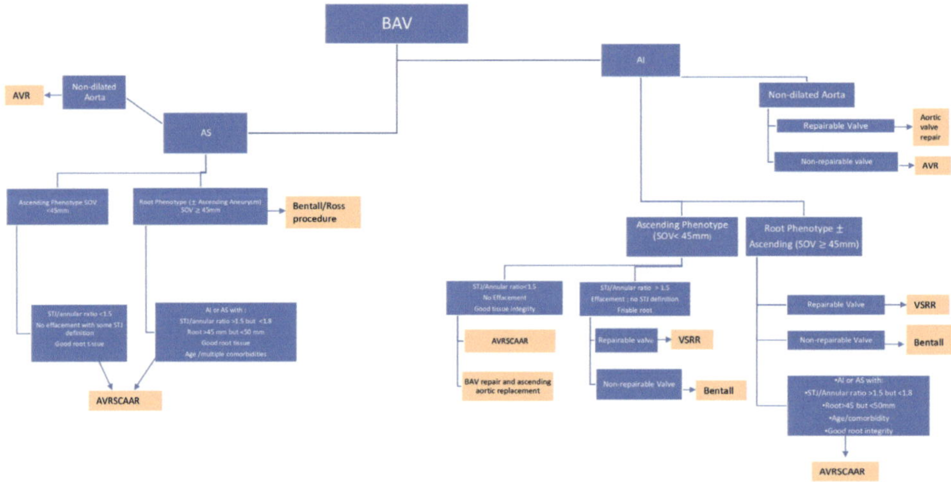

Figure 1.
Bicuspid aortic valve surgical management according to aortic phenotypes.

phenotype and aortic phenotype utilizing a specific algorithmic approach for variable aortic valve, aortic root, and ascending aorta pathophysiologies in BAV syndrome can provide good long-term functional and clinical results [4] (**Figure 1**).

2. BAV syndrome pathology and pathophysiology

The bicuspid aortic valve morphology has been characterized by raphe number and the position of cusps and raphes [8]. This morphology includes complete or partial leaflet fusion. The most common morphology in BAV patients is fusion of left and right coronary cusps. The next most common morphology in BAV patients is fusion of right coronary cusp with noncoronary cusp [8, 9]. The morphology of the bicuspid aortic valve has been described by various classification systems, most notably the Sievers classification [8–10]. Sievers Type 0 BAV has an incidence of 7% in the original Sievers and Schmidtke series and a BAV valve geometry of no raphe and 2 valve cusps [8, 11]. Sievers Type 1 BAV morphology is the most common and has an incidence of 88% in the original series with a BAV valve geometry of a single raphe and 2 valve cusps [8, 11]. Sievers Type 2 BAV has an incidence of 5% in the original series and is the rarest morphology of the three types in this classification with a BAV valve geometry of 2 raphe and 2 valve cusps [8, 11].

Patients with BAV are known to have high rates of various valvular pathologies in adult life [7], particularly aortic stenosis (especially in males) [12], aortic regurgitation [13], and infective endocarditis involving the aortic valve [14]. BAV is three to four times more frequent in men than in women. Approximately, 50–75% of patients with BAV will require aortic valve replacement procedure during their lifetime and up to 25% may require an aortic procedure often concurrent with their valve replacement [15].

BAV syndrome pathophysiology is associated with dilation of the aorta [2]. BAV may be associated with an ascending aortic aneurysm phenotype in around 26–50% patients or a root phenotype in up to 20–32% of patients [2, 3, 16]. These distinct phenotypes have been stratified into three categories. Type 1 is dilation of ascending

DOI: http://dx.doi.org/10.5772/intechopen.113315

aorta along its convexity and can involve root dilation. Type 2 is arch dilation and ascending aortic dilation with sparing of the root. Type 3 involves an isolated root phenotype and has been associated with a genetic causality [16–18]. BAV associated with aortic dilation increases the risk of dissection as the aorta dilates further. In BAV patients, aortic dissection has been observed to occur almost 5–10 times more commonly than trileaflet aortic valve population [19].

Aortic dilatation and aneurysm formation in BAV patients has been attributed to two different mechanisms: hemodynamic stress and the inherent aortic wall tissue abnormality. Hemodynamically, shear stress on the aortic wall due to blood flowing through a stenotic valve has been hypothesized to cause early dilatation of the aorta [20]. Abnormal flow patterns have been noted due to the configuration of the BAV even in absence of stenosis [21].

Dysregulation of the aortic wall can also contribute to aneurysmal dilation. Human and animal studies have identified that extracellular matrix dysregulation along with dysfunctional signaling pathways can contribute to hemodynamic effects observed in calcific aortic valve disease and regurgitation [22]. A recent study demonstrated newborns with BAV having aortopathy and dilated aorta even in the presence of relatively normal velocities across the valve [23] and this suggests inherent aortic tissue dysregulation as a factor which may impact the population of patients with BAV.

3. Embryology and genetics of BAV and associated aortic aneurysm

The aortic valve develops from endocardial cushions within the maturing heart tube and begins to form around the fifth week of embryonic development. In normal cardiac development, these cushions later divide into three distinct aortic valve leaflets. In patients with BAV disease, the cushions either fail to divide or fuse leading to the characteristic bicuspid morphology. It has been postulated that multifactorial variables including genetic/embryologic factors impact the formation of the bicuspid aortic valve.

There is a recognized genetic component to bicuspid aortic valve disease. It may occur sporadically or as an autosomal dominant disorder with variable penetrance [24]. And, it has been noted that some family members of BAV patients may present with isolated BAV, some with associated aortic (ascending/root) aneurysms and some may be carriers with no manifest disease. The spatial and anatomical sequences in development of congenital heart disease (CHD) continues to be defined. Outflow tract defects specifically those involving the aortic valve have been difficult to categorize as they appear to be multifactorial in origin with many signaling and transcriptional gene anomalies possible for the outcome. Autosomal dominant inheritance pattern has been described for BAV specifically involving the NOTCH1 gene pathway however, this is not exclusive [25].

The genetic mechanism for a majority of BAV cases remains unknown. Although these cases may seem ‘sporadic’ there is still a 10% increase in risk of having BAV in siblings and offspring based on epidemiological studies [26]. There is a similar rate of incidence of aortic aneurysms in family members with or without BAV demonstrating some role of shared environmental or genetic causes [27]. High number of genetic variants, associated with structural variation and mixed inheritance patterns of the disease have complicated the discovery of the BAV-associated genes [28]. Chromosomal mutations involving 9q have been linked to BAV disease [29]. Mutations at various loci on chromosomes 5, 15, and 18 are linked to familial BAV and aortic syndromes [24].

The occurrence of aortic aneurysm and coarctation in patients with BAV underlines a possible common genetic pathway for these disease entities. Microscopic examination of BAV associated aneurysm tissue has demonstrated non-inflammatory medial degeneration also known as cystic medial necrosis [30]. Dysregulation of the canonical (Smad2/Smad3) TGF-B signaling genes has been implicated to be a possible common defect for BAV and aneurysm formation. TGF-B signaling plays a role in cell migration and valvulogenesis that are pivotal in proper valve formation and functioning [30]. Similarly, Loeys-Dietz syndrome (LDS) is caused by mutations in genes encoding for TGF-B receptors. BAV along with thoracic aortic aneurysms are commonly found in patients with LDS.

With these multifactorial variables that impact BAV syndrome presenting as familial clusters and variable penetrance, screening is recommended in first degree relatives of patients with BAV disease [31]. An echocardiogram is commonly utilized to monitor the bicuspid aortic valvular pathophysiology. A CTA or MRA may also be utilized for monitoring the bicuspid aortic valve aortic phenotype.

4. Genetic syndromes with BAV

BAV is associated with several complex valvuloaortopathies and specific syndromes. Approximately 30–50% of patients with coarctation of the aorta have BAV [32–34].

Turner Syndrome is one of the most common genetic syndromes involving patients having a BAV phenotype [34]. The syndrome is associated with X chromosome monosomy in females. Approximately 30% of females with Turners can have a BAV [35]. The frequency of aortic aneurysms associated with BAV is also known to be higher in this group [36]. This observation along with the male predominance of BAV has led to the hypothesis that the X chromosome reduction maybe related to BAV incidence [37]. Generally short statured females with coarctation of the aorta should raise suspicion and lead to surveillance for BAV disease [38].

Loeys-Dietz Syndrome (LDS) is the second most common syndrome associated with BAV with approximately 10% of these patients manifesting the BAV phenotype [39]. TGF-B pathway gene mutations are known to be associated with the LDS. These mutations are common in non-syndromic thoracic aortic aneurysmal disease as well demonstrating a possible common pathway. Compared to non-syndromic patients, the LDS patients tend to present earlier in their life usually with symptomatic aortic regurgitation due to accelerated aortic dilation. Increased arterial tortuosity in major blood vessels and male sex have been determined to be associated with a higher risk of dissection in these patients [40].

Velocardiofacial Syndrome (DiGeorge Syndrome) is caused by deletions in gene 22; this syndrome involves cleft palate, immune deficiency, hypoparathyroidism, ventricular septal defect (VSD), and conotruncal defects of the heart (truncus arteriosus and tetralogy of Fallot). BAV and aneurysmal disease is more prevalent in this set of patients compared to the non-syndromic population [41]. The syndrome itself is a combination of genetic defects that are found in BAV disease demonstrating the multigenetic components that are involved in the BAV phenotype.

5. Surveillance of the aorta in BAV disease

BAV syndrome is a heterogenous disease presenting with variable aortic and valvular pathology over a spectrum of age groups. Asymptomatic BAV may be an incidental finding on imaging [32, 33, 38]. Patients with BAV syndrome require individualized treatment according to the degree of involvement of the aortic and valvular apparatus with patient comorbidities and age considerations. BAV patients should therefore undergo routine, periodic surveillance, to delineate the optimal timing of therapeutic intervention.

Surveillance for BAV syndrome patients is performed based on the pathophysiology of the aortic valve phenotype or aortic phenotype. Surveillance requires serial echocardiography for valvulopathy. The growth rate of the aorta in BAV patients can be 0.2–2.3 mm/year [16, 42, 43], and serial CTA or MRI should be performed to monitor the growth rate. For patients with ascending aortic and root dimensions within normal limits, imaging can be done every 3–5 years [35]. For dimensions ranging from 40 to 49 mm, imaging should be performed annually. For BAV patients with an aorta measuring 50–54 mm or with family history of aortic dissection or rapid growth of the aorta, imaging should be performed every 6–12 months [44].

5.1 Family screening

Current guidelines suggest family screening with echocardiography for all first-degree relatives with BAV probands. Relatives found to have BAV should have complete evaluation and CTA or MRA imaging [45]. When multiple signs of a disorder are present, genetic testing should be conducted for BAV patients especially those in their early years of life. Other high-risk features that should lead to genetic testing are family history of dissection or sudden death, congenital heart lesions, or other aneurysmal disease. Once identified, genetic counseling plays an important role in the holistic care for BAV patients. Due to the variable expression of causative genes, parents of BAV patients may not have a bicuspid aortic valve. Lifetime follow-up and aortic surveillance is also important as the timing of incidence of valve or aortic disease may be different amongst different family members.

6. Therapeutic strategies for bicuspid aortic valve syndrome

6.1 Aortic dilatation/aneurysm

The 2022 ACC/AHA guidelines for the diagnosis and management of aortic disease delineate the threshold for aortic repair in BAV patients without any other comorbidity or valvular dysfunction to be ≥50 mm [44, 46]. BAV patients who require cardiac surgery for any other pathology should undergo aortic repair if the diameter is ≥45 mm [44].

7. Aortic regurgitation

BAV has become the most common cause of isolated primary aortic regurgitation in the developed world. There may be mixed aortic regurgitation and stenosis; however, in approximately 5–10% of patients will have moderate-severe isolated primary aortic regurgitation [13]. Pathophysiology for aortic regurgitation in BAV usually includes leaflet deformities (size variation, prolapse, fenestrations, thickening or immobility), aortic root dilation (root phenotype), endocarditis or aortic dissection.

Patients with BAV syndrome are a younger population and therefore the long-term durability of surgical procedures and minimization of associated complications are critical outcome goals [4]. Decisions regarding the therapeutic interventions are based on aortic valve phenotype and ascending aortic/root phenotype (**Figure 1**).

Valve choice is an important decision. Currently, fewer patients are willing to alter their lifestyle or take the anticoagulation required for mechanical prosthesis, especially with TAVR options as a bridge. Equally important, consideration of therapeutic options and anticoagulation must be assessed for BAV women of childbearing age [4]. For these reasons a better understanding of the optimal surgical technique for BAV ascending/root aortic aneurysm disease is critical.

The **Figure 1** delineates the anatomic and pathophysiologic criteria utilized for decision making.

7.1 Aortic insufficiency (AI) phenotype

Indications for aortic valve intervention for AI and AS are delineated in the 2020 ACC/AHA Guideline [47]. Surgical aortic valve replacement currently includes either bioprosthetic or mechanical valve [4, 10].

There has also been a trend toward more reparative surgical approach for bicuspid aortic insufficiency. Primary cusp repair for patients with appropriate cusp pathology, although technically more complex than prosthetic aortic valve replacement, is becoming an attractive option as it may reduce the risk of Major Adverse Valve-Related Event (MAVRE) [4, 48]. Long-term outcome and follow-up studies will be important to monitor these patients.

7.2 Aortic insufficiency with aortic phenotype

For BAV syndrome patients with Aortic Valve Insufficiency phenotype and aortic root phenotype with sinus of Valsalva (SOV) measuring ≥45 mm, the **Figure 1** delineates the therapeutic options. The mechanical Bentall procedure has been a gold standard for multiple root pathologies with low morbidity and mortality [4, 49]. However, mechanical valves do not always carry 100% freedom from reoperation or a survival similar to age-matched controls [4]. Good long-term results for patients with a biologic composite root have been shown in a recent study and a meta-analysis of the Bentall procedure and revealed an annual linearized rate for late mortality of 2.02%, reoperation of 0.46%, bleeding of 0.64%, thromboembolic events of 0.77%, and MAVRE of 2.66% [4, 50]. This procedure can be performed for BAV aortic root and valvular pathologies with good long-term results [4]. A recent study in BAV patients undergoing Bentall procedure revealed a 5 and 10-year survival of 93% and 89% respectively, with freedom from reoperation of 100% and 1.9% stroke rate at 6 years [4, 51].

For patients with BAV aortic valve insufficiency phenotype and aortic root phenotype with a valve that is repairable, a valve sparing root replacement (VSRR) can be employed [4, 52, 53]. A study by de Kerchove reported 98.3% 5-year survival and 100% freedom from reoperation at 6 years in BAV patients undergoing VSRR [54]. Similarly, Kari reported 99% survival and 6-year 90% freedom from reoperation for BAV VSRR [55]. DeNino et al. demonstrated a lower aortic valve gradient and similar postoperative complication rates in the VSRR group compared to bioprosthetic valve conduit [56]. A study by Vallabhajosyula et al., in the isolated BAV insufficiency subpopulation noted a 5-year freedom from reoperation and survival for Bentall and VSRR at 98% and 100% versus 100% and 98% respectively [53]. These studies support the findings that primary repair with VSRR can be selectively utilized to treat BAV AI with root aneurysm [52–56]. This decision should be weighed against the risk of recurrent AI. The VSRR patients have been shown to have significantly lower mortality, stroke, and MAVRE compared to mechanical Bentall [4]. The results of recent studies may be utilized to inform young BAV patients interested in biologic conduit or repair options, especially those averse to taking anticoagulation and open to transcatheter valve options in the future. Long-term 15-to-20-year data will be important to better understand the role of biologic versus mechanical valves in BAV aortic root complex focused procedures. In patients with a non-repairable valve, Bentall procedure remains the standard of care [4].

7.3 AS and AI with mild-moderate root phenotype

For both BAV aortic stenosis and aortic insufficiency valve phenotype and mild-moderate root phenotype with ascending aneurysm and moderate dilatation (SOV 40–45 mm), the fate of the retained sinus segment and the effect of valvular pathology on post-operative sinus growth had been undefined. It has been proposed that the sinus segment in BAV aortopathies is at risk for future aortic events. Therefore, it has been advocated, by some, for removal of all aortic segments in patients with aortopathies despite moderate dilation [4]. A recent swing in the pendulum has occurred advocating for retention of the sinus of Valsalva for moderate root aneurysms [56, 57]. This change results from studies reporting a slower growth rate for the sinus segment and a less aggressive aortic event rate for the preserved moderately dilated aortic root [4, 56–58]. Peters et al. found the sinus segment growth rate was only between 0.27 mm and 0.5 mm per year requiring an average of 29.1 years for the sinus segment to become aneurysmal after AVRSCAAR Please do not use an abbreviation without first defining it [58]. For patients with either BAV aortic stenosis and aortic insufficiency with ascending aneurysm and moderate dilatation (40–45 mm) AVRSCAAR can be performed as a therapeutic option with good long-term results (Consort Diagram **Figure 1**) [4, 56–58].

7.4 Aortic stenosis

Aortic valve stenosis occurs in approximately 50% of adult patients with BAV valve phenotype that requires aortic valve replacement [12, 59]. Progression to critical aortic stenosis pathophysiology resulting in therapeutic intervention in BAV patients often occurs at a younger age than patients with trileaflet aortic valves.

7.5 Aortic stenosis valve phenotype

For patients with aortic valve phenotype, but no aortic aneurysm phenotype, aortic valve replacement with a prosthetic aortic valve is the therapeutic option (**Figure 1**). Additional trials are needed to delineate the optimal anatomy, sizing, and implantation techniques for TAVR [60, 61].

The Ross procedure (pulmonary autograft to replace the aortic valve and homograft to replace pulmonic valve) can also be considered as an option to replace the stenotic aortic valve. In patients with the appropriate pulmonary and aortic annular anatomy, good long-term durability has been noted [62].

7.6 Aortic stenosis with root phenotype

In patients with BAV aortic stenosis phenotype an unrepairable valve and aortic root phenotype with a sinus of Valsalva ≥45 mm, a mechanical or bioBentall procedure is a therapeutic option (**Figure 1**). This involves replacing the aortic valve and ascending/root aorta as a composite and reimplanting the coronary arteries to the tubular graft. This can be either mechanical or bioprosthesis (BioBentall).

For patients with BAV aortic stenosis phenotype an ascending aortic aneurysm and moderate sinus of Valsalva (SOV) dilation (40–45 mm), aortic valve replacement and supracoronary ascending aortic replacement (AVRSCAAR) can be performed thereby preserving the root. Studies have shown that the aortic root remains stable over long-term [4, 56].

Figure 1 delineates the surgical procedure for AS phenotype and the associated aortic phenotypes.

8. Management of BAV in pregnancy

Patients with known BAV should be counseled regarding the risks of heritable disease, risk of aneurysm dissection or rupture during pregnancy, and complications of valve related disease. Valve related management is achieved keeping in mind the risk of anticoagulation during and after pregnancy. Pregnant patients with BAV and aneurysm disease are at a higher risk of spontaneous aortic dissection or rupture [63]. Pregnancy associated hemodynamic changes are associated with this increased risk along with the inherent intima media weakness attributed to BAV patients. The highest risk is during the 3rd trimester or postpartum [63]. Aortic aneurysm >40 mm and increase in aortic size during pregnancy have been demonstrated to be common factors in patients who had Type A dissections pre- or post-partum [64]. Contemporary management of BAV and ascending aortic disease has reduced the significant maternal and fetal risk associated with these entities. Contemporary guidelines suggest surveillance of any aortic dilatation in pregnant patients with echocardiography every month during pregnancy if the diameter is >40 mm and every 12 weeks if there is dilation of the aorta but the diameter does not exceed 40 mm [65]. Current guidelines recommend avoidance of pregnancy if the known aortic diameter is >50 mm in BAV patients [65, 66]. Blood pressure control is the mainstay for general management in pregnant females with any thoracic aortic dilation. Surgery during pregnancy is generally avoided due to the high maternal and fetal risk involved; however, it would be indicated in severe valve dysfunction if transcatheter approaches are not an option.

9. Conclusion

1. BAV syndrome presents variable aortic valve phenotype and aortic phenotype.

2. Bicuspid aortic valve patients present with a spectrum of valvular, ascending aortic, and aortic root aneurysmal pathologies.

3. This variable spectrum has mandated the development of an array of surgical procedures to be able to tailor an individualized approach to BAV syndrome for a typically younger BAV population in whom long-term outcomes are especially relevant.

4. Patients with bicuspid aortic valve syndrome require personalized management based on the level of involvement of the aorta and age at presentation. Care can be provided an utilizing an algorithm-based approach delineated in **Figure 1**.

5. For patients who undergo isolated valve surgery for BAV related structural valve disease surveillance is important for ascending aortic disease in the future.

6. Family surveillance of known BAV patients requiring surgical care is also important with consideration of heritable characteristics of this disease.

Author details

Syed Usman Bin Mahmood, Prashanth Vallabhajosyula and Rita Milewski*
Division of Cardiac Surgery, Yale School of Medicine, New Haven, CT, United States

*Address all correspondence to: rita.milewski@yale.edu

IntechOpen

© 2023 The Author(s). Licensee IntechOpen. This chapter is distributed under the terms of the Creative Commons Attribution License (http://creativecommons.org/licenses/by/3.0), which permits unrestricted use, distribution, and reproduction in any medium, provided the original work is properly cited.

References

[1] Fedak PW, Verma S, David TE, Leask RL, Weisel RD, Butany J. Clinical and pathophysiological implications of a bicuspid aortic valve. Circulation. 2002;**106**:900-904

[2] Hahn RT, Roman MJ, Mogtader AH, Devereux RB. Association of aortic dilation with regurgitant, stenotic and functionally normal bicuspid aortic valves. Journal of the American College of Cardiology. 1992;**19**:283-288

[3] Michelena HI, Della Corte A, Prakash SK, Milewicz DM, Evangelista A, Enriquez-Sarano M. Bicuspid aortic valve aortopathy in adults: Incidence, etiology, and clinical significance. International Journal of Cardiology. 2015;**201**:400-407

[4] Karianna Milewski RC, Habertheuer A, Bavaria JE, Suhail M, Siki M, Hu R, et al. Long-term outcomes of aortic root procedures for heterogenous ascending aneurysm disease in bicuspid aortic valve syndrome. The Journal of Thoracic and Cardiovascular Surgery. 24 Nov 2022:S0022-5223(22)01256-9. DOI: 10.1016/j.jtcvs.2022.09.068. PMID: 36631305 [Epub ahead of print]

[5] Braverman AC, Güven H, Beardslee MA, Makan M, Kates AM, Moon MR. The bicuspid aortic valve. Current Problems in Cardiology. 2005;**30**(9):470-522

[6] Michelena HI, Prakash SK, Della Corte A, Bissell MM, Anavekar N, Mathieu P, et al. Bicuspid aortic valve: Identifying knowledge gaps and rising to the challenge from the International Bicuspid Aortic Valve Consortium (BAVCon). Circulation. 2014;**129**(25):2691-2704

[7] Michelena HI, Desjardins VA, Avierinos JF, Russo A, Nkomo VT, Sundt TM, et al. Natural history of asymptomatic patients with normally functioning or minimally dysfunctional bicuspid aortic valve in the community. Circulation. 2008;**117**(21):2776-2784

[8] Sievers H-H, Schmidtke C. A classification system for the bicuspid aortic valve from 304 surgical specimens. The Journal of Thoracic and Cardiovascular Surgery. 2007;**133**(5):1226-1233

[9] Fernandes SM, Khairy P, Sanders SP, Colan SD. Bicuspid aortic valve morphology and interventions in the young. Journal of the American College of Cardiology. 2007;**49**(22):2211-2214

[10] MichelenaHI, CorteAD, EvangelistaA, Maleszewski JJ, Edwards WD, Roman MJ, et al. International consensus statement on nomenclature and classification of the congenital bicuspid aortic valve and its aortopathy, for clinical, surgical, interventional and research purposes. Radiol Cardiothorac Imaging. 2021;**3**(4):e200496

[11] Ridley CH, Vallabhajosyula P, Bavaria JE, Patel PA, Gutsche JT, Shah R, et al. The Sievers classification of the bicuspid aortic valve for the perioperative echocardiographer: The importance of valve phenotype for aortic valve repair in the era of the functional aortic annulus. Journal of Cardiothoracic and Vascular Anesthesia. 2016;**30**(4(August)):1142-1151

[12] Roberts WC, Ko JM. Frequency by decades of unicuspid, bicuspid, and tricuspid aortic valves in adults having isolated aortic valve replacement

for aortic stenosis, with or without associated aortic regurgitation. Circulation. 2005;**111**(7):920-925

[13] Roberts WC, Morrow AG, Mclntosh CL, Jones M, Epstein SE. Congenitally bicuspid aortic valve causing severe, pure aortic regurgitation without superimposed infective endocarditis: Analysis of 13 patients requiring aortic valve replacement. The American Journal of Cardiology. 1981;**47**(2):206-209

[14] Fenoglio JJ Jr, McAllister HA Jr, DeCastro CM, Davia JE, Cheitlin MD. Congenital bicuspid aortic valve after age 20. The American Journal of Cardiology. 1977;**39**(2):164-169

[15] Michelena HI, Khanna AD, Mahoney D, Margaryan E, Topilsky Y, Suri RM, et al. Incidence of aortic complications in patients with bicuspid aortic valves. Journal of the American Medical Association. 2011;**306**(10):1104-1112

[16] Verma S, Siu SC. Aortic dilatation in patients with bicuspid aortic valve. The New England Journal of Medicine. 2014;**370**(20):1920-1929

[17] Schaefer BM, Lewin MB, Stout KK, Byers PH, Otto CM. Usefulness of bicuspid aortic valve phenotype to predict elastic properties of the ascending aorta. The American Journal of Cardiology. 2007;**99**(5):686-690

[18] Girdauskas E, Disha K, Rouman M, Espinoza A, Borger MA, Kuntze T. Aortic events after isolated aortic valve replacement for bicuspid aortic valve root phenotype: Echocardiographic follow-up study. European Journal of Cardio-thoracic Surgery: Official Journal of the European Association for Cardio-thoracic Surgery. 2015;**48**(4):e71-e76

[19] Braverman AC. Aortic involvement in patients with a bicuspid aortic valve. Heart. 2011;**97**(6):506-513

[20] Della Corte A, Bancone C, Quarto C, Dialetto G, Covino FE, Scardone M, et al. Predictors of ascending aortic dilatation with bicuspid aortic valve: A wide spectrum of disease expression. European Journal of Cardio-thoracic Surgery: Official Journal of the European Association for Cardio-thoracic Surgery. 2007;**31**(3):397-404; discussion –5

[21] Entezari P, Schnell S, Mahadevia R, Malaisrie C, McCarthy P, Mendelson M, et al. From unicuspid to quadricuspid: Influence of aortic valve morphology on aortic three-dimensional hemodynamics. Journal of Magnetic Resonance Imaging. 2014;**40**(6):1342-1346

[22] Wu B, Wang Y, Xiao F, Butcher JT, Yutzey KE, Zhou B. Developmental mechanisms of aortic valve malformation and disease. Annual Review of Physiology. 2017;**79**:21-41

[23] Sillesen AS, Vogg O, Pihl C, Raja AA, Sundberg K, Vedel C, et al. Prevalence of bicuspid aortic valve and associated aortopathy in newborns in Copenhagen, Denmark. JAMA. 2021;**325**(6):561-567

[24] Loscalzo ML, Goh DL, Loeys B, Kent KC, Spevak PJ, Dietz HC. Familial thoracic aortic dilation and bicommissural aortic valve: A prospective analysis of natural history and inheritance. American Journal of Medical Genetics. Part A. 2007;**143A**(17):1960-1967

[25] McKellar SH, Tester DJ, Yagubyan M, Majumdar R, Ackerman MJ, Sundt TM 3rd. Novel NOTCH1 mutations in patients with bicuspid aortic valve disease and thoracic aortic aneurysms. The Journal of Thoracic and Cardiovascular Surgery. 2007;**134**(2):290-296

[26] Huntington K, Hunter AG, Chan KL. A prospective study to assess

the frequency of familial clustering of congenital bicuspid aortic valve. Journal of the American College of Cardiology. 1997;**30**(7):1809-1812

[27] Glick BN, Roberts WC. Congenitally bicuspid aortic valve in multiple family members. The American Journal of Cardiology. 1994;**73**(5):400-404

[28] Martin PS, Kloesel B, Norris RA, Lindsay M, Milan D, Body SC. Embryonic development of the bicuspid aortic valve. Journal of Cardiovascular Development and Disease. 2015;**2**(4):248-272

[29] Garg V, Muth AN, Ransom JF, Schluterman MK, Barnes R, King IN, et al. Mutations in NOTCH1 cause aortic valve disease. Nature. 2005;**437**(7056):270-274

[30] Tadros TM, Klein MD, Shapira OM. Ascending aortic dilatation associated with bicuspid aortic valve: Pathophysiology, molecular biology, and clinical implications. Circulation. 2009;**119**(6):880-890

[31] Stout KK, Daniels CJ, Aboulhosn JA, Bozkurt B, Broberg CS, Colman JM, et al. 2018 AHA/ACC guideline for the management of adults with congenital heart disease: A report of the American College of Cardiology/American Heart Association Task Force on Clinical Practice Guidelines. Journal of the American College of Cardiology. 2019;**73**(12):e81-e192

[32] Masri A, Svensson LG, Griffin BP, Desai MY. Contemporary natural history of bicuspid aortic valve disease: A systematic review. Heart. 2017;**103**(17):1323-1330

[33] Brown ML, Burkhart HM, Connolly HM, Dearani JA, Cetta F, Li Z, et al. Coarctation of the aorta: Lifelong surveillance is mandatory following surgical repair. Journal of the American College of Cardiology. 2013;**62**(11):1020-1025

[34] Corbitt H, Morris SA, Gravholt CH, Mortensen KH, Tippner-Hedges R, Silberbach M, et al. TIMP3 and TIMP1 are risk genes for bicuspid aortic valve and aortopathy in Turner syndrome. PLoS Genetics. 2018;**14**(10):e1007692

[35] Bravo-Jaimes K, Prakash SK. Genetics in bicuspid aortic valve disease: Where are we? Progress in Cardiovascular Diseases. 2020;**63**(4):398-406

[36] Carlson M, Silberbach M. Dissection of the aorta in turner syndrome: Two cases and review of 85 cases in the literature. BML Case Reports. 2009;**2009**:bcr0620091998

[37] Prakash SK, Bosse Y, Muehlschlegel JD, Michelena HI, Limongelli G, Della Corte A, et al. A roadmap to investigate the genetic basis of bicuspid aortic valve and its complications: Insights from the international BAVCon (Bicuspid Aortic Valve Consortium). the American College of Cardiology. 2014;**64**(8):832-839

[38] Fuchs MM, Attenhofer Jost C, Babovic-Vuksanovic D, Connolly HM, Egbe A. Long-term outcomes in patients with turner syndrome: A 68-year follow-up. Journal of the American Heart Association. 2019;**8**(11):e011501

[39] Patel ND, Crawford T, Magruder JT, Alejo DE, Hibino N, Black J, et al. Cardiovascular operations for Loeys-Dietz syndrome: Intermediate-term results. The Journal of Thoracic and Cardiovascular Surgery. 2017;**153**(2):406-412

[40] Morris SA, Orbach DB, Geva T, Singh MN, Gauvreau K, Lacro RV.

Increased vertebral artery tortuosity index is associated with adverse outcomes in children and young adults with connective tissue disorders. Circulation. 2011;**124**(4):388-396

[41] Putotto C, Pulvirenti F, Pugnaloni F, Isufi I, Unolt M, Anaclerio S, et al. Clinical risk factors for aortic root dilation in patients with 22q11.2 deletion syndrome: A longitudinal single-center study. Genes (Basel). 10 Dec 2022;**13**(12):2334. DOI: 10.3390/genes13122334. PMID: 36553601; PMCID: PMC9778342

[42] Avadhani SA, Martin-Doyle W, Shaikh AY, Pape LA. Predictors of ascending aortic dilation in bicuspid aortic valve disease: A five-year prospective study. The American Journal of Medicine. 2015;**128**(6):647-652

[43] Della Corte A, Bancone C, Buonocore M, Dialetto G, Covino FE, Manduca S, et al. Pattern of ascending aortic dimensions predicts the growth rate of the aorta in patients with bicuspid aortic valve. JACC: Cardiovascular Imaging. 2013;**6**(12):1301-1310

[44] Borger MA, Fedak PWM, Stephens EH, Gleason TG, Girdauskas E, Ikonomidis JS, et al. The American Association for Thoracic Surgery consensus guidelines on bicuspid aortic valve-related aortopathy: Full online-only version. The Journal of Thoracic and Cardiovascular Surgery. 2018;**156**(2):e41-e74

[45] Guntheroth WG. A critical review of the American College of Cardiology/ American Heart Association practice guidelines on bicuspid aortic valve with dilated ascending aorta. The American Journal of Cardiology. 2008;**102**(1):107-110

[46] Isselbacher EM, Preventza O, Hamilton Black J 3rd, Augoustides JG, Beck AW, Bolen MA, et al. 2022 ACC/AHA Guideline for the Diagnosis and Management of Aortic Disease: A report of the American Heart Association/American College of Cardiology Joint Committee on Clinical Practice Guidelines. Circulation. 2022;**146**(24):e334-e482

[47] Otto CM, Nishimura RA, Bonow RO, Carabello BA, Erwin JP III, Gentile F, et al. 2020 ACC/AHA guideline for the Management of Patients with Valvular Heart Disease. A report of the American College of Cardiology/American Heart Association Joint Committee on Clinical Practice Guidelines. Circulation. 2021;**143**:e72-e277

[48] Ehrlich T, de Kerchove L, Vojacek J, Boodhwani M, El-Hamamsy I, De Paulis R, et al. State-of-the art bicuspid aortic valve repair in 2020. Progress in Cardiovascular Diseases. 2020;**63**(4):457-464

[49] Hagl C, Strauch JT, Spielvogel D, Galla JD, Lansman SL, Squitieri R, et al. Is the bentall procedure for ascending aorta or aortic valve replacement the best approach for long-term event-free survival? The Annals of Thoracic Surgery. 2003;**76**(3):698-703

[50] Mookhoek A, Korteland NM, Arabkhani B, Di Centa I, Lansac E, Bekkers JA, et al. Bentall procedure: A systematic review and meta-analysis. The Annals of Thoracic Surgery. 2016;**101**:1684-1689

[51] Etz CD, Homann TM, Silovitz D, Spielvogel D, Bodian CA, Luehr M, et al. Long-term survival after the Bentall procedure in 206 patients with bicuspid aortic valve. The Annals of Thoracic Surgery. 2007;**84**:1186-1193; discussion 1193-4

[52] Coselli JS, Hughes MS, Green SY, Price MD, Zarda S, de la Cruz KI, et al.

Valve-sparing aortic root replacement: Early and midterm outcomes in 83 patients. The Annals of Thoracic Surgery. 2014;**97**(4):1267-1273; discussion 73-4

[53] Vallabhajosyula P, Szeto WY, Habertheuer A, Komlo C, Milewski RK, McCarthy F, et al. Bicuspid aortic insufficiency with aortic root aneurysm: Root reimplantation versus Bentall root replacement. The Annals of Thoracic Surgery. 2016;**102**(4):1221-1228

[54] de Kerchove L, Boodhwani M, Glineur D, Vandyck M, Vanoverschelde JL, Noirhomme P, et al. Valve sparing-root replacement with the reimplantation technique to increase the durability of bicuspid aortic valve repair. The Journal of Thoracic and Cardiovascular Surgery. 2011;**142**:1430-1438

[55] Kari FA, Liang DH, Kvitting JP, Stephens EH, Mitchell RS, Fischbein MP, et al. Tirone David valve-sparing aortic root replacement and cusp repair for bicuspid aortic valve disease. The Journal of Thoracic and Cardiovascular Surgery. 2013;**145**(S35-40):e1-e2

[56] DeNino WF, Toole JM, Rowley C, Stroud MR, Ikonomidis JS. Comparison of David V valve-sparing root replacement and bioprosthetic valve conduit for aortic root aneurysm. The Journal of Thoracic and Cardiovascular Surgery. 2014;**148**:2883-2887

[57] Vendramin I, Meneguzzi M, Sponga S, Deroma L, Cimarosti R, Lutman C, et al. Bicuspid aortic valve disease and ascending aortic aneurysm: Should an aortic root replacement be mandatory? European Journal of Cardio-thoracic Surgery: Official Journal of the European Association for Cardio-thoracic Surgery. 2016;**49**(1):103-109

[58] Milewski RK, Habertheuer A, Bavaria JE, Siki M, Szeto WY, Krause E, et al. Fate of remnant sinuses of Valsalva in patients with bicuspid and trileaflet valves undergoing aortic valve, ascending aorta, and aortic arch replacement. The Journal of Thoracic and Cardiovascular Surgery. 2017;**154**(2):421-432

[59] Mohler ER 3rd. Are atherosclerotic processes involved in aortic-valve calcification? Lancet. 2000;**356**(9229):524-525

[60] Park CB, Greason KL, Suri RM, Michelena HI, Schaff HV, Sundt TM 3rd. Fate of nonreplaced sinuses of Valsalva in bicuspid aortic valve disease. The Journal of Thoracic and Cardiovascular Surgery. 2011;**142**(2):278-284

[61] Yoon SH, Lefevre T, Ahn JM, Perlman GY, Dvir D, Latib A, et al. Transcatheter aortic valve replacement with early- and new-generation devices in bicuspid aortic valve stenosis. Journal of the American College of Cardiology. 2016;**68**(11):1195-1205

[62] Vincent F, Ternacle J, Denimal T, Shen M, Redfors B, Delhaye C, et al. Transcatheter aortic valve replacement in bicuspid aortic valve stenosis. Circulation. 2021;**143**:1043-1061

[63] Mazine A, El-Hamamsy I, Verma S, Peterson MD, Bonow RO, Yacoub MH, et al. Ross procedure in adults for cardiologists and cardiac surgeons: JACC state-of-the-art review. Journal of the American College of Cardiology. 2018;**72**(22):2761-2777

[64] Anderson RA, Fineron PW. Aortic dissection in pregnancy: Importance of pregnancy-induced changes in the vessel wall and bicuspid aortic valve in pathogenesis. British Journal of Obstetrics and Gynaecology. 1994;**101**(12):1085-1088

[65] Immer FF, Bansi AG, Immer-Bansi AS, McDougall J, Zehr KJ, Schaff HV, et al.

Aortic dissection in pregnancy: Analysis of risk factors and outcome. The Annals of Thoracic Surgery. 2003;**76**(1):309-314

[66] Regitz-Zagrosek V, Roos-Hesselink JW, Bauersachs J, Blomstrom-Lundqvist C, Cifkova R, De Bonis M, et al. 2018 ESC Guidelines for the management of cardiovascular diseases during pregnancy. European Heart Journal. 2018;**39**(34):3165-3241

Section 7

Patient Perspective

Chapter 13

Perspective Chapter: Complication Using TAVR – A Patient

Philip Hutchens

Abstract

This is the story about a person now in his 80s. He was born with a congenital aortic valve defect. Over his lifetime, the diagnosis and treatment of heart disease improved dramatically. Recently, the author corresponded with a number of patients undergoing heart valve replacements today and found all to be concerned about how long they would live and complications they would have with a replacement valve. The author's experiences should help put valve replacement recipients' minds at ease and help physicians address their patients worries and concerns. He describes procedures from the patient's perspective for implanting a pacemaker, getting an ablation, and being evaluated for a TAVR. The author is living in the third year with his replacement valve. He is on his 40th year with a pacemaker. He found modern medicine and physicians to be miraculous in many ways and is grateful for the added years given to his life.

Keywords: TAVR, aortic heart valve defects, pacemaker, ablation, echocardiogram, catheterization

1. Introduction

Recently, I corresponded with a 71-year-old physician who had just received a replacement aortic valve using a Transaortic Valve Replacement (TAVR) procedure. Instead of being happy for a successful procedure, the physician complained about the procedure. First, he complained about the cost – that he estimated at about \$140,000, even though his procedure was fully covered by his insurance. He said that \$140 K could treat a lot of people in a third world country for a lot of different medical conditions. He added, "I feel guilty having the money spent on me when so many others are going without medical attention." A part of me admires his desire to help others. However, another part of me feels his reasoning was a little like my mother telling me when I was a child to "Eat your peas. There are children starving in China." Even as a child, I reasoned to myself that eating my peas, or not eating my peas, would not affect starving children in China. My older brother and I finally confronted our mother on her peas-exhortation, and she soon quit with the message. Had the complaining physician declined the TAVR procedure, I doubt it would have resulted in any more patients being treated in a third world country: at least not directly.

IntechOpen

Second, the complaining physician said, "I do not expect that a new valve will extend my life more than three to six months." He made this inaccurate and rather startling statement even though he had no other underlying health concerns or conditions. Obviously, the cardiovascular system was not his specialty. A recent aortic valve durability study showed valves doing well after 8 years in younger patients (under 65 years of age), regardless of whether the valve was a surgical aortic valve replacement (SAVR) or a Transaortic Valve Implantation (TAVI – also referred to as a TAVR) [1]. This is an important finding for older folk because replacement valves tend to last longer in older patients than in younger patients.

I was corresponding with this physician because I, also, had been evaluated for an aortic heart valve replacement using a TAVR procedure. I wrote about my aortic valve experience in a popular medical journal, and as a result of that article, I have corresponded with several TAVR recipients or prospective recipients. All of us seem to have some concern about how long we might live with a replacement valve. The good news is that TAVR aortic valves are made from the same biological tissue as surgically replaced valves and should last about as long as a Surgical Aortic Valve Replacement (SAVR). Just this past week I talked with a 90-year-old retired physician whose 94-year-old sister had been living with a SAVR for 25 years – the same valve for all 25 years, and she still was having no issues with her valve.

A few months ago, I corresponded via email with a retired military officer who was soon to have a replacement aortic valve at age 69. He, too, was worried about how long his valve would last. He was scheduled to have a TAVR procedure, and he asked me about how long a replacement valve would last. He was hoping to live into his 90s. He had been reading on the internet and had come to believe that replacement valves do not last too long. He asked me about what might happen if he needed a new valve in about 10 years. I reminded him that I was not a physician but that I had been reading about new procedures involving "re-valving" or "valve in valve" procedures. He then wanted to know what would be done if he had a valve-in-valve procedure around age 80 but then needed a third replacement valve at around age 90. I discussed the durability of today's valves, and that is where our correspondence ended. However, I was impressed with his optimism and zeal for a longer life.

About a year ago, I corresponded via email with a psychologist whose 59-year-old brother was scheduled for an aortic valve replacement using the TAVR procedure. Primarily, she was concerned about the safety of the procedure, and her brother primarily was concerned about how much shorter his life would be with a replacement aortic valve. I explained to her the process a TAVR patient would go through as I understood it, and that seemed to put her mind at ease. In follow-up correspondence, she described how well her brother was doing and that he was back at work full-time following his procedure.

I have come to believe physicians should avoid discussing the length of time someone might live when talking with patients about a valve replacement. Instead, I believe it is better to discuss how much improved valves are and how durable they are. For example, I was 80 years old when I was being evaluated to determine if I was a viable candidate for a replacement valve. Since the average longevity for males in the U.S. is about 78 years of age (or less), why discuss with me how much longer I might live with or without the need for a replacement valve? I had already passed the average age for longevity. The good news is that there have been tremendous advances over the past 50 years in the treatment of diseased aortic heart valves. That's the story I believe prospective heart valve recipients need to hear. If patients are *not* reassured about the high quality of today's valves, then we may tend to start looking for ourselves on the internet about longevity with replacement valves, and we may be subject to gaining a lot of misinformation and outdated information. Bad information can lead to poor decisions regarding our health and cause us unnecessary stress. Additionally, it stands to reason that physicians will be better at their treatment of patients if they have a better understanding of what the patient is going through. We've all heard stories about physicians who were ill and reported they were better at their profession after their illness and recovery – after they had gone through the experience of being a patient. Physicians are used to being in control, and you lose most of your control when you are a patient for a replacement heart valve. My intent in writing this chapter is to show a little bit about what it means to be a patient based on what I went through with my aortic heart valve. In Section 2, I share my early experiences with my congenital heart valve defect. In section three, I share my experiences with pacemakers and my evaluation for a valve replacement. Also, I share the possible kinds of issues facing any heart valve recipient.

The process of replacing someone's aortic heart valve always will have worries and possible complications. My story about the complications I went through with my aortic heart valve follows.

2. My aortic heart valve history (the first four decades)

I was born in 1940 with an undiagnosed aortic heart valve defect. When I was 4 years old, my granddad gave me a two-wheeler bicycle. I considered myself to be a pretty good athlete based on my interactions with my buddies in the neighborhood, but I quickly noticed that I did not have the stamina to ride my bike up hills. However, all the other kids in the neighborhood had no trouble riding up hills. I knew something was wrong, but being a little kid, I thought very little about it.

In 1951, General Dwight David Eisenhower (Ike) was elected President of the United States. I was 10 years old. Ike served two terms as president from 1953 until 1961. My grandfather was a devout supporter of Ike, and his devotion to Ike caused me to pay special attention to Ike's health, especially from 1955 until Ike's death in 1969. In 1955, Ike had a massive heart attack. In the 1950s and 1960s, there was little being done for cardiac infarctions. Nevertheless, a legendary and highly respected physician by the name of Paul Dudley White was rushed to Ike's side [2]. White was a pioneering cardiologist and advocate for preventive medicine. Ike's cardiac team prescribed long term use of anti-coagulants (non-traditional treatment at the time). In addition, White prescribed light exercise, cessation of Ike's heavy smoking, and a revised diet. White remained Ike's cardiologist, and over the remainder of his life, Ike had at least four other myocardial infarctions, a stroke in 1957, and 14 other cardiac arrests. Ike's case is an amazing example of a strong-willed leader who benefited from having complete trust in his cardiologist. White successfully used his public forum as Ike's cardiologist to educate the public about heart health. Little did I know at the time, but Paul Dudley White's path and my path would 1 day cross.

Early in my freshman year in college, 1958, I decided to try out for the college's freshman basketball team (I was 17 years old). In those days, freshmen were not allowed to join a varsity team. The physician conducting the physical was concerned about my heart and referred me to a heart specialist before he would approve me joining the team. The referral cardiologist listened for quite a while to my heart with his stethoscope and suggested it might be best if I did not play competitive sports. However, he wrote a permission slip for me to play if I felt strongly about it. He told me that I had a loud aortic valve murmur, but he could not tell what the cause might be. He felt it better not to stress my heart with the rigors of competitive basketball. I played college basketball for one semester and then dropped out. I would sometimes need to leave the court and throw up, and frequently I did not feel well after vigorous exercise.

Later in my freshman year in college, but now 18 years old, I had my tonsils removed. The physician performing the tonsillectomy also listened to my heart. He told me he had heard many heart murmurs in his career, and he felt certain I had a bicuspid valve. He told me I would not live much past my early 40s and that I should plan my life accordingly. Today, his warning might seem overly harsh and misguided, but remember, that was 1959. The first mechanical replacement valves did not take place until the 1960s [3]. The physician was advising me based on what treatments were known to him to be commercially available at the time.

Growing up, our family was attended by a General Practitioner (GP), but that physician never mentioned a heart murmur to my parents or to me. I asked him about my heart murmur when I was 22 years old, and he told me lots of people have heart murmurs and he did not think it was overly significant. A couple of years later I saw another GP, and he referred me to a cardiologist who listened intently to my murmur and suggested I just wait and see what might happen and recommended I take no further action for the time being. However, occasionally I would have angina or angina-like discomfort, and that discomfort was always worrisome to me.

In 1967, now 26 years old, I moved from the West Coast to the East Coast and started being treated by an Internist specializing in the treatment of heart disease. The internist sent me to a local clinic for an x-ray in the hope that it might show calcification on the aortic valve if such calcification in fact existed. The results of the x-ray did not clarify much about my condition. The x-ray showed extensive calcification in the heart, but it could not be determined exactly where it existed in my cardiovascular system. However, the radiologist believed that the calcification likely was in the aortic valve area. Remember, MRIs and CT scans were not yet in use at that time [4].

I told my internist about my chest discomfort, and he prescribed nitroglycerin sublingual tablets to ease my discomfort. He told me to always carry the tablets with me and to dissolve one under my tongue whenever I had angina discomfort. I put a couple of the tablets in a small envelope and carried them with me in my wallet for several months. I used them a couple of times and did not like the way I felt when using the drug, and besides, I did not notice any improvement in my angina. After a couple of years, my internist told me it would no longer be necessary to use the nitroglycerin tablets.

When I was 28 years old, my internist sent me to a major hospital (near where I was living) for a heart catheterization. That procedure did not go well. I was taking a full aspirin at the time (on a daily basis) for my migraine headaches and because my internist thought that aspirin also might be helpful for my heart. The hospital did not give me any instructions about ceasing the aspirin before the catheterization. In fact, I had heard that a possible side effect of the catheterization could be a blood clot. So, I mistakenly took two full aspirins on the morning of the procedure. The two physicians performing the procedure gave me blood thinner, and after they wheeled me back to my room, I internally bled an estimated two pints of blood into my groin and leg. The hematoma on my groin, and the black and blue discoloration of my entire leg did not clear up completely for about 5 months. The good news for me, however, was that the cardiologists performing the procedure did not see any need for further medical intervention involving my heart condition.

When I was 30 years old, my Internist referred me to another Cardiologist at a different major university hospital in the area where I was living. The Cardiologist performed a heart catheterization (my second). The next morning after the catheterization, the Cardiologist asked me if he could present my case at his rounds, and I agreed. Around 11 a.m. I was wheeled out of my hospital room, down a corridor and through a door leading directly onto the stage of an auditorium with about 300 people in attendance. The cardiologist was presenting data from my catheterization to the audience when I arrived in the theater. There were two other physicians sitting in chairs on stage, but they were located off to the side of the stage. One of the two other physicians appeared noticeably older than the physician sitting beside him on stage. Clearly, the cardiologist who performed my catheterization was center-stage and appeared to be fully in command of the audience. I was very surprised. I had expected "rounds" to mean I might meet and discuss how I was feeling with maybe a handful of young physicians. The cardiologist briefly introduced me to the audience, and then he continued with his explanation of the blood pressures in my heart chambers and connecting blood vessels as determined by the catheterization.

At first, he spoke about how he had found no blockages in the arteries feeding my heart muscle, and that made me feel pretty good. He then began to discuss the calcification he had found on the aortic valve. Again, reviewing the pressure numbers from the catheterization, he said that he was recommending that I immediately be scheduled for a replacement valve. Remember, I'm 30 years old and being told in front of an audience of 300 people that I need open heart surgery. My jaw dropped. With great aplomb and apparent satisfaction with his diagnosis, the cardiologist took a seat in an empty chair next to the older physician still sitting onstage. The older physician then rose to address the audience.

His comments were brief. He said, and I will never forget his words, "This patient may surprise you. I do not recommend surgery at this time." No sooner had he uttered that statement than all hell broke loose on the stage and in the audience. Apparently, it is rare for one physician to contradict another physician, and especially in front of an audience of 300. There were murmurings and wild conversations throughout the audience. The cardiologist who had been presenting my case jumped up and began yelling about how he had been misunderstood. Someone, who I did not see, walked up being me and whispered in my ear, "You listen to Dr. White, he's God to you." Bingo! All of a sudden, it became clear to me that the older physician on stage was none other than Paul Dudley White, the physician who had attended President Eisenhower. The cardiologist who had performed my catheterization was jumping around on stage like a wild man and ordered that I be removed from the stage and taken back to my room immediately. A nurse quickly pushed me in my wheelchair out the backdoor of the stage. I do not know how ordered was restored, but it was a wild time for all involved. I doubt there has been anything like it since.

The cardiologist who performed my catheterization visited me in my room later that day. He repeated to me that I needed a replacement value urgently, and that I should not listen to Dr. White because he was old and did not understand modern medicine. I told the cardiologist that I had decided to postpone the heart valve replacement, and I went home the next morning. The cardiologist wrote a letter to my internist and told him I needed valve replacement surgery and told him I should get a Multigated Acquisition Scan (MUGA) every 3 months to check for changes in my ejection fraction or to check for any other changes in the heart functions.

Dr. White's advice not to rush into surgery clearly influenced my decision to put off surgery. Also, there were a couple of other reasons that informed my decision not to replace my aortic valve at that time. One, I was working for a publishing organization, and while we did not publish medical journals, we were the recipients of a regular medical journal that I read religiously when it crossed my desk. The journal frequently contained articles about heart valve surgery with pictures of failed "ball-cage" or "ball in cage" valves removed from cadavers. Frequently, a metal prong from the cage was broken, or in some instances the ball was missing. I could see why it would not be a good outcome for a piece of metal to be loose inside the cardiovascular system let alone for the ball to break free and travel through an artery until it became stuck. Surgical replacement using tissue valves had been introduced at this time, but they would not last very long primarily because it was not known how to adequately preserve the tissue valves. Another reason I decided to delay surgery was that I had read an article written by a surgeon who said to "remember that absent strongly compelling evidence to the contrary, the best heart valve is the one you are born with." In any event, I knew about all the shortcomings of replacement valves at that time and was both relieved by Dr. White's advice and most willing to follow his advice.

My decision to delay surgery was made overnight as I lay on my hospital bed. However, from that time forward I thought of my life as being pre-and-post heart valve surgery. I was convinced that I would need surgery at some point and that that point might not be too far away. Assuming the likelihood of surgery not being too far off impacted all decisions about my personal life for the rest of my life.

In the early 1970s, I began my MUGA scans every 3 months. These scans required the injection into a vein in my arm of a radioactive chemical called technetium-99 m-pertechnetate (Tc-99 m). I would lie on my back and a special camera would take pictures of my aortic valve as the blood pumped through it. At the end of the exam table were bicycle pedals I could pump to elevate my heart rate. For some exams I pumped the pedals and other times I did not [5].

My ejection fraction (EF) was always around 60%. This meant that 60% of the blood in my left ventricle would pump out each time my heart took a beat. A normal heart will have an ejection fraction of about 50–75%. This meant that my EF was perfectly normal. There was one anomaly: when I pumped the bike pedals and my heart rate increased, my EF did not increase. The only way my heart could deliver more blood when needed was by pumping faster. My EF never rose above 60%. For a normal heart, the EF goes up with increased heart rate. However, this was not a factor in determining whether or not to replace the valve. The MUGA scan every 3 months went on for several years with no change in my EF, and my internist eventually decided to scan every 6 months, and the six-month scans went on for several years with no change in my EF. Eventually, my internist agreed with Dr. White and ceased all scans. After every scan I was told to go home and drink plenty of water to flush the radiotracer out of my system; and I did as I was directed.

In case you were wondering, the echocardiogram (echo) was just beginning to be used in the early 1970s [6]. An echocardiogram is totally noninvasive: there is no radionuclide injected into the blood. In the early 1970s, the pictures from an echo were not as clear as they are today. In addition, the results from an echo were not as accurate as the results from a MUGA especially involving EF data. Use of the echo has grown in popularity, and over seven million echocardiograms are now performed annually in North America. However, the MUGA scan is still widely used today as well.

3. Pacemakers to the rescue

When I was 43 years old, I had some periods of time when I just did not feel well, and I felt like my heart was skipping beats at times and getting extra beats at other times. The results from an electrocardiogram caused my internist to outfit me with a Holter monitor for 24 hours. The results of the Holter monitor test showed I had developed intermittent left bundle branch block. Although it was impossible to tell for sure what was causing the left branch block, it seemed very likely that calcification in the aortic valve was pressing on the nerve going to my left ventricle and causing the nerve to periodically misfire. My internist referred me to a major hospital in the area for evaluation for a pacemaker. The cardiologist at the hospital insisted I needed both a valve replacement and a pacemaker. When he saw that I was not willing to undergo valve replacement, he recommended a pacemaker be implanted but insisted I would need a replacement valve within 2 years at the longest.

I got my first pacemaker when I was 44 years old. It was implanted by a semi-retired surgeon who told me he got too tired standing during open heart surgeries but that implanting pacemakers was perfect for him because he did not need to stand very long during the procedure. I laid on the operating table and he gave me an injection of pain killer in my upper right chest. Then he entered the superior vena cava vein going from my right arm into my heart, and he strung the pacemaker leads through the vein into my heart. Once the wires were in place, he made an incision on my chest, forced open a "pocket" under my skin, connected the pacemaker wires, and slid the pacemaker into the pocket. Final steps in the procedure were the stitches and placement of a bandage over the wound, and I was sent home the next day.

The pacemaker was set at 55 beats per minute, and this rate was to cause me problems for many years to come. I found out many years later that the natural pace of my heart was 57 beats per minute. However, the pacemaker setting proved to be too close to my natural pace. Pacemakers are designed to wait and see if the heart will beat on its own. If the heart does not beat, then the pacer sends a signal for the heart to beat. My pacer was a dual pacer, so that the pacer would send a signal both to the top of the heart and to the middle (and lower sections) of the heart as needed. My upper sinus mode always worked well, but the signal had difficulty going through to the lower chambers of the heart. The heart has a sinus node both at the top and middle of the heart, and sometimes my pacer would send a signal for the lower sections of my heart to beat just as the natural signal from my heart was sending a signal. Thus, I frequently got double beats in the lower sections of my heart. Remember, all of this is happening in a fraction of a second, because the average heart will naturally beat 50 or more times per minute. Getting my pacemaker settings in concert with my natural beat settings was an issue for my physicians starting with that first pacemaker.

A few days after getting my first pacemaker, I needed to fly on a business trip from the East Coast to the Mid-West. The first evening of my business trip, my right arm swelled up to about double size. I called my internist back on the East Coast, and he directed me to the Emergency Room (ER) of a hospital near me. Two ER physicians examined me and could not tell what was causing my arm to swell. Out of an abundance of caution, they put me on a mild dose of antibiotics and told me to see the surgeon who had implanted the pacemaker as soon as I returned home. Besides being swollen, my arm had a slightly reddish color to it, but I was not in any pain. Back home and during my visit to the surgeon, he quickly advised that the wires from my pacemaker into my heart had blocked the vein returning blood from my right arm to my heart. We decided to make no medical intervention, and after about 6 weeks, my cardiovascular system grew new veins around the blockage and my arm size and coloration returned to normal. You can still see a lot of "extra" veins in my right chest.

I had one other scare with my first pacemaker about 10 days after it had been implanted. I was attending a professional basketball game with my sons. We were watching the game when my name was announced over the loudspeaker system of the stadium saying I was to contact my pacemaker physician immediately. I went to the stadium office and called the physician at the hospital as directed. The physician told me they had been reviewing my pacemaker data and felt they had made some incorrect settings on the pacemaker and wanted me to come in right away so they could correct the settings. The next morning, they made a number of changes in the pacer parameters. My understanding was that they changed the time the pacemaker would wait to see if the heart was getting a natural signal to beat. I could not feel any difference. They left the pacemaker beats per minute at 55.

My first pacemaker was needed by my heart only intermittently and remained in place for about 16 years. By then, I had semiretired and was scheduled to take a vacation trip from the East Coast of the United States to Australia. Although the battery had some charge remaining, my internist felt it best to swap out the old pacemaker for a new one and not take any chances on a pacemaker failure being so far from home and in a foreign country. I got my second pacemaker when I was 59 years old. Apparently, I was becoming more dependent on the pacemaker, because my second pacemaker lasted less than 5 years.

When I was 62 years old, the internist who had been tending to my heart issues for 35 years, retired for health reasons. He was having a rough time with his hip replacement. His first hip replacement was recalled, and after his second surgery, he got an infection and had to have the second hip removed. He needed to be home in bed and on antibiotics for a month awaiting a third hip surgery. Interestingly enough, he told me before he retired that he would have been a better physician had he been a patient earlier in his life. He felt he had lost control over all of his medical care, and he did not like the feeling of losing control.

A friend recommended a cardiologist to me who was taking new patients. This gentleman made a strong effort to go over my heart valve history, and he was especially interested in any discomfort I might be having in my chest. I told him that occasionally I had angina-like discomfort when I exercised, especially when it was cold, and especially after I had been sitting at my desk at work for a long period of time and then walked several blocks to the subway to go home at night.

This new cardiologist ran a few tests in his office and told me I had a blocked artery in my heart. He showed me a picture from his in-office tests confirming the blockage. He said he could not be certain which artery was blocked, but he was scheduling me for a heart catheterization to determine how much blockage existed and where. He told me that most likely I would be needing bypass surgery. He, personally, did not perform catheterizations, but he recommended a colleague of his, and the next week, I was in the hospital with his colleague performing my third catheterization. The technician assisting in the procedure said to me after the procedure: "In my twenty years of medicine, I have never seen anyone with larger and more wide-open coronary arteries than yours. You will not be needing bypass surgery anytime soon if ever." A few days later, back at my new cardiologist's office, he said he had misread the test data. He said he did not know that the fraction of a second delay in the pacemaker sending a signal for the lower chambers of my heart to beat would cause the tests to be invalid. He apologized profusely for having me undergo a totally unnecessary catheterization. He unceremoniously dropped his office test results in the trash can next to his desk. He placed the catheterization results in my file as he explained that whatever chest dis-comfort I was having was not due to blocked arteries.

I received my third pacer when I was 64 years old. The placement of my third pacer did not go entirely as planned. I was not sedated for the procedure. The physician implanting the pacer and the technician assisting him started arguing about the size of the pocket and who would close my wound after the replacement pacer was in place. One of them pushed on the pacer when it was in my chest and the leads coming out of the pacer bent around the edge of the pacer. The technician stormed out of the procedure room and the physician closed the wound. Unfortunately, there was a significantly raised area around the pacer where the lead wire for the pacer was bent around the pacer and pushing up my skin above the pacer. The area became puffy in just a couple of days. My pacemaker physician had gone on vacation, and I was scheduled for a business trip from the East Coast to the West Coast. I consulted a different physician, and he believed the puffiness would eventually subside, and it did subside after several weeks. My third pacer lasted about 5 years.

I still have my third pacemaker in my right chest even though it is now inert, and the lead wires still push the skin up around the pacemaker. The reason for leaving the pacemaker in place is interesting. When I got my *fourth pacer*, I was 69 years old, and the leads to the old pacer were deteriorating. I was still semiretired and had moved from the East Coast back to the West Coast, and my new pacemaker cardiologist decided to put in a whole new pacer system on the left side of my chest – new pacemaker and new leads into the heart. He told me that one worry they always have when implanting pacemakers and wires is that an infection might occur on the pacemaker itself or on the wires. If he removed the old pacemaker on the right side at the same time he installed a new pacer system on the left side, and if I got an infection, he would not be able to tell whether the infection was on parts of the old wires still remaining in the right side of my chest, or if the infection was on the new system on the left side of my chest. Removing old wires, especially when they have been screwed into the heart muscle can be life threatening, and in cases like mine, the old pacer is usually removed, but the wires going into the heart are left in place. Hence, he made the very wise decision to leave the entire old system in place (pacer and wires) even though the old pacer was turned off when the new system was implanted.

The new pacemaker system on my left side required the new leads to go through the vein from my left arm into my heart. The procedure was similar to what I had gone through when I got my first pacer, it was just on the opposite side of my chest. The most significant difference was that this physician insisted upon me being under anesthesia for the procedure. Also, this was the first time I was told that I had become "pacemaker dependent." I was told not to worry, however, because the pacemakers were space-age technology. I did not find the space-age language comforting given all the problems that can and had occurred in space. A couple of my friends asked if it was difficult for me to live with the knowledge that if my pacer stopped working, I would die in a matter of seconds. Those questions were not reassuring to me as well. In the long run, I just had to shut out of my mind any worry about whether a pacemaker might stop working.

As mentioned, I received my fourth pacer when I was 69 years old. However, my luck was improving regarding battery life. My new pacemaker physician, working with the pacemaker company representative, decided to set my beats per minute at 50 in order to try and eliminate my double beat problems. That adjustment did work for a number of years. My fourth pacer lasted for 7 years, and I received my fifth pacer when I was 75 years old. The double beat issue still was not a problem.

As mentioned, I had moved from the East Coast back to the West Coast, and my new cardiologist advised that in addition to my aorta issues, I had a prolapsed mitral valve. He explained that when someone, like me, has a large amount of blood flowing back into the left ventricle of the heart because the aorta valve does not close properly, that it puts pressure on the mitral valve and eventually may cause it to become prolapsed. He believed this was my situation. This is the first time I had been told I had a prolapsed mitral valve.

When I was 79 years old, I had an incident where I felt like I was going to pass out. The incident lasted for about 12 seconds. I saw my pacemaker physician a few days later, and fortunately, the newer pacemakers make a recording of any unusual disturbances in heart rhythm. This was not my first episode of feeling faint. I remember talking to a different physician years earlier about feeling faint, and he told me it was probably the pacer sending a wrong message to my heart. He told me to go into a limp position whenever I had that feeling, and I remember going limp on a few occasions in the past. The faint feeling always went away in a few seconds.

My pacemaker physician informed me that I had suffered a short run (14 seconds) of ventricular fibrillation (VF). He consulted with my cardiologist, and I checked into the hospital that night. The next morning, my pacemaker physician removed my fifth pacemaker and implanted a new combination pacemaker and defibrillator. I was informed that VF is a rapid life-threatening heart arrhythmia. It is sometimes referred to with a married male patient (like me), as "the widow maker." It can be that serious because when the heart is in VF, it cannot pump blood throughout the body. Fortunately, all my runs of VF had been short lived and self-corrected. It is when the VF continues for more than a few seconds that it becomes most dangerous. With the new combination pacemaker and defibrillator, I am now protected against the "widow maker."

While I was still 79 years old, I began having more extra beats and a return of the double beat problem – a worsening of a condition I had off and on since my early 40s. It was determined that I not only had extra beats but that I had atrial flutter as well. Atrial flutter occurs when the heart's electrical system tells the heart to beat faster. My pacemaker physician, in consultation with my cardiologist, recommended I undergo an ablation using a radio frequency procedure to burn out the extra signals. The ablation procedure itself is amazing to me. I was treated by a physician who specialized in such procedures. Using a grid that overlays the heart, the physician was able to determine where in my heart the extra signals were originating. A Radio Frequency (RF) catheter was inserted through my right groin femoral artery and into my heart. In my case, it turned out that the extra beats were coming from one spot in the annulus of the right atrium. The signal would originate in a nerve in the annulus and then travel in a circle around the annulus and cause the same originating nerve to fire again in a continuous loop. The physician burned or ablated the nerve where the extra beat was originating. In addition, he ablated another spot on the annulus just in case the originating nerve was not completely ablated. He did this to prevent any unwanted electrical signal from going in a circle and starting the extra beats to repeat as in the past. As it turned out, this was a smart move by the physician because subsequent tests showed the original unwanted firing of the nerve was still taking place on an intermittent basis. Now, however, the signal was blocked by the second ablation, and the repeated beats ceased. I still get an occasional extra beat, but nothing like before. Also, the physician was able to locate the source of the atrial flutter, my right atrium, and ablate the offending nerve. The atrial flutter has not returned.

My pacemaker physician set my new pacer at 70 beats per minute (bpm). This faster bpm stopped the double beat issue, and any serious problem with double beats has gone away. At first, I felt like my heart was racing. After all, I had been set at 50 bpm for many years, and I could tell the difference. My physician said to try the rate of 70 bpm for 3 months and we would go from there. For a while, I felt like my heart was working overtime and I seemed more tired. By the time 3 months rolled around, I was feeling better, and the double beats had largely subsided. Only occasionally now do I get extra beats that are bothersome. My bpm remains at 70.

4. The right time for a heart valve replacement

While still 79 years old, my cardiologist was beginning to be concerned that the time was getting right for a replacement aortic valve. I was having more angina-like discomfort in my chest when I went for my daily walks. The echocardiogram (echo) showed that my ejection fraction had dropped from its previous reading of 55 to 45. Also, the valve opening had narrowed, due to calcification, to a dangerously narrow number using echo readings. Finally, the valve had become stenotic, that is, it was not opening and closing as it had previously. However, to my way of thinking, my cardiologist seemed slow to pursue valve replacement. He put me through a whole series of tests, including my fifth catheterization (not counting the ablation). In a discussion with him about the procedure, he explained that a team of three physicians, including himself, had been put together to access my situation. All three physicians had concerns about how successful an aortic heart valve procedure might be in my case. Some of the following parts of my story that follows at times involve my assumptions and projections about what happened, so none of the physicians involved can be held to account exactly for my views as stated below.

The surgeon on the team had determined that surgery was not an option. I met with her, and I do not recall her using the term "inoperable," but someone may have used it at least once. In any event, my understanding was that she ruled out surgery due to the extensive calcification of the valve. This is concerning because a part of her role is to be present during the TAVR procedure in case something goes wrong, and it becomes necessary to move me from the procedure room directly into the operating room. So now I'm uncomfortable knowing that if something goes wrong during my TAVR procedure that surgery is not a promising backup plan. However, the surgeon did agree that a TAVR procedure was the best option for treating my condition. Not doing anything about the valve was not a good option either. One physician estimated I had only 6 months to a year to live given the condition of my valve and the deteriorating condition of my heart as shown in the echo results.

In addition to the team's concern about surgery not being an option, the team had five other concerns about implanting a new aortic valve in my heart using the TAVR procedure. Any one of the five would be a good reason for not performing the procedure, so I'll discuss each of the five and explain why each was problematic in terms of a favorable outcome.

4.1 The size of my existing aortic valve was unusually large

My team planned to use a replacement valve they regularly used for such procedures, but the largest valve made by their preferred maker of TAVR valves was 20 percent smaller than my valve opening (i.e., the largest valve was only 80 percent in size of what they preferred). Using the right sized valve is critically important to the success of the procedure. If the replacement valve is too large for the patient's aortic valve opening, it could severely damage the heart muscle and even cause death right there on the table. If the replacement valve is too small (my case), it could slide out of position and have a fatal outcome.

A process called hemodynamics [7] helps hold the stent supporting the valve in place in the aorta. As a normal heart pumps blood out through the aortic valve, it does so with a fair degree of velocity and force, but there is not a lot of pressure on the valve itself because the cusps are open, and the blood is flowing right through the open valve. Likewise, when the valve closes, there is not a lot of backflow pressure because the backflow of blood is not being pumped, it is simply stopped from flowing back into the heart. Still, replacement valve slippage is a concern.

Also, a process known as reendothelialization (where cells lining the blood vessels grow in and around the stent) helps hold the valve in place [8]. Finally, the metal valve frame or stent will be pressing out against the old tissue valve which is squeezed between the stent or frame of the valve and the lining of the aorta, and this will help hold the valve in place. Despite all this, a valve can slip out of place, and therefore, proper size is important. The nearest thing I can compare the importance of valve size to is clothing, a new pair of shoes for example. Even when we buy "our size" in a different shoe it can be too long, or too short, or too wide, or too narrow, or have the wrong arch support or just not feel right. For these reasons, we usually try on a new pair of shoes before we buy them to make sure they are the right size. The same goes for a pair of gloves and other clothing items. The outcome of an improperly sized replacement heart valve may come with more deadly consequences. During a catheterization procedure, physicians carefully measure the size of the old valve opening in choosing the proper replacement size. Interestingly, the replacement valves are not made to order. They are premade in a very limited number of sizes and are either available from the maker or stocked in the TAVR Centers where implantation will be taking place.

My team knew that another maker of aortic heart valves happened to make a larger size valve that would be much better for my situation. The team contacted the maker of that replacement heart valve and described my case to the maker and explained why the team wanted to implant the larger valve in my heart. The maker of the larger valve declined to allow their valve to be placed in my heart fearing that my situation was too dangerous for a replacement valve to be successful.

If the team was to go ahead and attempt my aortic valve replacement procedure, they would need to use a valve they regularly used and had access to even if the valve was too small. There were a couple of advantages in the team's favor. The valve they usually used had a section in the middle of the frame that allowed for expansion of the valve using a balloon catheter. In other words, once the valve had been deployed in my heart, they could then insert a balloon catheter into the valve and expand it outwards in the middle of the valve. However, they could not make up being 20 percent too small. In addition, the valve comes with a "skirt" designed to expand and lessen blood around the outside of the frame. The "skirt" could prove helpful should they go ahead with the procedure. Finally, the team reasoned that the extensive calcification would likely hold the valve in place even if all else failed.

4.2 My aortic valve had an unusual shape prone to leakage

As opposed to being round or somewhat oval shaped, like most aorta valves, my valve is elongated and shaped more like a football. My team was worried that if they

DOI: http://dx.doi.org/10.5772/intechopen.112120

put a round replacement valve inside an elongated space that there would be an unacceptable amount of blood leaking back into the heart around the frame of the valve. This is commonly referred to as regurgitation or aortic insufficiency (AI). My team did not want to operate and create a new major issue due to an unacceptable amount of blood leaking back into the heart with each heartbeat.

4.3 The cusps of my valve were deformed

The newer and higher quality echo device at the hospital where my cardiologist performed my last echocardiogram to help determine if I was a candidate for a TAVR for my aorta valve, finally showed the deformity of my valve from birth. Typically, the aorta valve has three cusps that open and close with each heartbeat. I only had two cusps. The third cusp was missing. I was not a classic bicuspid valve case. In addition, my two cusps were fused together, so I really had only one double-sized cusp that was opening and closing with each heartbeat. Instead of the valve opening and closing normally, it was moving more like a small door opening and closing in a large door frame. The team was concerned about how compliant the large and fused cusps might be when the replacement valve was deployed.

4.4 My aortic valve had extensive calcification

My team was especially concerned about how pliant the calcification in the aortic valve would be. They were worried that if it was too hard that it might damage the heart muscle when the replacement valve was deployed. However, as previously mentioned, the team thought the calcification might help hold the undersized replacement valve in place.

4.5 My aortic valve had a piece of heart muscle blocking the implantation of a replacement valve

The last echo showed a piece of heart tissue protruding into the aorta valve right where the replacement valve would be placed. Proper positioning of the replacement valve is critical for success. You do not want it too far inside the left ventricle, and you do not want it too far into the aorta itself. In fact, during the TAVR replacement procedure, the team has to agree that the valve is properly placed, and they have to agree to implant it. Unfortunately, the piece of tissue was right in the way. The replacement valve can be moved slightly, but only slightly, and there was no way to avoid the extra tissue. It might distort the frame of the valve, or it might push into the heart muscle and cause issues. The team would have to put the replacement valve over the extra tissue and hope for the best should they decide to go ahead with the procedure.

Given all the above: my unusually large aortic valve opening; my football shaped valve; my missing cusp and my fused cusps; my extensively calcified valve; and the piece of tissue blocking implantation of a replacement valve, it was fully understandable that my team was having second thoughts about replacing my valve. Obviously, they did not want a patient to die on the table, nor would they want to be accused of being reckless in going ahead with a risky procedure. However, I did not appear to have too long to live. As mentioned earlier, my EF was dropping, and it had dropped from its long held 55–45%. the opening area of the valve for the blood to flow out of the heart was narrowing to a critical point (due to calcification), and the valve had become stenotic (described to me as a lack of movement due to calcification forming around the cusp). The risks against a successful procedure were significant, and the risks were discussed with me. I could live out my life as best I could, maybe even have a few years if lucky, or I could have a replacement valve, maybe live many more years, and maybe live a much more satisfying life than otherwise would be the case (i.e., feel better and be more active). The choice was mine. The team was willing to go ahead if I wanted them to do so. I chose a replacement valve, and I was assigned to a scheduling nurse to arrange for the procedure. The scheduling nurse had to reserve the procedure room, schedule all three physicians on my team to be there, of course get me there, and schedule the assistants and assure all necessary supplies are in place, including some replacement valves, and schedule the operating room in case I needed to be moved from the procedure room into surgery. She was able to set it all up for a procedure date in about 4 weeks.

5. Do not forget the dental work

Unfortunately, on the day of the scheduled procedure, I woke up with a significant tooth ache. I tried to call the scheduling nurse and my doctor for guidance, but no one was answering their phone. I went to the hospital and went through the preparatory steps, but the procedure wound up being canceled. I was told it would not be a good idea to proceed if I had an infected tooth and there was any danger of the infection spreading to my new valve. I was told to get my dental work done and then reschedule. Interestingly enough, I began to feel like I had a little more energy. I even commented to my wife, “maybe I don’t really need a replacement valve after all.” I would later find out why I was having a little more energy, and I will report on that matter in a section below.

There was another issue of concern. My procedure was scheduled during the height of the COVID-19 pandemic. My wife could not accompany me to the procedure. She dropped me off in front of the hospital and wished me luck. It is difficult to imagine how stressful a procedure like a heart valve replacement is for loved ones. All medical members need to be mindful to stay in touch with the listed contact for the patient.

I thought my teeth were in good shape. I regularly visited my dentist, had my teeth cleaned, and had dental work completed as necessary. It turned out that the tooth that was aching on my scheduled procedure day was cracked down to the root and needed to be extracted. That was followed up with an implant and crown. Additionally, I had one other tooth that needed a root canal; another tooth needed a bone graft, and one other tooth needed to be re-filled because the previous filling was leaking. All the dental work took about 3 months, and the scheduling nurse was not able to get me rescheduled for another couple of months. Five months after my original procedure date, I again reported to the hospital for TAVR.

6. The actual procedure

The actual procedure started out in an interesting fashion as I was lying on the procedure table. One technician set up the echo machine and flashed an image of my aortic valve on a large elevated screen. The first thing that the technician and I both noticed was that a huge section of my aortic valve had torn loose and was being held by just a thread of tissue. On the echo, the large piece of torn valve looked like a flag flapping in a hurricane. It moved out straight with every heartbeat and appeared as though it could tear loose at any moment. Who knows what my fate would have been had that large piece of valve torn loose. At least I now knew why I had a little more energy. My heart no longer needed to pump blood through a tiny opening in my stenotic valve. The opening was now bigger and apparently my heart was not straining as much. The physicians had not yet entered the room, and the technician's and my eyes met in response to seeing the big piece of valve torn loose and hanging by a thread. She looked at me and said, "Oh, you're in the right place." That was some of my last recollections in the procedure room as the anesthesiologist had entered and was administering my anesthesia.

It's amazing to me to think that a large replacement heart valve could be collapsed down to the thickness of a lead pencil, be inserted into my heart through my groin artery, and then blown up to full size. The frame of the valve, or stent, is a metal mesh made from cobalt and chromium. It is strong yet flexible. The tissue in my replacement valve was bovine (i.e., made from tough pericardium tissue from a cow's heart). The manufacturing of a bovine aortic replacement valve requires hundreds of stitches to form the leaflets of the replacement valve. The tissue is treated with a chemical that sterilizes the tissue, kills any live cells, and preserves the tissue for endurance purposes. It is treated with an anti-calcium building solution to reduce the chance of future stenosis. Finally, it is tested for quality assurance, because the leaflets will be opening and closing around 70 times a minute for many years to come.

The bovine valve is very different from using a pig (porcine) replacement heart valve. When using a pig valve, the entire valve is harvested and implanted as a whole valve. Some people argue about which is best, but the bottom line is that they are both good.

Everything went as planned during the procedure until my team implanted the valve into the heart. At that point, the metal frame of the valve bent around the calcification in my heart and about half of my blood was leaking around the outside of the valve and then leaking back into my heart after every beat. My team was now finding out why they had been reluctant to perform the procedure. They were not sure what to do. I was alive, and if they did nothing more, I probably would live another 6 months to a year. However, I would most likely be wheelchair bound and have no energy for daily activities. If they tried further intervention, I could die on the procedure table, and they certainly did not want that. Also, they ruled out taking me to the operating room. My cardiologist remembered from our prior discussions that I had told him I did not want to live as an invalid. I had always been active, and I wanted to return to my normal active life.

Based on my previously stated wishes, they decided to insert a balloon catheter into the valve and try to force the frame into a normal straight shape. Apparently, the tension was palpable. Too much force and the heart could rupture, and I would be gone on the spot. Using a balloon catheter, they were able to expand the collapsed frame of the valve back into a straight alignment. There was no damage to my heart. The calcification had been pressed out of the way. Some blood leakage existed, but it was minimal. They abandoned any plans they might have had of expanding the valve to minimize any leakage around the outside of the frame. It was working, and they decided to leave well enough alone. Using a smaller valve turned out to be fortuitous. Later, my cardiologist told me I was very lucky. There was a lot happening during the procedure that could have gone wrong but did not. I went home a new person the next day following the procedure.

7. COVID-19

Despite all my precautions, I contracted COVID-19 just short of 2 years following TAVR. At first, I was not too sick, but after day four I did not feel at all well for another week. I tested positive for 12 days. My general practitioner (GP) felt it was not necessary for me to be treated with antiviral medication. In hindsight, antiviral medication might have both speeded and eased my recovery. I had received all the recommended vaccines and boosters, and that no doubt helped me avoid serious illness of hospitalization. My cardiologist told me the replacement valve was likely important to my being able to fight the virus. My biggest complaint post-Covid-19 has been a loss of energy, but my energy level finally began returning to normal about 5 months since I stopped testing positive for COVID-19.

8. Conclusion: life after a TAVR replacement aortic heart valve

I visit my pacemaker physician every 4 months. I am told that of all his patients, I have been living the longest with a pacemaker – almost 40 years. Unfortunately, his next patient living the longest with a pacemaker is a 42-year-old man who received his first pacer when he was 6 years old. I say unfortunately, because it makes me feel very lucky to not need my first pacer until I was 44 years old.

I am now in my third year following TAVR. I would describe my life as normal, or like it was before I became symptomatic with heart issues. In fact, if anything, I have a little more energy now with less discomfort when I exercise. I walk twice a day (about two miles total). I have been able to vacation on the Central Coast of California for up to a month at a time. This is my favorite vacation. I do not feel that the money spent on my procedure was wasted nor do I feel guilty about the cost of the valve and implantation procedure that was fully covered by my insurance (i.e., in the neighborhood of $150 K). I fully realize that life is uncertain and that I was lucky. However, I give thanks every day for the skill of my medical team and their staff and for the extra days (now years) I have been given.

I received my TAVR 50 years after Paul Dudley White said I might surprise the cardiologists in the room who wanted to operate, and that he could not recommend me for valve replacement at that time. I thank Dr. White for his clinical expertise and experience. I sincerely hope that hearing my version of my heart valve experience will aid and be of comfort to other patients and physicians in the future.

Author details

Philip Hutchens
Independent Scientist (Retired), La Mesa, CA, USA

*Address all correspondence to: khutchp@aol.com

IntechOpen

© 2023 The Author(s). Licensee IntechOpen. This chapter is distributed under the terms of the Creative Commons Attribution License (http://creativecommons.org/licenses/by/3.0), which permits unrestricted use, distribution, and reproduction in any medium, provided the original work is properly cited.

References

[1] Goel SS, Reardon MJ. Indication creep in transcatheter aortic valve implantation—Data or desire? JAMA Cardiology. 2023;**8**(6):519-520. DOI: 10.1001/jamacardio.2023.0674

[2] Lee TH. Seizing the teachable moment—Lessens from Eisenhower's Heart Attack. New England Journal of Medicine. 2020;**383**:e100. DOI: 10.1056/NEJMp2031046

[3] MacIsaac S et al. How did we get here?: A historical review and critical analysis of anticoagulation therapy following mechanical valve replacement. Circulation. 2019;**140**:1933-1942

[4] Injury Care Center. The History and Use of MRI and CT Scans. Glenolden, Pennsylvania: Injury Care Center; 31 Jan 2020

[5] Odak M, Kayani WT. MUGA Scan. Treasure Island, FL: StatPearls Publishing; 2023. Available from: https://www.ncbi.nlm.nih.gov/books/NBK564365/

[6] Di Franco A, Ohmes LB, Gaudino M, Rong LQ, Girardi LN, Sarullo FM, et al. Serendipity and innovation: History and evolution of transthoracic echocardiography. Journal of Thoracic Diseases. 2017;**9**(Suppl 4):S257-S263. DOI: 10.21037/jtd.2017.03.90

[7] Secomb TW. Hemodynamics: National Library of Medicine. Bethesda, Maryland; 15 Mar 2016. DOI: 10.1002/cphy.c150038

[8] Wang X et al. The combined contribution of vascular endothelial cell migration and adhesion to stent re-endothelialization. Frontiers in Cell Developmental Biology. 2021;**2021**:9. DOI: 10.3389/fcell.2021.641382